IMMACULATE DECEPTION II
Myth, Magic & Birth

ALSO BY SUZANNE ARMS:

A Season to Be Born

Adoption: A Handful of Hope

Bestfeeding:
Getting Breastfeeding Right for You

The original *Immaculate Deception* was in print for two decades. It continues to be required reading in many medical schools and nursing programs. SUZANNE ARMS was an early champion of midwives and birth centers, and founder of The Birth Place in Menlo Park, California. Her film "Five Women, Five Births" is considered a classic in childbirth education.

Text and Photographs by
S U Z A N N E   A R M S

IMMACULATE DECEPTION II

Myth, Magic & Birth

C E L E S T I A L   A R T S
Berkeley, California

For Molly

The publisher assumes no liablility for any injuries or other problems sustained in conjunction with following the advice, therapy,
or treatments described in this book. Individuals are cautioned
that this material appears for informational use only and may not
be appropriate for their individual needs.

Suzanne Arms can be contacted at (303) 884-4090
P.O. Box 1040, Bayfield, CO 81122

CELESTIAL ARTS
P.O. Box 7123
Berkeley, California 94707
(510) 559-1600

Photographs by Suzanne Arms
Cover and text design by Nancy Austin
Typesetting by Wilsted and Taylor, Oakland
Production by Catherine Jacobes

Library of Congress Cataloging-in-Publication Data
Arms, Suzanne.
   Immaculate deception II
              p.   cm.
   Includes bibliographical references and index.
   ISBN 0-89087-633-9
   1. Childbirth. 2. Mothers--Interviews.
   3. Obstetricians--Interviews. 4. Midwives--Interviews.
   I. Title.
   RG525.A792   1994
   618.4--dc20   92-23355
                                            CIP

FIRST PRINTING 1994
Printed in the United States of America

4   5   6   7   —   04   03   02

Contents

Foreword

Suzanne Arms was sneaking into labor and delivery wards across the United States at the same time as I was being educated—and indoctrinated—in them. The first *Immaculate Deception* had just come out when I was finishing medical school in 1975. Then, when I was in my obstetric residency, I cared for a few patients who, as a result of reading it, had brought a birth plan with them to the hospital.

I went through medical school at Dartmouth, and many of our obstetric patients were well-educated women who gave birth as naturally as was possible at the time, which I later discovered wasn't natural at all! We had thought then that because we didn't give women enemas or pubic shaves we were being progressive. And, for the times, we were.

During my ob/gyn residency in Boston, at one of the venerable old hospitals, I was introduced to "twilight sleep" for maternity patients. This involved the injection of Seconal and Scopalamine into the laboring woman so she wouldn't feel or remember her labor. Ironically, it was when they began to use electronic fetal monitors that these same obstetricians saw the effects of twilight sleep on the baby and finally stopped the practice, replacing it with drugs such as Demerol for labor and spinal anesthesia for delivery.

When the occasional woman in labor came into the hospital carrying her birth plan, I listened and made every effort to help her achieve her desires, but it wasn't always easy to do so within the medical system. Even we doctors who were progressive and who thought, as I did, that much of what we were being taught was incomplete still believed that Suzanne Arms had overstated her case. It wasn't until much later, after I had been out of obstetrics for several years, that

I finally understood how the medical system acts like a dysfunctional family in the way it keeps its members in line. It was also then that I recognized how women's need for their obstetricians' approval was only an extension of their dependence upon, and need for approval from, their husbands.

Our system for birth flows seamlessly out of the values of the technologically driven, materialistic society we live in, a society that is too often cut off from nature's wisdom. I've often said that I would go back into obstetrics if and when the whole system changes, but this will only happen when a critical mass of people begin to question their fears and need for control. Then the insights gained must, of course, be applied to their daily lives.

Most of us, men and women alike, are trained with a "don't just stand there—do something!" mentality, and this mind-set favors the view that birth is a crisis requiring intervention. Yet, when a woman is centered in her own power while giving birth, the men around her are awed and (most of them) will naturally support her. It is only when we doubt ourselves and our ability to birth and care for our babies that we unwittingly set ourselves up for intervention and complications.

I've learned that women and men who have a great deal of self-confidence and self-trust can go into most situations and get their needs met. One of the key ways a woman can develop a sense of trust in her own power is through birth, but most women today lack confidence in their bodies. Given the history of women and their health care in Western cultures, this is understandable. Consequently, even those who have read books such as *Immaculate Deception* are apt to lose their sense of self in the hospital OB ward, perhaps more than in any other setting. Fear is *so* contagious, and that particular fear is fueled, in part, by the unresolved birth trauma of everyone present at a birth. To whom do we turn for guidance?

Immaculate Deception II is a treasure! Suzanne Arms tells the truth, and she does it with great clarity and compassion. Her photographs are compelling and heart-centered, and show the healing of birth and the nurturing qualities of both men and women. I also love the quotes from female physicians whose experiences, like mine, have led them to question the system that trained them. These awakened women healers are pioneers—they understand and support women's power in birth and what it means to trust nature, a view not all women physicians share.

The health care system as we have known it is in chaos, and this includes maternity care. The system and the mind-set that created it are going through a painful and dysfunctional labor—struggling to stay in control. Suzanne Arms's vision, put forth so compellingly in this book, can help midwife this system right now. Like all good birth attendants, Suzanne understands the nature and power of support, understanding, and compassion. Those qualities help a woman, and even a health care system, to let go and allow the new creation to emerge.

Christiane Northrup, M.D., O.B.

This is an extraordinary book. For many, like myself, it will be a hard book to read. For physicians, it will be hard to read about our shortcomings, our inability to deliver the illusion of perfection we claim to offer, and our failure to provide safe, gentle passage to each new life placed in our hands. For women who have given birth, it will be hard to see the ways in which we failed ourselves and our babies by not asking for more—more information, autonomy, and care from our families, caregivers, and culture. Still, it also offers illumination and the possibility of a different way to bring new souls into the world; until we can see a different possibility, we will never change.

For physicians who have seen the problems with our high-tech obstetrics and feel trapped by the malpractice attorney, the third-party payer, and the patients who want "the best medicine science has to offer" and mean "the most intervention possible," this book will be a friend.

For women who are willing to take their fate into their own hands, to make hard decisions and take responsibility for them in order to create a better birth and a better world, *Immaculate Deception II* offers encouragement and well-researched information. Anyone involved in the sacred task of bringing new life into the world would do well to read this book.

Bethany M. Hays, M.D., Obstetrician, FACOG

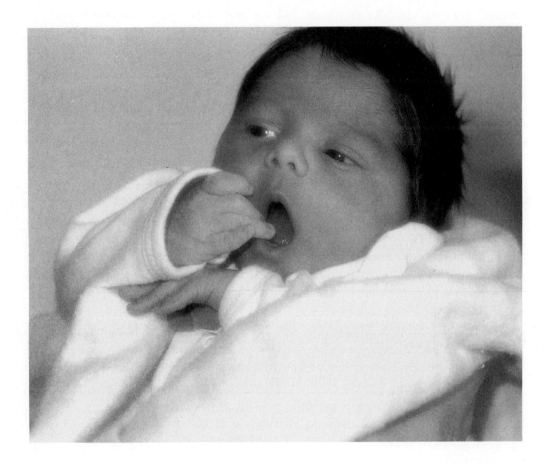

Acknowledgments

In the long process of writing this book many people have helped and taught me. I want to thank a few who have been instrumental for their wisdom, inspiration, and unwavering support:

Faye Gibson, who calls herself a "domiciliary" midwife and has been attending women in their homes for fifteen years, who from 1991–1992 waged a long but successful legal battle for the privilege, and who has been my research assistant extraordinaire as well as the friend with whom I honed many of my ideas;

Roxanne Potter, lay midwife turned nurse-midwife, my dear and long-term friend who has freely shared her experiences and special insights, who has always gifted me with her passionate, compassionate, and humorous observations, and who insisted I was the only one who could write this book;

Kate Bowland, a pioneering lay midwife who, in the early 1970s, followed the call to train herself and assist women having home births in her community whom doctors had turned their backs on, and who is today a senior wise woman and practicing home-birth midwife;

Don Creevy, obstetrician, who for two crucial decades (1970–1990) provided openhearted backup for dozens of midwives across four counties because he believes in the right of birthing women to make their own choices, who is a skilled practitioner in the art of gentle and minimal medical intervention, and yet who insists that he learned all he knows from birthing women and midwives;

Michael Witte, a rare pediatrician and family physician who has dedicated his life to creating working models of effective, personalized health care, and who practices his egalitarian belief that physicians are no better than nurses, midwives, and physician assistants, who provided apprenticeship training in the 1970s for a number of midwives, and was one of the few physicians in North America to openly go into practice with midwives;

Michel Odent, French surgeon and obstetrician, who single-handedly transformed an entire hospital's approach to birth, who listened to midwives, who dared to question what physicians do to birthing women, who pioneered the use of warm-water baths to facilitate birth, and who ultimately left the confines of a hospital and turned to a home-birth practice in London, shedding all the preconceptions of his profession;

Chloe Fisher, British midwife, special wise woman friend and mentor, who shares my passion about women and childbirth, who opened my eyes to the politics of breast-feeding, who has dedicated her life to bringing women back to their senses without ever judging them for their choices, and who has managed to remain in a system that is both rigid and narrow-minded, carrying her light and good-heartedness wherever she goes;

Inke Schwaab, birth educator and VBAC mom, who insisted I write this new edition and provided candid feedback; Sharilyn Hovind, the editor who caught my passion for this book and shepherded the manuscript through various editors and several revisions; Ellen Umansky, for her insight and knowledge of women's issues; Suellen Miller, C.N.M., Ph.D., for her expertise in childbirth and careful work; Nancy Austin, a gifted book designer who actually reads the books she designs and discusses her ideas with authors; David Hinds, my patient publisher and friend;

my dear and long-term friend Susan Berthiaume, who has always believed in me and been there when things got rough, and whose own beliefs have inspired and strengthened my own; my ex-husband, John Wimberley, for providing patience and a serene home to write in when I was struggling with my demons; my friend Jesse Suber, for his honest editorial feedback and for the solid ground he provided when I was at sea in my passion over this subject;

and finally, my daughter, Molly Arms, who had no choice but to make personal sacrifices in her childhood so that I could do this work, who sometimes accompanied me on my nightly journeys to witness and photograph a birth, and who today carries on my beliefs and represents an even stronger generation of women who will not be fooled into giving up their bodies.

IMMACULATE DECEPTION II
Myth, Magic & Birth

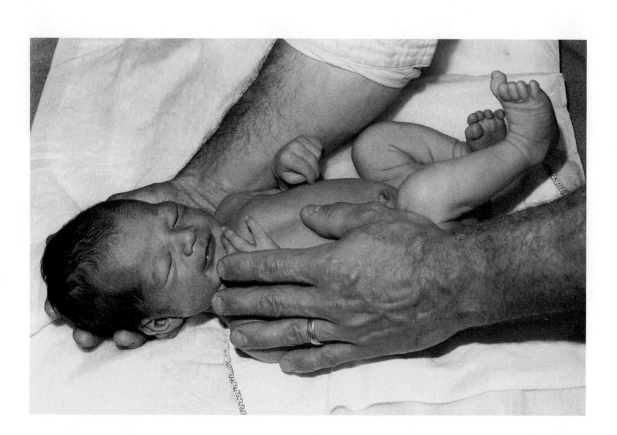

Immaculate Deception

I WAS BORN IN 1944, a time when hospital birth had just been established as the norm in North America. In the hospitals, laboring women were routinely drugged unconscious and often didn't wake up until a nurse brought their babies to them. Nurses were under strict orders to call the doctor only at the very end of labor, but it was imperative that he (virtually all doctors at the time were men) be there for the delivery—nurses were not allowed to deliver babies themselves. Women in those days often had their legs held or even tied together to keep them from delivering before the doctor came, and unknown numbers of babies were permanently brain-damaged from being forcibly held back.

Because I came faster than expected and my doctor was enjoying a night out, he did not come quickly enough. My mother was alone with the nurse: she was not allowed to have any friends or family members with her, according to hospital policy. (Her own mother, a petite deaf woman from Russia, had actually been locked in a hospital room to go through labor alone during World War I, with the excuse that there was a shortage of nurses.) Although drugged, my mother was awake when I was born. When my head began to show and the doctor had not yet arrived, the nurse placed a sanitary napkin between my mother's legs and pressed my head back each time a contraction forced it out, until the doctor finally came and "delivered" me.

It was routine to separate mothers and babies after birth in U.S. hospitals. Most mothers weren't conscious to see and feel their babies emerge. When my mother first saw me, three days after I was born, she did as her doctor instructed and fed me formula from a bottle without attempting to put me to her breast.

That was modern childbirth in 1944.

*　　　　　　　*　　　　　　　*

In 1970, at the age of twenty-six, I gave birth to my first and only child, my daughter, Molly. I was terribly afraid and did not trust either the process of birth or my body. My mother had told me nothing of the ways of the female body, just as her mother had told her nothing. The film I was lucky enough to have seen in pregnancy had seemed unreal, and my birth teacher spoke of labor as if it were some kind of sports event, with the father as the coach and the doctor as the general manager.

Although I lived at the time in California, where some women were daring to have births at home instead of in a hospital and other women were daring to assist them, I'd never seen a birth and didn't know what it was all about. Despite being a college graduate, I was ignorant. Docile and frightened, I labored for one whole day in a bed in a tiny, windowless room in the hospital basement (which was where many hospital obstetric units were then located). I was fortunate in that my child's father was permitted to be at my side, holding my hand, but I was still miserable. Hour after hour, I stared at the large clock on the wall at the foot of my bed, trying to cope with the seemingly endless contractions.

It was an all-too-typical birth, I found out later: admitted to the hospital too soon; put to bed instead of being encouraged to remain upright and active; given a shot of narcotic every few hours to sedate me, an artificial hormone to make contractions stronger, then shots of anesthetic to numb me, then more stimulant. Nurses came and went, but were too busy to stay; they told me I wasn't "progressing" well enough and threatened me with a cesarean. And so it went, for twenty-three hours, without my ever seeing the sun or moon or breathing in fresh air to remind me that all was well, I was simply having a baby.

My body must have been confused by all of the drugs, for my cervix didn't dilate easily and, despite my pushing in every possible position, the baby did not move down the short distance of the birth canal. Finally, a doctor pulled her out with forceps. I held her and cried.

Because I was drugged, my memory of Molly's birth is not complete, but I remember several parts of it clearly. I recall a nursing instructor stopping by to teach her students how to give back massage on a woman (me) whose baby was facing posterior. It felt incredibly good to have her hands on my aching body, but she had to leave after half an hour. I remember the second of the three doctors who were "managing" my labor in shifts. He only stayed the few minutes it took him to sketch a picture on a little blackboard he'd brought, to show me how my uterus wasn't "doing what it should." I felt ashamed. I remember the anesthesiologist trying nine times to get a needle into the right spot along my spine, while I lay as instructed, curled on my side, a position that caused excruciating pain during contractions. He swore and stomped out of the room, and a second anesthesiologist had to finish the job. An hour later, numb from the waist down, I listened patiently to the first anesthesiologist's explanation when he returned to apologize and complain of the bad day he was having. I was the obedient, grateful patient I'd been taught to be. I listened to everyone but myself.

∗   ∗   ∗

During Molly's birth, decision making and control were taken from me. Trusting so little in my innate knowledge of this natural process, I bent to the authority of those who "knew best." They—the doctors and nurses—had ostensibly done everything they could to help me and to make the birth safe. Why, then, was it such a difficult and traumatic experience?

Looking back now, I see that we had all been caught in a web of confusion, untruths, misappropriated power, and miscommunication—a large-scale deception resulting from centuries of interference in natural childbirth by an entrenched, patriarchal medical community. The doctors, nurses, and I were just doing what we had been taught. They didn't know any better—and neither did I. But that experience opened my eyes.

The overall effect was shattering. Molly's birth did not show me my strength, it made me question my abilities as a woman and as a mother. My recovery was slow and I had a headache that lasted two weeks, a side effect of the spinal anesthetic. No one suggested that birth might have been traumatic for Molly as well. She cried inconsolably whenever I tried to lay her down. Doctors said, "It's just colic," but her pain and my exhaustion made me feel desperate.

As I recovered, I went about the days, tired but awed and filled with Molly's presence. I felt the love and trust a newborn baby brings and I rose to meet the challenge of so much love and need. It wasn't until Molly's first birthday that I began to feel the sorrow and anger from the birth, and with that came the driving need to do something about it. I had been deceived, and I was determined not to be deceived again.

I set out to discover what had gone wrong, not just in my child's birth, but in the American way of birth, for I quickly discovered my experience was typical.

I had a burning need to know why modern childbirth was so unnatural, and why so many women were so afraid and passive that we literally handed over our bodies—and our babies—to medical experts and hospitals.

My quest for knowledge took me to other countries, where I found physicians and midwives who knew how to keep birth normal and uncomplicated, and where I met expectant mothers who looked on birth without the extreme anxiety so common in North America. I also attended dozens of home births in this country and discovered that having a baby doesn't usually require either a physician or a hospital, only a midwife to stay with the woman once labor is active. I found that, while birth can sometimes be physiologically complicated and is often made unnecessarily traumatic, it can also be an ordinary, fulfilling, or even transcendent experience.

I wrote the first *Immaculate Deception* in 1975 to try to understand this paradox and to discover what I and so many other women had missed in giving birth. When I began writing, the book burst from me like water from a broken dam; I hardly knew what I'd started. Soon the book was published, and I was being introduced on television and radio shows across the country as an "angry young mother." I was discussed in the press as a radical who was against hospitals and doctors.

Yet what I'd written and what I had to say struck a deep chord in women. I received hundreds of letters and phone calls thanking me for "waking them up" and for "telling the truth." That original book sold 250,000 copies, and many more people than that read it, as women passed their copies on. New mothers wrote me long, intimate letters recounting birth experiences that made them— and me—furious, and I felt their sorrow as well as their outrage.

For doctors and nurses, what I had to say seemed to provoke mostly anger. *How dare you?* they wanted to know. I recall a rare invitation by an appreciative nursing director to speak to her staff at lunch. Most refused to come, and, of those who did, half turned their chairs so their backs were facing me. I also remember a chance encounter with a renowned physician-researcher during a large childbirth conference. I respected him because he had dared to publish research results that were among the first to question the usefulness and safety of electronic fetal monitoring. When I introduced myself and began to thank him for his courage, he turned a fierce face on me and spit out, "I know who *you* are! You have destroyed women's trust in doctors!"

But there were also nurses and physicians who expressed gratitude at my outspokenness and my book; who brought me their hospital birth statistics and grieved over what they saw and what they had to participate in; who stood staunchly on the side of natural childbirth and a woman's right to give birth at home—even though this attitude usually cost them their peers' approval, often their career advancement, sometimes even their jobs.

*   *   *

There have been many positive changes in American culture since *Immaculate Deception* first appeared in 1975. A childbirth movement has come into existence. There are now more than one hundred birth centers across the United States. Women midwives are once again handing down wisdom to the younger generation, sharing the knowledge of how to give birth normally. Some fine films and videos have been made of home births as well as hospital and birth center births so that parents and others can see what they are like and make more informed decisions (see Resources).

Yet despite all this, despite all the childbirth books that have been written, despite all the birth conferences that have been held, it is surprising how little has really changed. In fact, women in the United States are more afraid of birth than ever before and with good cause: there are higher rates of cesareans, premature births, low-birth-weight babies, and infant mortality in this than in any other industrialized nation, and complications surrounding birth have risen steadily in the last few decades. In my experience witnessing births and interviewing mothers in North America, only about 10 percent of women today have what I consider a straightforward, normal childbirth.

The information about birth that was lacking in the mid-seventies is now readily available, yet information alone does not create positive change or transform people's way of thinking. Without an appreciation of the natural process, many women are demanding to be anesthetized for labor; parents watch, without protesting, as their babies are taken to intensive care nurseries for "observation." Families leave the hospital just hours after birth, when mothers should be resting, and women receive no postpartum care when they return home. Fewer women are breast-feeding, and more are having problems when they do. Many mothers go back to work within weeks of giving birth—by choice as well as need—and their infants have no choice but to accept this separation.

Unfortunately for mothers and newborns, family and cultural ties today are stretched thin, often to the breaking point. Little in our modern machine- and money-driven culture supports the developing bonds of love and the healthy interdependence so necessary during and after a birth. And although more men are doing their part to help their partners and babies, many of them are unsupported in the vital role of fathering.

*   *   *

Immaculate Deception II is my best effort at making sense of the complexity of childbirth today: the issues, the history, the problems, and the possibilities. The subject still fires me with passion—though I hope it is now tempered with greater compassion and understanding. For twenty years, I have been able to witness and participate in births. I've always brought my camera and a pad and pen or tape recorder, and in places as diverse in their routine practices as a huge public hospital in New York City, a tiny private hospital in rural Kentucky, a respected teaching hospital in Los Angeles, as well as people's homes and local birth centers, I have photographed and I have listened.

I have interviewed countless nurses and many, especially those who have been midwives in other countries, tell me how they hate what they have to do to women and babies. As one nurse put it: "So often I feel like an accomplice to a crime, not a healer." Most nurses and doctors I have talked to, however, feel *good* about what they do and are candid in saying that women in labor "can't be trusted to make good decisions" and that couples who choose home birth are "child abusers" who care only about their own feelings, not their child's welfare. I think the majority of doctors and nurses really believes that artificially stimulated labor is no different from natural labor, that medical intervention in childbirth is necessary, and that babies can't feel pain in birth and certainly don't remember it.

I continue to be appalled by many of the routine practices I see, in even the "best" hospitals. I've never fully understood the numbness with which most people—even mothers themselves—accept whatever is done to laboring women and babies as "good medical care." I have watched helplessly as a nurse took a rough sterile scrub brush, held a brand-new baby under a tap, and vigorously scrubbed its delicate head, then wrapped the whole baby in sterile paper. I have seen nurses run for the doctor to perform an episiotomy, when the woman in labor was doing fine pushing the baby out and in no danger of tearing. I was once shoved up against a wall for saying to a resident cutting into a newborn's vein, "You need to ask the father's permission before doing that. He's right here." So many times I've felt like grabbing a laboring woman or a baby in the nursery and fleeing with them—but I'm usually the only person besides the parents who thinks something is wrong. It's crazy-making.

I am happy to report that not all is bad. I have witnessed many wonderful birth experiences, mostly—but not all—in homes and birth centers. I meet caring people in every setting without whom I could not continue my work. They have given me a vision of what birth *can* be like: health workers laboring to keep birth natural and uncomplicated; parents refusing to have their babies taken from their arms and insisting on holding them during procedures; families creating a cocoon of privacy at home for the first days and even weeks, drinking in the sweetness and love that a newborn brings to the world; fathers and mothers changing their priorities and schedules to be with their babies in the first year of life.

*   *   *

Birth affects each of us, strongly. We come to it—as mothers, as fathers, as helpers—in various states of consciousness, with different capacities, holding different versions of what we seek. I am convinced that the circumstances of a person's life in the womb, birth, and first hours—through the first eighteen months—have a tremendous impact, for good or for ill. Beginnings matter profoundly.

In this book, I have attempted to go underneath the fear and denial surrounding modern birth to find what has caused it to be such an unnatural and problematic experience for so many mothers and babies. Certainly one can make a case that it is simply power politics (or economics, or an arrogant patriarchal system) that controls birth and alters what is essentially a normal, healthy process. But to me the trouble is far more complex: it is all of these factors and many others as well. There is no clear target for blame and no easy way to change things. I have tried to provide a look at the whole picture: the history of birth in the Western world, particularly the United States; cultural traditions in other countries that Americans can learn from; personal accounts from mothers, fathers, midwives, doctors, and nurses. I also include many photographs of natural births that I hope will dispel fear and challenge prevailing notions of what birth should be like.

I offer *Immaculate Deception II* in the spirit of hope, with the belief that if we can relearn to trust our instincts, we will have a much better chance of creating an optimal birth for our babies and ourselves. I do not claim to be impartial on this subject, and any book written with passion should be read cautiously. No matter what your personal conclusions, however, I want you to leave this book with your eyes opened. Choose to see what's going on. Let yourself feel the full implications of birth. Take responsibility for the birth of your children.

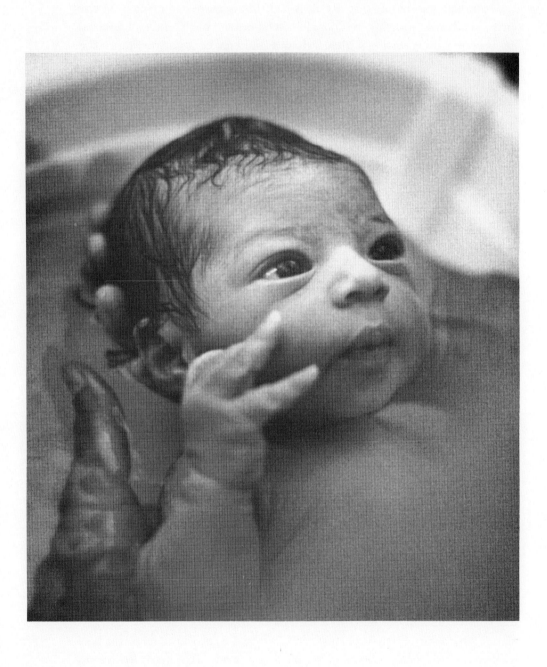

CHAPTER ONE

Childbirth from the Beginning

Your Sister Has a Baby Girl

Imagine your ancestor, a young woman living at the edge of a forest near a broad, meandering river. Her tribe is nomadic during the warmer months, traveling in small bands and living off the food they gather, sleeping in hammocks strung between trees. In the colder months the tribe comes together in a circle of simple huts whose doorways face a central firepit.

Imagine that this young woman, your ancient sister, is pregnant with her first child. She has a mate, an older man from a neighboring tribe, and she has been living with his people; but as she neared term she returned to her own family, as is the custom, to live with her mother and other women kin. After the baby is born, she will remain there until one full cycle of the moon is completed, being fed and massaged and cared for by the women and resting from her daily obligations. The discharge from her womb will have ceased before she returns to her husband and their home. She will be received with a special ceremony accorded a new mother.

Meanwhile, it is early autumn. The days are still warm, but the nights are chilly. Your sister and five other young women are tending the winter crops in the land cleared just beyond their circle of huts. Only a few old men are in the village today; the rest of the men and older boys are away on a hunt to bring back meat that will be cured and eaten during winter. When families are foraging in the warm months the roles of men and women are not strictly defined; everyone does what is necessary for survival. When the tribe is in the village, however, gender roles become defined. There, women and men lead largely separate lives, yet everyone realizes that their survival is dependent on every other member of the tribe.

The life of the tribe follows the rhythms of nature. Days are punctuated with prayers and chants, and the change of seasons is marked with special ceremonies. Other rites are performed when someone dies or is born, and the spirits of the ancestors are continually acknowledged for their ongoing part in the tribe's well-being. It is believed that all of these rituals must be observed in the prescribed manner. In these ways heaven and earth, plants, and animals are kept in balance and chaos is avoided.

For the women, the ceremonies and daily observances center primarily around the phases of the moon, to which their cycles are linked. Because they live in such close contact, they ovulate and menstruate at the same time each month, following the fullness and darkness of the moon. The older women pass on what they know to the younger women when they become pregnant: how to stay healthy while a baby is growing in your body; how to prepare yourself for labor; how to tend the stump of the umbilical cord until it falls off; how to get the baby to suckle; and how to care for the baby. They are the ones who conduct the special ceremonies to prepare a woman for her first labor, to imbue her with strength and remind her of all her ancestors who have made the same journey.

Your ancient sister has learned the ways of the women well. She knows how to take care of children, tend the animals and the garden, prepare food, tan the hides used for winter clothing and bedding, and make the simple clay pots used for storing food. As she grows older, the other women will share with her the secrets of the medicinal herbs that have been passed down for generations. Already she knows all the special chants and prayers women offer up for a safe birth and a healthy child, and she is confident that she and her child will be protected from harm as long as she follows the rhythm of the seasons, the cycles of the moon, and the customs of the tribe.

Like her mother, her mother's mother, and every woman before her, she has been taught to be careful in pregnancy, to eat certain foods—such as the slippery pulp under the skin of a broad-leafed plant, to ensure that the baby will come easily—and to refrain from eating other foods that are thought to cause a difficult birth or a deformed or stillborn baby.

Your sister knows she is fortunate to be giving birth during the months when the tribe is in the village, for she will not be alone and if there is a problem (something that rarely occurs when a woman is healthy) she has not only the experience of the wise woman of the tribe but also the magic of the shaman to rely on. If her childbirth occurred during the months of foraging for food, she would not have the comfort of a hut to birth in, or the presence of her mother and other women. But she has been taught how to deliver her own baby. She knows how to clean any fluid from the baby's mouth or nose if it has difficulty breathing; how to cut the cord that unites her and the baby; how to wipe the end of the cord with the juice of a certain plant to stop its bleeding; how to chew a piece of her own afterbirth if she bleeds too much; and how to protect the baby from the chill of night. She knows the chants for labor that are said to keep the baby in good position and the contractions strong and useful, and the ones that coax the baby from her body if it does not come with ease. All this she can do, just as countless women before her have done. She has heard the stories, and she has confidence and trust in the ancestors who guide her. Your sister says prayers to quiet her occasional pangs of fear. She believes, as she has been taught to believe, that it is unwise to spend much time giving voice to fears.

Your sister does not expect to need any herbs for the discomfort of labor. If the labor were to go too slowly, or if she were to bleed excessively afterward, she knows which herbs to use. However, the elder women say one should never take any substance that dulls the pain and aching, for it might also harm the baby or make the birth difficult for the mother. This makes sense to her. Birthing a child is an ordinary part of life, not a sickness.

Your sister knows that not all babies survive the journey of birth, and that a few others will die before they begin to walk, of a sickness marked by diarrhea. After that, accidents or disease can claim a child's life. Still, in her tribe, most women have two or three children they can count on to help them in their old age, and many can boast they have never lost a child. Sometimes— it is not known why—a baby comes too early. These babies are small and frail and do not always survive. But few babies die at birth. On rare occasions, when a baby is born deformed or the mother has nearly died in giving birth, the baby will not be allowed to live. Your sister has heard of one case like that. The baby's legs were strangely twisted and a bubble of flesh was protruding from its spine. One of the older women took the baby into the forest and put her hand over its face to stop its breathing, then buried it far from the village. It was believed this had to be done to protect the entire tribe.

Listening to other women tell their birthing stories in the women's circle around the evening fire, your sister has gained confidence. She has been present for half a dozen labors. It is customary for children to wander in and out of a hut where a woman is giving birth, and it is a tribal custom that every child, both girls and boys, witness at least one birth and one death, so that they will respect both life and death and be afraid of neither. Only the men stay away, to protect themselves from what is considered the extraordinary power of a birthing woman, stronger even than the power women have when they bleed each month. It is believed that men are weakened by the sight or touch of women's blood.

*   *   *

It is midafternoon. Your sister works slowly, bare-breasted, her full, high belly making her normally graceful movements somewhat awkward as she stoops and squats. The women are singing in unison as they work, to make the work go easier. As she sings, your sister wonders when her baby will come, what the birth will be like, and whether it will be the son everyone hopes for. A boy as a first child is believed to be a special blessing, an assurance that there will be another hunter and protector of the tribe. The old women, who sit working skins for winter clothes and bedding, have kept their eyes on your sister over the past few days. They whisper and tell jokes, and they tease her. They know the infant will soon arrive, and their intent is to keep her spirit light so the baby will be happy to go through its journey from the spirit world into this world.

For a week your sister has felt new sensations in her abdomen, different from the churning or kicking movements of the baby that she often feels when she is resting. There have been frequent sharp twinges deep inside her groin. At first she was frightened about them, but she asked her aunt and was reassured that they were only a sign that the birth was near and that her body and the baby were getting ready. She has drunk a special tea daily during the last cycle of the moon, ever since the tribe returned to the river. It is a tea that women often take late in pregnancy, when they can find the right plant, and it is said to strengthen a woman's body and to make a first labor easier.

Today she has a new feeling, a dull aching in her lower back, which in the past few hours has slowly spread around toward her abdomen. She is thirsty and drinks water frequently from a gourd she carries slung over one shoulder, and she goes off many times into the trees to urinate.

Several times she stops in her work to stand and rub her aching back. She thinks about the childbirths she has seen. She has watched her mother give birth to her two younger siblings, and she suddenly recalls the moist, sweet smell of the hut during those times, her mother's moans, then her panting, then her low grunting as she squatted in the semidarkness on a bed of moss.

Suddenly your ancient sister feels a sharp, quick tugging inside, down very low. She is immediately alert. After a few minutes it is followed by another and, in rhythmic sequence, a third, then a fourth. As the setting sun marks the end of the day, the sensations become a regular pattern, and she walks back to her hut slowly, singing along with the other women to keep herself calm, but unable to keep up with them when the aching, pulling sensation is at its peak. When she stops to catch her breath the women turn around and tease her; they know it is her time and they want to make her spirit laugh. Her two younger sisters come running to meet her and, seeing the expression on her face, stop and eye her with curiosity. They are aware that her time is near and they want to know what is happening, for they will experience it one day, too.

She calls to her aunt, who is outside the hut with her mother, preparing the evening meal at the fire pit. It is growing cool. Your sister goes inside and wraps a soft, tanned skin around her shoulders, then comes out to sit by the fire alongside her mother and her aunt. She wants to be close to them. Birds sing in the dimming light.

During the evening the rhythmic tugging and aching turns into a stronger pain that rises and falls. It tires her, but there is time in between to rest and empty her mind. After dinner, inside the hut, she listens to her mother and her aunt tell stories. They know the baby will likely come this night, so most of their stories are to give her courage and to keep her spirits up. Some are of their own birthings, and they laugh at some of the memories and sometimes turn to tease her so she will laugh and forget the gripping inside her. Mostly she is too engulfed by these sensations to respond, but she smiles at moments of rest. When her mother and aunt begin the familiar labor chants, she joins in. The two she likes the most are one that says to be strong and courageous like a warthog, and one about a large bird that soars, strong and free, above the earth.

The younger sisters watch from their mats until they cannot keep their eyes open any longer and they fall asleep. There is a fire, and in its light your ancient sister's face now looks dazed. Between the intense sensations that erupt deep within her, she tends the fire, carefully banking it so that it will burn slowly through the night and keep the hut warm for the baby. She is hot now, too hot to wear clothes.

It has only been a few hours since the contractions grew close together and strong and long enough to cause her difficulty in speaking and chanting. Now she feels heavy and tired and wonders when it will be over. Occasionally, anxiety fills her mind between the pains, and at those times she prays and is comforted by the voices of her mother and aunt. They know she needs to do this part alone. No position feels comfortable, not standing or walking or crouching. So she squats, then stands, then leans against the doorway of the hut. Now her mother goes to stand by her, allowing her daughter to lean her weight against her body.

The night outside the hut is cool; crickets are singing. Your sister is suddenly very restless; she paces back and forth across the hut between contractions, going to the open doorway each time to look at the rising moon. She chants a prayer for strength, but her voice seems far away and her eyes have a wildness in them, like that of a doe trapped in a thicket. Although the older women feel all is going well, her mother now asks the aunt to fetch the wise woman. She is called to help first mothers, for her years of attendance at births have given her a special wisdom and calmness.

The wise woman knows all of the special medicinal herbs of the region, the ways of bringing a pregnancy on, or preventing or even stopping one. She has gleaned some of her knowledge from talking to the women of other tribes and finding out how they handle certain situations. She is well versed in all aspects of a woman's sexual life, and knows how to care for any injury or wound. But, most important, she knows how to keep birth normal and what to do if something goes wrong. She carries a special root that she will steep in heated water and give to your sister to drink if there is too much bleeding after the baby comes. She even knows how to turn a baby who cannot be born because it is lying sidewise in the womb. She can tell if this is the case by observing the shape of the abdomen. She was taught by the wise woman before her how to turn a baby by carefully yet firmly massaging the area. If what she knows is not sufficient, the wise woman sends for the tribe's shaman. He performs special incantations and does magic and, if none of that works, it is understood that no more can be done, and that this mother and baby are now in the hands of the spirits.

The wise woman arrives with a small pouch of implements: a sharp piece of rock for cutting the cord and a slender length of sinew for tying it off, as well as the dried root to be brewed in case of bleeding and another to be chewed if the mother needs extra strength. She checks to see if a pallet has been prepared for your sister and the baby. It has, and a fresh, extra-soft, extra-thick animal skin has been rolled up alongside the mat. There is also a pile of fresh moss by the doorway. The wise woman teases your sister when a contraction slowly fades, in order to ascertain how relaxed she is, then makes herself comfortable by the fire, letting your sister handle the contractions in her own way. She knows not to interfere when things are going well, and she judges that this baby will come on its own shortly.

With each contraction now your sister drops into a hunched position on the floor, her feet apart and her buttocks on her heels, letting her head fall back or rocking it from side to side as she exhales heavily. Frequently she moans as her abdomen mounds into a hard peak. With the onset of the next contraction she lets out a loud cry, then, during the next visible bulging of her abdomen, she grunts a bit.

The contractions come quickly one after another, with little time in between. Your sister's gaze seems farther away, and the pupils are slightly rolled up so that the whites show underneath. She is breathing quickly, almost panting, at the peak of each contraction, and she is perspiring heavily. Sometimes she calls out to the spirit of the baby to give her strength, sometimes to the spirit of her women ancestors. Several times during the evening she leaves the hut to urinate. Much earlier in the day her bowels emptied, and she has not been hungry since, though she continues to reach frequently for water from a gourd near the doorway and sometimes chews on a particular root to give her energy. The older women, sitting by the fire, brew tea and chant prayers to the spirits to make this passage safe and gentle for mother and baby. The sounds of insects can be heard outside, and a light wind has come up.

It is not long before the rhythm of her labor changes again, and the frequency with which her belly mounds lessens a bit. Now your sister has a longer time to rest between contractions. During these contractions she squats, but between times she leans forward onto her hands and knees. Her mother and aunt assist her in squatting when she grows tired and turns to one or the other of them. She is now straining and grunting each time her belly grows hard. After ten or maybe twelve more of these bearing-down times, a small, round, wet area of dark hair appears between her open legs. Your sister is now upright on her knees over the pile of moss. Two more grunting pushes and a head slips out, then the body, and the baby drops onto the moss. Your sister sinks back onto her heels, exhausted and dazed.

Slowly she turns her gaze to the infant lying on the moss and moving slightly. After a minute or so, she reaches down and slowly picks up this warm, wet baby girl. The cord that dangles between her legs is thick and pulsing, ending in the baby's abdomen. She picks up her daughter and cradles her against her flaccid stomach. No one in the hut moves or says a word. It is the mother's voice a baby must hear first. Slowly the baby begins to change color from bluish red to red, and her eyes slowly open in the semidarkness. She turns her head toward the face of her mother, who is looking with amazement into her clear, dark eyes.

The two younger girls are wide awake now and staring from their beds. Your sister shivers slightly, and her mother picks up one of the newly tanned soft skins and places it gently around her shoulders. Suddenly, out of the silence in which only the baby's first squeaking sounds are heard, the new mother begins to sing. It is not a song she has learned, but one that comes from deep within her. What she sings is her baby's song. Each child is said to come into this world with its own song, a song that only its mother knows. Even she does not know it until it arises from her, at the first sight of her child. Singing it shows a baby who it is.

Your sister is now holding her daughter against her body. The baby opens her mouth and begins to turn her head toward the nearest breast. With one arm under the baby's upper back, and the fingers of that hand cradling the warm, wet head, your sister brings her up onto her breast, where the baby begins to suckle. After a few sucks, your sister grunts once more and a large, wet, dark-red mass slips from her body to the moss. The child's cord is attached to it. The wise woman takes her sharp stone and severs the cord, and the aunt moves the afterbirth and the bloody moss to the other side of the hut. Tomorrow it will be buried far from the hut. Now there is nothing to be done but to wipe away the small amount of blood and fluid on your sister's skin and to cover her and the baby to keep them warm.

Throughout the next morning the other women and children come to the hut to see the new baby. She is usually at her mother's breast, sometimes asleep with her mouth half open, other times suckling, sometimes just looking out at the world from the warmth and safety of her mother's arms. If your sister were alone she would, of course, have had to find the strength to rise from where she lay and take her baby back to her companions, but this time

IMMACULATE DECEPTION II

she has the luxury of being in a warm hut, with others there to take care of all her needs. She will have no responsibilities for many days except to feed her baby, who already suckles strongly, drinking in the nourishment from her mother's body.

*   *   *

For the first year or more, your sister's daughter is in almost continual physical contact with her mother's body, either in her arms or in a sling across her back or at her hip. She will take milk from her mother's breast for many months before she is given any other food. She will continue to suckle—from both her mother and, when her mother is not near, from other mothers—until she is three or four. Mostly she is carried. It is believed that a child should not be put down on the ground until ready to walk, lest an evil spirit bring it harm. This child is thus protected from all danger by being carried, and by sleeping with her mother until she is old enough to sleep with cousins or a younger sibling.

Your sister resumes her daily activities after one full cycle of the moon has passed. Carrying the baby with her, she learns to recognize her daughter's needs and particular moods as well as she knows her own. When walking, she will stop to shift her daughter from her back to her breast, or to hold her body away from her and out a little distance to let her urinate or defecate. The baby's first year is a time of physical comfort and security in the almost constant presence of her mother or another familiar member of the tribe.

Your sister is now a woman, the mother of a thriving child, and she is connected to all the women who came before her and to all those who will come after. She feels a sense of well-being. One day, if she lives long enough, she will become an elder and pass along all that she knows to her daughter and help her become a woman. And so it will continue.

How Has Childbirth Changed Since Ancient Times?

FOR A NUMBER OF REASONS, childbirth was probably easier for most women in early cultures, especially in hunter-gatherer societies, where everyone was accustomed to physical labor and supple and fit from daily activity. This is confirmed by archaeological remains and contemporary anthropological research on extant Stone Age cultures. Women and men in these societies lived close to the earth, and their lives were part of the natural rhythms of the sun and moon and the changes of the seasons. A woman's body was not tightly bound in any restrictive way, and she walked straight and tall, with her feet flat on the earth. She did not spend hours sitting, but she often squatted. Her diet contained no processed foods or chemical additives and was full of fiber, so she seldom suffered from constipation or hemorrhoids. The air she breathed and the water she drank were usually clean. Life had its harsh aspects but, unless she lived where long-term drought or severe climate made food supplies inadequate, or unless she met with an accident, she usually was in good health. As is the case with indigenous peoples around the world, we can assume that members of early societies who were not in good health were not able to reproduce or didn't survive to pass on unhealthy genetic traits, such as diabetes.

Women evolved over the ages—both physically and psychologically—to give birth successfully. A high level of physical activity during pregnancy helped to keep babies head down and well positioned for birth. During labor, though women may have been apart from the rest of their tribe, they were on their feet and active until the actual delivery. As the baby descended the birth canal and the mother felt the overwhelming urge to bear down, she naturally assumed a squatting or kneeling position.

Modern scientific research into the effects of the various positions a woman can assume in labor and during the expulsion stage—and reports from women themselves—show that there is a great benefit in being upright and moving around during labor, and being upright, squatting, or on hands and knees during delivery. Labor is made longer and contractions are made more painful and generally less effective when a woman is inactive or lying down. This was as true for your ancient sister as it is today; that is why women left to their own devices have instinctively, the world over, chosen to be upright and active long into labor and why the most common position for delivery has been some form of upright squat. Yet, until the last few years, modern women have been routinely kept in bed for labor and on their backs for pushing and delivery. Only recently have the persistent efforts of a few childbirth advocates finally resulted in women being "permitted," or even encouraged, to be on their feet during labor and in a squatting position for birth.

Except for epidemics of disease, which have periodically swept through large parts of the world, your ancient sister was not likely to have encountered the numerous degenerative diseases associated with civilization and modern life. Rickets, the disease caused by vitamin D deficiency, deformed many women's pelvic bones as recently as just a century ago, and for hundreds of years this made childbirth difficult or even impossible. Rickets flourished in the polluted cities of Europe in the Middle Ages through the Industrial Revolution, where there were few fresh fruits and vegetables; it was virtually unknown in traditional societies where people managed to eat sufficient amounts of fresh fruits, seeds, and vegetables and were exposed to sunlight.

Although we see almost no cases of rickets in industrialized societies today, many of the things we do, ingest, or breathe strain our bodies and can affect our births and the health of our babies. In ancient times, however, it was highly unlikely that a woman with a serious condition would carry a pregnancy through to term, especially since women had ways of preventing or aborting pregnancy. And, since it was the only way to feed them, it would have been impossible for a baby not to be breast-fed for at least a year or two, if not by its birth mother, then by another woman.

Anthropological evidence shows that the average hunter-gatherer woman had only three or four pregnancies in the course of her life, probably because her physically active life delayed puberty and because her low percentage of body fat lowered the amount of estrogen in her system throughout her life. These two factors, combined with the practice of breast-feeding each child for an average of three years, meant babies were naturally well spaced. (Breast-feeding tends to suppress ovulation.) This corresponds with the theory that a woman's body takes three years or so to fully recover from its pregnant and birthing states.

Women in hunter-gatherer cultures also found it easier to care for their babies because they did not have to do it alone. Child rearing was a group responsibility, and for as long as people's lives took place in proximity to other members of the community, mothers did not find infant care a burden. Tribal life should not be idealized. There were real dangers, from severe weather to predators. People did not have sophisticated medical techniques. Some tribes even engaged in such brutal practices as genital mutilation of children. However, normal physiological functions such as birth and breast-feeding were respected. Although life in hunter-gatherer cultures was different, and ancient women in general were in better health than women are today, their bodies are fundamentally the same and giving birth remains the same elemental process.

HAVE BABIES CHANGED?

The reason it takes most humans much longer than other mammals to birth their young, even in traditional societies, is physiological, not pathological. It has mainly to do with the internal dimensions of the female pelvis and the angle of the pelvis, which shifted when humans first stood upright. Therefore, physical effort on the part of the uterus is required to push the baby through and out.

This tight fit through the birth canal is functional for a baby. The continual squeezing and pushing by the uterus first enlarges the cervix, which is the opening of the uterus, the strongest muscle in the human body. The uterus then changes shape, with the greatest mass of that muscle contracting toward its top, creating a powerful piston that propels the baby down through the birth canal. The action of the uterus in labor also stimulates the baby's entire body, readying its nervous system and brain for the new world it will live in once it is out of the mother's body. Because this is a world of air and gravity, the baby's body must make a tremendous adjustment in the first few minutes. The baby must exchange its own oxygen, or breathe, for the first time. It must control its own blood pressure and keep its body warm.

Labor, and the descent through the birth canal, prepares babies for their life outside the womb in a way that nothing else can duplicate. It is this action that stimulates the baby's adrenal glands to produce the hormone that allows the baby's body to do on its own all the things that were up until now done for it in the womb. This stimulation does not occur in the event of cesarean surgery, in which the baby's own efforts to be born are cut short and the baby is pulled out from above, usually without having had any benefit of what is known as "the pushing phase" of labor. Because they don't go through this, cesarean-born infants are more likely to have initial problems clearing their lungs and getting breathing established. For the baby, as well as the mother, birth can be exhausting, but it serves a vital function. During this first journey of its life, a child is not meant to be helpless or passive. It is meant to be awake and aware, a fully active participant.

It is true that human beings have undergone some physiological changes over time. The average size of babies may appear to have increased, especially during this past century, as women's caloric intake has increased and their physical activity has decreased. However, birth records show that in the past it was quite normal for healthy Caucasian women in North America to give birth to babies weighing eight or even ten pounds. And the structure of the female pelvis allows the successful birthing of even large babies. This is because the human pelvis is not rigid bone but flexible and jointed. The female pelvis is made of three plates of bone, joined by cartilage. During pregnancy, this cartilage becomes softened, due to the secretion of a hormone known as relaxin. The fetal head is also constructed of plates of bone. These plates can freely ride over each other in the course of its tight journey down the birth canal and then spread out again after birth. This ability of the baby's head to "mold" before delivery makes birth easier for the mother as well as for the baby. Even babies weighing ten or twelve pounds can usually be born without intervention. We have ample proof of this fact, since it is not unusual for a woman who has had one cesarean childbirth (because her pelvis was believed to be too small to accommodate her baby's head, a condition called cephalopelvic disproportion, or CPD) to vaginally deliver a second baby that weighs a full pound or more than the first!

Babies' health has not changed very much over the centuries, either. They have always been more likely to be born in good health when their mothers were healthy throughout pregnancy. They have always benefited when birth was normal and uncomplicated and have been more likely to suffer when the birth was abnormal and placed added stress upon them. Infants have always gained added special protection by a combination of being breast-fed for many months, by being held or worn against an adult's body and carried until they could walk, and by sleeping alongside one of their parents. All three of these practices were the norm until fairly recent times, when such practices have been devalued.

Today, a baby sleeps in its own room, is routinely carried around in a plastic container or pushed in a stroller, and is fed out of a bottle. Some people actually believe independence can be fostered by treating babies this way from the start.

Of course, in the past, not all babies survived the journey of birth. That is still true today; however, if we look to modern-day hunter-gatherer societies, we find that most of the infant deaths do not occur during or immediately after birth. Instead they occur weeks or months later, notably at the time when the infants either are weaned or have their diet supplemented with coarse gruel meant for older children and adults but from which their undeveloped bodies cannot extract enough nourishment. Death is also more likely to occur when babies are able to crawl and walk and are no longer receiving the protection of being carried. At this point, they become subject to infections, parasites, and accidents.

A striking example of what can happen when we stray too far from spontaneous human behavior with regard to childbirth and the care of babies occurred during World War II. Newborn babies had been routinely separated from their mothers for days, beginning right after birth, because mothers who had been given general anesthesia during childbirth were incapable of caring for their babies. Suddenly, outbreaks of infant diarrhea began to spread through newborn nurseries all across North America. Many babies died and many others got very sick, because dehydration resulting from diarrhea is life-threatening to a newborn. There were no antibiotics at the time, so there was little effective treatment.

At first the response in hospitals was to keep babies quarantined in the newborn nursery, so that their mothers could not see them at all. Only a chronic shortage of hospital nurses forced staffs to change that practice and replace it with the one of putting all healthy-seeming newborns alongside their mothers for the entire seven- or ten-day hospital stay, so that the few nurses there could care for the sick babies in the nursery. Nurses and doctors were shocked to discover that the epidemic of infant diarrhea virtually ended with this one simple change of hospital routine.

Breast-feeding, instead of the then-routine practice of feeding babies artificial formula, would have further strengthened those newborns. The short-term and long-term benefits for babies of suckling the breast and of having a diet exclusively of breast milk are now well known. Scientists are also beginning to understand the complexity of the relationship between mothers and babies, and the risks of separating them, especially in the first days following birth. One factor now believed to be significant in sudden infant death syndrome is that some babies need to be in physical proximity to the mother's (or another person's) heartbeat while sleeping, in order to keep their hearts beating regularly. Only as the child grows does its own body eventually take over this function so it can be on its own.

In traditional cultures it would have been almost unheard of for a mother and baby to be out of sight or sound of each other, unless another mother-surrogate in the tribe were available to take the mother's place. It would have been unthinkable, and far too dangerous, for babies to sleep apart from their mothers, or to spend many hours without being held and touched.

We now have a mass of scientific evidence that shows how vital stimulation and affection are to most aspects of human development, from the development of language to the development of self-esteem, the ability to give and receive affection, and the ability to maintain intimate relationships. Traditional ways of caring for babies, which extended the world over for tens of thousands of years, have proved to be optimal, because a human infant is born physiologically immature and is in need of constant physical care.

One little-considered fact that supports the value of maternal and infant bonding is that human infants take nine months or more to develop to the stage that most larger mammals reach within just twenty-four hours after birth! Newborn cows, sheep, goats, and horses are on their feet, able to search out the mother's milk and even to follow their mother across a field within minutes or hours after birth. The human infant has important vestiges of these abilities, such as being able to tell the scent of its own mother's milk from any other woman's milk within days of birth, and being able to recognize the sound of its mother's voice from a group of voices, but human infants still need almost constant care and protection.

CHILDBIRTH AS WOMAN'S ACHIEVEMENT
THEN AND NOW

Birth is woman's work, a natural part of female sexuality and creativity. Prehistoric fetishes of the pregnant female body tell us that in ancient times, birthing women were revered by other women and by men for their ability to create life. This was acknowledged and honored, even when women were feared for that same power.

The physical effort involved in childbirth is not inherently different for a tribeswoman in the Amazonian jungles today than it was for a woman in New Guinea thousands of years ago. Nor need it be much different for today's modern woman. For women everywhere, childbirth—especially a first birth—has always been a tremendous achievement, one for which a woman's body must make a tremendous effort. In order to give birth, her body must vastly proliferate its blood supply, her abdominal muscles must stretch considerably, her back must bear the added weight of the baby, and her uterus—the strongest muscle in the body, stronger even than the heart—must expand to twenty times its normal size!

The cervix, which must be tightly closed throughout pregnancy to keep the baby in the uterus, must soften and thin, then stretch to accommodate a head the size of a grapefruit. The vaginal tissues must unfold and stretch to accommodate the baby's shoulders. The perineum—the tissue between the outlet of the vagina and the rectum—must also soften, thin, and stretch to allow the baby to pass through without tearing.

Even when women are physically fit and relaxed, labor may still involve great discomfort and a good measure of pain, especially with a first baby or one that is quite large for the mother's pelvis or is not lying in the normal head-down, back position. But this pain is functional. It is due to tremendous physiological changes—the stretching of tissues, the work of muscles not ordinarily used—and is not a sign that anything is wrong. Labor ordinarily proceeds without serious complications. The process is designed in such a way that the woman and the baby can rest in the intervals between contractions. In fact, labor creates an altered state of consciousness as a normal part of the process. Women sometimes even fall asleep between pushes at the end of labor, due to a combination of being tired and the body releasing hormones that diminish the sensation of pain.

Anthropological research shows that the most important difference between modern women and our tribal ancestors is that in tribal cultures women do not suffer from mistrust or fear of the body and of the natural process of childbirth. Such cultures have never believed that life is meant to be free of all discomfort or pain. Modern people, however, believe that we ought to be able to shape our environment and our lives to avoid pain and even death.

Fear is a normal human response to the unknown, especially when there is any possibility of harm or death. However, the level of fear and anxiety traditionally felt by women at childbirth could not have been anything like that felt by women in the filthy, disease-ridden cities of Europe from the Middle Ages up through the early years of the Industrial Revolution. Nor could it have been anything like the anxiety and fear experienced by so many modern women, who may be privileged to live in physical comfort but still carry the legacy of those times, the belief that childbirth is too dangerous and painful for women to endure without medical intervention.

The attitude a woman has toward her body and its ways, and the attitude of those around her—especially in the medical professions—has affected the birth process so that it bears little resemblance to its normal, natural state. The modern attitude of asserting control over and attempting to "manage" a birth is the antithesis of trust in the body and the normalcy of childbirth.

What *can* women do to make childbirth more normal? We could choose to live healthier, less stressful lives, at least during pregnancy and when we are caring for our babies. We could choose to live more closely connected to the earth, to find more time to be out in nature, and to make our bodies more fit. Our health workers—doctors in particular—seldom recommend living a more naturally wholesome life and practicing a more positive attitude toward our bodies as the best ways to ensure a normal pregnancy and birth. Yet those are the very things that will make a difference! Most women, even if they have been poorly nourished prior to conception or have been doing harmful things to their bodies, can bring themselves to a state of reasonable health in the course of a pregnancy and then give birth normally to a healthy baby.

And a positive attitude is important, too. Nature is not prepared to handle inordinate fear and self-doubt. We hear so much today about the harmful effects of cocaine and other drugs on babies in utero, but we hear nothing about the harmful effects of our bodies being constantly flooded with stress hormones that weaken our immune system and inhibit normal birth. If, in addition to making our bodies fit, we do as much as we can to learn about birth as a natural process, we will do much to alleviate unnecessary fears and be able to face birth with calm and courage.

*   *   *

There is much we can learn from looking at what birth has traditionally been like for women the world over. For one thing, it is unlikely that our ancient sisters would have resisted or fought the process of childbirth, and that is important. Acceptance of the process—of the contractions, of the pain—results in fewer complications. There is very little of that kind of acceptance today. Instead, women comply with medical procedures: then *give up* responsibility for childbirth rather than *giving in* to the process.

In the past, childbirth was an event young women witnessed and quite possibly assisted with. Women's knowledge of the birth process—as well as of menstruation and menopause—came through stories, observation, and direct experiences. Their attitude toward birth was largely unquestioning, un-self-conscious, uncomplicated, and full of trust mixed with a healthy respect and awe for the risks involved.

Women in all types of societies have routinely gathered to share their daily life experiences with one another. Young women have traditionally received knowledge, comfort, and courage from being part of the community of women. Once, there was no shame about the normal processes of the female body and no reason to hide them from young girls. Feelings of shame about the female body, its natural functions and its sexuality, are not something that occurs spontaneously. They come from outside, from what girls are taught. Traditionally, girls heard birthing stories of women's strengths, prowess, and endurance, not of their difficulties and suffering. Since all of life took place immediately around them, in the next hut and down the path, they shared freely in the experiences of women.

Today, however, young girls in the United States inherit a toxic legacy of attitudes about childbirth that poisons their natural self-esteem. They grow up fearing and not understanding what it means to have a baby. What separates most birthing women today from women in the past is the loss of familiarity with the birth process, the loss of community with other women, and the loss of traditional feminine wisdom.

Fortunately, not everything has been lost. A healthy view of childbirth is alive and well in some families and among a few religious communities—such as the Amish, Mormons, and Seventh-Day Adventists—who all believe in and continue to practice normal childbirth. And it is alive and well in what is called "the alternative birthing community" (see chapter 5). It can be found virtually anywhere where there are practicing midwives, and especially where there are women who plan home births and share their experiences with other women. This subculture of childbirth maintains the view of women as inherently strong, courageous, and competent in birth. This view is different from that of the mainstream because it does not focus on pain, fear, and suffering, and does not cause women to think of themselves as helpless or as victims of a faulty process.

Remember this: Birth is a process that nature has successfully refined through tens of thousands of years. The knowledge of how to give birth without outside intervention lies deep within each woman. Childbirth is as natural as pregnancy or sexuality. Like those natural states, what successful childbirth depends on is an acceptance of the process.

All that most women need in order to do this is the belief that birth works and will work for them. But this is no small thing to hold on to. We are in the midst of an era of high-tech, managed childbirth. Women must reclaim childbirth themselves, for themselves. In the process, I believe we will reclaim an important part of womanhood and do a great service to our children.

The Main Problem with Childbirth Today

Ironically, the main difficulty with childbirth today is that modern medicine has been *too* successful in its attempts to rescue mothers and babies when something goes terribly wrong. The problem is that an entire system of care has been built that focuses on disasters and *expects* them to occur. It is a system based upon fear: the expectation is that anything that can go wrong will go wrong. Traditionally, human beings were not able to exert much control over the natural process because of technical limitations. Now, because technical innovations make interventions possible, people are constantly on guard for the worst. They have lost their trust in the birth process and in the natural capacity of women and babies to conduct their own births successfully. Unfortunately, this means a situation more likely to create problems than to support normalcy.

Upon entering a modern hospital maternity and newborn unit today, especially in the English-speaking world, we can see that the unit is not organized to reduce problems by supporting normalcy; it is organized so as to treat every laboring woman and her baby as potentially in jeopardy. Worse than that, many hospital units are guided by the unspoken—or even spoken—belief that a birthing woman is "a problem," especially if she does not go along with the way things are done; only passivity is rewarded. Yet in nature, it has always been a woman's assertiveness, actions, and resourcefulness that have served her best both in childbirth and in protecting and caring for herself and her child.

Women today do not believe that their bodies know what to do, much less that their babies also know what to do. Because they are afraid and feel like they lack knowledge, they are often reassured rather than anxious when they enter the hospital. At least at the conscious level, they believe that all will be well within those walls. They believe this because they trust that someone else will know what to do if something goes wrong. The authority has been transferred to someone outside. But the body doesn't lie, and that is why, despite a feeling of comfort in the hospital, many women still find that their labor slows or stops on admission to the maternity unit. It is also why so many women harbor nagging doubts about the necessity of many of the procedures done—to them and to their babies—in the name of helping. It is why so many women—and most health workers today—do not know the difference between intervention and support. Unfortunately, birthing woman has not only lost touch with her body and with her ancient female lineage. She has also lost her voice to speak up, to question intervention, to ask for support, to demand respect for the work of giving birth and caring for her infant. When she finds that voice, she will regain a vital part of her creativity and power as a woman.

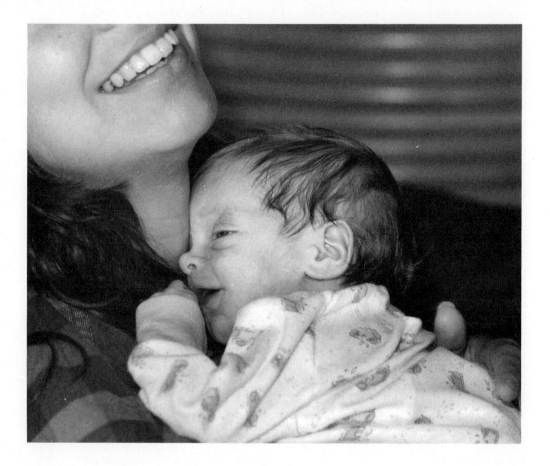

CHAPTER TWO

Women, Childbirth, and the History of Medicine

Your Sister Has a Baby Boy

Spring came late to Boston in 1853. Sarah Hanley had almost given up on ever seeing the cherry tree flower outside the parlor window. She was feeling so tired, so heavy, that she thought she could not go on one more day. Yet the doctor said there were still two weeks to go in her pregnancy. She had not walked outside her Boston townhouse in nearly three months; instead she took her exercise each day by making circles around the parlor. Women in her condition were not seen in public; it wasn't proper. With nothing but the same four rosebud-papered walls to look at, she often wanted to scream.

Of course, a well-bred young woman would never allow herself to make a fuss. The most Sarah allowed herself was an occasional stamping of her feet, and she tried to do that only when her husband, Charles, was not home. He would call Dr. Lewiston if she got into one of her "fits," as he referred to them, and Dr. Lewiston would make one of his evening house calls. He and Charles would stand conferring with each other and looking at her as sadly as if she were a china doll who'd fallen from the shelf. Anyway, it only resulted in her being put to bed and having to take a bitter tonic the doctor brought to calm her.

If this baby ever came, Sarah would be twenty-three when the baby was two months old. This was her and Charles's first child. There had been one miscarriage, last year, which had come early in the pregnancy. She had bled a lot afterward and had had to stay in bed for several months. It had taken a long time to regain her strength.

"How do working women like Mary do it?" Sarah wondered. Mary, the servant girl, was only twenty-one and already had two children. She had somehow managed to work for Sarah and Charles right up until the week she delivered each baby, and she took only a few weeks off before returning to their household. Sarah had seen the children several times, and they both looked healthy. Mary talked about breast-feeding each of them in the hours she was off-duty, and Sarah supposed Mary had a woman friend nurse them the rest of the time.

But Sarah had no intention of allowing her own body to be used like a cow's. She and Charles had interviewed and selected a wet nurse for her baby, a woman who had recently lost one of her infant twins, and so had ample milk for another. In addition to the wet nurse, they had hired a monthly nurse, who was to live in for a few weeks before the baby was due, to get the household organized for the baby. The monthly, as she was called, had already moved in, taking the bedroom on the third floor. She would be with Sarah in labor until the doctor came, then stay on to care for the baby for several months until Sarah was "well enough" to take over the care of her baby.

*   *   *

"Dr. Lewiston is a kind man," Sarah thought. He'd been a friend of Charles's in school, before Charles went on to study law. William Lewiston had gone to Ireland to do his medical training, at the famous Rotunda Hospital in Dublin, a highly respected place for a young man to train. The chief of service at that time, Sarah recalled hearing him once say, was a man named Aberdeen, renowned for his pioneering work in discovering the communicable and infectious nature of childbed fever.

Sarah shivered at the very thought of childbed fever. Women died of it within a few days of giving birth, even very healthy women. Even women her age. Sarah was not all that healthy; she had regular fainting spells, she didn't sleep all that well, and her appetite had never been good.

Right there in middle-class Boston, just as in other North American cities and in Europe, childbed fever was a grave danger for all birthing women. It was commonly believed that it was caused either by the bad temper of the mother, by her being unfaithful to her husband, or by her being exposed to cold air during or immediately after the birth. Women who gave birth in hospitals, who were the poor women who lived on the streets and had no homes to go to, died by the thousands of childbed fever. It was rumored that of twenty women in a large ward, nineteen might die, each in the order in which she was examined.

Oliver Wendell Holmes, Sr., an American physician and writer who lived near Charles and Sarah, was recommending that physicians begin washing their hands thoroughly before and after examining a birthing woman. Sarah had read in the newspaper of the controversy Dr. Holmes's suggestion had brought about and had mentioned it to Charles over dinner one night. He had said, "You mustn't worry your lovely head, my sweet. This doesn't have to concern you. William is a family friend and a brilliant doctor. He would never do anything that might hurt you or the baby."

Still, she sometimes did worry, and she wondered. None of the servant girl Mary's friends in the crowded slums of Boston ever seemed to contract the fever. They had all been delivered by midwives, women who could not even read. Mary said these midwives knew a lot about what to do to help a woman have a baby. Sarah once raised the idea to Charles. "What if I had a midwife, Charles? Mary seems to know a very competent one. I'd like to meet her. Couldn't we?"

Charles had scoffed. "You can't be serious! A midwife! They're dirty, illiterate old women. How could you possibly think I'd allow anyone like that to be near you at such an important time? I'm surprised at you, Sarah. Where has your common sense gone? Dr. Lewiston went all the way to Ireland to study. He knows everything there is to know about having a baby!"

Sarah never brought the subject up again to her husband, and when she mentioned it to one of her women friends with whom she'd gone to school, the friend was equally shocked. Midwives, she said, might be acceptable for immigrants and low-class women, but they certainly weren't fitting for a lawyer's wife.

Sarah tried to keep from brooding, but with so little to do except embroider and play the piano, she couldn't help it. Sarah had many fears about giving birth. Her mother, like most women in her class, had not told her anything about it. And the women in her circle never talked about it at all, except to say that it was a horrible experience. The only people she had to turn to when doubts and anxiety plagued her were Mary and Dr. Lewiston. Dr. Lewiston had a way of making her feel like a child if she expressed any concern or asked any questions, even though he was only eight years older than she was.

Thank God for Mary. Mary, it turned out, was full of information and was quite willing to talk. She was also confident that Sarah would do just fine. "After all, Missus," she would say, "we women have been having babies since the beginning of time. Sometimes all by ourselves. Sometimes out in the woods. How do you think people would have survived if having babies was all that terrible?" Yes, it hurt, she would never deny that. But the pain was different from the kind of pain you have when you are injured, she told Sarah. "The pain of labor has a purpose. It doesn't mean something is wrong with you. It just means your body is working hard."

Mary's words made Sarah feel a lot better than Dr. Lewiston's. Sometimes when she awoke in the night with fear of what lay ahead, she would go over and over Mary's words. She would try to imagine what it would be like and to picture everything going well; but it was so hard to imagine a baby coming out from between her legs. There just didn't seem to be enough room. She couldn't tell Mary that fear. It wasn't proper.

When she was four months pregnant and still able to conceal her rounding figure with a tightly laced corset, Sarah had gone to an evening lecture with two women friends on the subject of the populist health movement. It was mostly women like Sarah who attended, and the talk was about the virtues of a healthy life: getting vigorous exercise, eating healthy foods, and using natural herbal remedies to treat illness. The speakers espoused the belief that the human body worked well, was intended to be in perfect health, and would function perfectly if people would treat it well and give it the rest, nourishment, and exercise it needed. They talked about what women were doing to their bodies by lacing themselves up in tight corsets, eating less than would nourish a child, and staying inside to keep their skin milky white and their hair in place. They ridiculed what fashion had done to women's bodies, and said that women were turning themselves into invalids by their daily habits and that trying to have a wasplike waist was the cause of women's frequent fainting spells.

They told the audience that women the world over were capable of hard physical labor, that upper-class women were no different in their anatomy than working-class women or women who lived in tribes in Africa and Asia, and that those tribal women actually were healthier than many of the women in the audience.

Sarah couldn't help but nod her head, as she shifted uncomfortably on the chair, suddenly very conscious of how constricted she felt in her corset and heavy, tight dress with whalebone stays. She did feel light-headed a lot of the time, and wondered if that really might be due to her clothes, and to how little she ate and how little exercise she got. The books she had read about women and birth told women to remain indoors during the last months of pregnancy and for months afterward, and to walk around the parlor a dozen times a day for exercise.

"Modern life is ruining women's health." The words rang in her ears for days after the lecture. She had several interesting conversations with Charles about the ideas she'd heard, but she had to agree with him that, although the bloomers these women suggested should replace corsets might be comfortable, one simply could not fly in the face of convention and do whatever one felt like. What would people say? They had both laughed at the idea of Sarah going out of doors, with her ungainly figure a sight for everyone to gawk at.

*   *   *

Sarah went into labor one Wednesday morning, after her typical breakfast of black tea and toast with marmalade. She had had several days of fitful sleep, awakening often, feeling small tightenings and occasional sharp twinges deep in her groin. She had been too excited to sleep much but didn't want to keep Charles awake; he worked so hard at the office. She did tell Mary and got very excited when Mary assured her that what she was feeling was certainly a sign that labor was not far away. Mary told her she needed to eat a lot and not to pay much attention to the contractions, as they were called, but just to keep on with her normal life. "That way you won't focus on the pain so much when they begin, and the time will go much faster. You'll see," Mary said.

Sarah didn't call Charles. She felt quite strong and didn't want to bother him or Dr. Lewiston until it was necessary. Mary stuck close by her all afternoon; she kept reassuring her and helping her to keep her mind clear of fearful thoughts. By late afternoon both women were sure that Sarah was in labor. Mary had insisted that Sarah wear a loose-fitting shift, and when she changed she saw that her drawers were stained with a red mucus.

"That's a very good sign, Missus; it means you'll have this baby by dawn for sure," Mary said. Mary would have liked to let Sarah get along by herself during this early phase of labor; that's what the women she knew did, staying upright, going about their regular business, foregoing reassurance and comfort until late in labor when they became confused from all the contractions. The women she knew didn't take to their beds until they could feel the pressure of the baby's head at the opening of their vagina. But Sarah wasn't like the women she knew, and Mary responded by giving her almost constant attention and praise for how strong she was and how everything was going just right. Together they managed quite well, and in Mary's company Sarah somehow felt she would be able to have this baby.

The pains were coming every five or six minutes by the time Charles returned from the office. He was shocked and concerned that Sarah had spent the day by herself and immediately sent for Dr. Lewiston. He told Sarah she needed to be in bed, to rest herself. Mary had told her it was important to keep walking, that walking would make the baby come down in the right position and would make the birth happen faster. Sarah tried a compromise, sitting during several of the contractions, then lying down on the chaise in the parlor. It seemed to hurt more when she was lying down than when she was standing and walking, but Charles's will prevailed, so Mary helped Sarah up the stairs and into a nightgown and put her to bed. Mary brought Sarah some hot tea with honey and some toast and promised her that she would not leave her side again until the baby was born. Charles, meanwhile, paced the parlor, deeply concerned about how his slender wife would do in birth.

Across the city in his carriage, Dr. Lewiston was worrying about the same thing. "After all, we have made some advancements in the past two hundred and fifty years," Dr. Lewiston thought to himself. There was a time when, if a woman labored on and on with no sign of the baby coming, a doctor had only two choices: to let labor continue, in which case the mother might die of exhaustion, or to kill the baby by inserting instruments into the vagina to crush its skull and then remove its body in pieces, hoping to save the mother's life by doing so. "Thank God I don't have to do that very often these days," thought the doctor.

When Dr. Lewiston reached the house, Charles greeted him with a per-spiring hand, and they spent a few minutes talking about Sarah's condition. Then the doctor went up to her bedside, leaving his black bag in the parlor. In this bag Dr. Lewiston carried smelling salts, various bromide medicines, and several different sizes of forceps made from long-handled metal spoons fitted together. These he had to use often, as many of the women in his care suffered from the long-term effects of childhood rickets, which resulted in various kinds of pelvic deformities. Dr. Lewiston couldn't understand why so many modern well-to-do women should have rickets. Nor did he understand why so many genteel women in Boston had such protracted labors and difficult births. "It wasn't that way with the Irish women in the slums whom I attended during my training," he thought.

In Dublin, Dr. Lewiston had learned the valuable skill of podalic version, or how to turn a baby lying crosswise in the womb by reaching up inside the mother, grabbing hold of the baby's feet, and pulling it down. This had worked miraculously in many cases and was one of the reasons for the doctor's fine reputation in Boston. It was a risky procedure, however; it was done without anesthesia, which resulted in a level of pain that could put the mother into shock. If that didn't kill her, subsequent infection might. Dr. Lewiston certainly did not wish to have to use this procedure with Sarah.

Sarah labored in bed all evening and into the night and grew more discouraged and afraid with each hour that passed. Charles continued to pace back and forth downstairs, too worried to eat. Mary kept Sarah drinking a lot of hot tea with honey, but it was hard to keep her spirits up, she was in such pain lying there curled up like a sick child. Even Mary began to worry. "The women I know have first labors that take eight or ten hours at the most, and they don't pay much mind to the first hours," she thought. "Why should Missus Hanley be having so much trouble?"

Mary suspected the problem lay in the sedentary nature of Sarah's life, her skimpy diet, and all those waist-cinching clothes. "It's just not good for a woman," she told herself. By dawn, Sarah was still struggling to get through every contraction and was convinced she was going to die. Dr. Lewiston consulted with Charles. Together they decided it might be time to use the forceps. Dr. Lewiston would not have considered taking Sarah to a hospital. They were places of disease and fit only for the poor, who were used as training material for physicians. So it fell to him, and him alone, to respond to Sarah's anguished cries of "Do something, do anything!" Before removing the forceps from their sterile wrapping, he had Mary boil water and used some of it to thoroughly wash his hands. He agreed with Aberdeen that physicians themselves might be the cause of women's deaths when they failed to make sure their hands and their instruments were clean before placing them in a woman's body.

Fortunately, Sarah's cervix was fully dilated when Dr. Lewiston began, or serious tearing would have resulted. He had to place the forceps correctly on the baby's head by feel alone, first reaching in with his fingers to learn which way the baby was facing. Then, when placing the forceps on the baby's head, he tried to avoid catching an ear or an eye, and he carefully and slowly turned the head just slightly so that it would fit more easily through the outlet of the pelvis. He then slowly drew the baby down and out, praying that his instruments had not torn Sarah's vaginal wall in the process.

Sarah and Charles's son came out looking vigorous and let out several strong cries, assuring everyone he was in fine health. Sarah perked up immediately, although she was weary to the bone. Mary had stayed the night alongside her and had been an invaluable presence, even Dr. Lewiston agreed. The monthly nurse had not been asked in until toward the end, to act as an assistant to Dr. Lewiston. It was she who first held the baby, and she cleaned and wrapped him before placing him in Sarah's arms. Charles came in as soon as Sarah had been cleaned up, the bedding had been changed, and Sarah was lying in a fresh gown on clean sheets under a warm comforter.

Mary saw to it that Sarah was fed a nourishing breakfast, and over the next weeks she personally tended to her every need, leaving her own children in the care of others. Sarah did not contract the dreaded childbed fever, and the forceps had not torn her inside tissues. There was a large tear at the outlet of her vagina, however, which Dr. Lewiston had carefully stitched up. It caused Sarah a great deal of discomfort, so Mary gave her hot poultices of a particular herb she said the local midwives always used in such cases. They decided not to tell Charles about this. Between applications, Mary had Sarah lie with her legs apart so the wound could dry, and slowly it began to heal.

Sarah regained much of her strength after a month. Her baby, whom they named Andrew, grew steadily at the wet nurse's breast. The monthly nurse took care of the child between feedings and brought him to Sarah to play with when he was fed and clean. Sarah loved her son and looked forward to the time when she would be able to care for him herself. The cherry tree outside the parlor window bloomed plentifully that spring.

The Beginnings of Modern Childbirth

SARAH HANLEY WAS a product of the culture in which she lived—as we all are—and that culture viewed the process of childbirth as innately dangerous and a threat to the life of every woman who had to go through it. Few people questioned why this should be the case. Because so many women had arduous labors and complicated births, women and men assumed this was normal. Living in polluted, crowded cities, cut off from the land and the growing of their own food, many people had no connection with the earth. Even the changes of the season meant little except a change in fashion and the heating or cooling of homes.

This disconnection from the earth and from bodily processes brought about a profound ignorance and fear regarding childbirth. Fear was a breeding ground for self-doubt, passivity, and helplessness, and it led to dependency on outside authorities who told women what was going on in their bodies and how to care for their babies. For upper-middle-class women such as Sarah, the authorities in birth were exclusively men, men who were themselves for the most part also ignorant and fearful in regard to childbirth and women's bodies. Sarah was lucky to be attended by Dr. Lewiston, who had studied within another culture and who was very careful to sterilize his equipment and to be cautious in his use of it.

Women today are in many ways products of nineteenth-century city culture in their approach to childbirth. And physicians are still in the grip of the nineteenth-century belief that childbirth is too risky and painful, and women too fragile, for birth to be allowed to proceed on its own. The fears of women and the fears of physicians have been playing off each other right up to the present day, and the underlying belief in the inadequacy of women feeds the fear.

Childbirth is viewed to some extent as women's Achilles' heel, where they are the most vulnerable. But why should this be true? Giving birth is a powerful and creative experience, a basic and reaffirming part of women's sexuality. In other areas of life, women since 1850 have made tremendous strides. They have gained more self-determination and personal power in practically every area in life except childbirth. Why is childbirth not a center of women's power today? To understand this we must recognize that childbearing, and the suckling of a baby, is a fundamental part of a woman's sexuality, and we must look at the relationship between female sexuality and power.

Organized Western Religion and the Position of Women

Where did women like Sarah—and like so many birthing women today—learn that there is something inherently inadequate in their ability to bear children? If we look at the history of Western civilization, we will see that a number of factors have played a part in fostering this belief.

Most anthropologists today believe that as many as ten thousand years ago all religions centered around a mother goddess who was linked to the fertility and vitality of the earth. This goddess was both procreator and destroyer, nurturing mother and sexual consort. She held final power in life and death, and she was both worshiped and feared. In art she was often shown as an ample-breasted, full-hipped, and often pregnant woman.

It is not known for sure what caused the worldwide shift among early cultures from seeing the power at the center of life as female and fertile to viewing it as male and paternal, but we do know this: that shift began the loss of balance between the sexes and the declining status of women that has continued unchecked for thousands of years and is only now beginning to change back. The shift to a male-centered religion and society coincided with a change from hunting and gathering food to growing it through farming and breeding domesticated animals. This change resulted in an excess of goods to be stored, exchanged, and protected. The material wealth and power created by the accumulation of goods and property resulted in gender and class distinctions. Women began to be seen as property and means of production as men took control of decision making.

With the rise of Western religions, which all began in the Middle East, people—apparently for the first time—began to worship a single, male god. A few centuries after the death of Jesus, Christianity began to embrace the concept of a split between God, who held dominion over all that was good, and the Devil, who ruled the kingdom of evil. This view of all life as divided into two ever-opposing forces was the legacy of an earlier Middle Eastern religion known as Zoroastrianism. This religion promulgated the view that God was in an eternal cosmic struggle against the forces of evil. The principle of evil had long been accepted by human beings, but now it was seen as an outside force forever attempting to pull humankind into its sphere.

Religious and philosophic beliefs in the Far East had never viewed life as a split between good and evil, nor did they consider the source of life—God, if you will—to be exclusively good. Life was seen to consist of both the dark and the light, and human beings were also seen to contain both. They existed in balance, and one did not have supremacy over the other. In fact, it was considered as impossible for good to exist without evil as it was for day to exist without night. When Western religions declared life to be split into two opposing parts, human beings began to look for someone or something outside themselves to blame for evil events. Thus developed the idea of the scapegoat, originally a real goat on which all the sins of the village were said to be placed, so that it could then be cast out.

Several hundred years after the murder of the prophet Jesus, the Christian Church was organized into a patriarchal institution. The various books containing the teachings of Jesus and his disciples were gathered into one book called the New Testament. Gospels deemed not in agreement with the dictates of this new church, especially ones referring to the direct experience of knowing God, were omitted.

Control and leadership of this new church were in the hands of a few men. Church fathers based their theology upon the doctrines of Paul, who based his beliefs largely upon the Greek notion of a split between the physical and spiritual dimensions, where the physical (embodied by women) is antithetical to the spiritual (embodied by men). God was given a gender, and it was exclusively male. The ancient, earth-based, mother goddess of previous Western religious expression was suppressed by this new Church. Holy days were intentionally set to replace ancient seasonal celebrations and churches were built on top of consecrated places of goddess worship to convert people to Christianity.

By the Middle Ages, the human body with its innate sexuality was sin-filled. Christians were warned to avoid things that gave pleasure to their senses. The ovulating, menstruating, and procreating female body had always frightened men as it was a source of special power. Yet, whereas men had traditionally respected, feared, and stood in awe of women and their unique powers, they now found their inescapable physicality sinful. In fact, women were made the carriers of all human passion (both hers *and* his) and so Christian men did not have to take any responsibility for it. *Anything* that demonstrated a woman's power or wisdom—understanding and using herbs for healing, holding property or having political influence, or having mystical experiences—was considered the work of the Devil. If a man demonstrated one of these same powers, it was the work of God.

In virtually all cultures dominated by institutionalized religion, women are still viewed as objects to be controlled, with their natural tendencies toward impulsivity, self-indulgence, and sinfulness. Christianity, combined with Western medicine and technology, has warped the concept of childbirth. Is it any wonder that as birth was pushed out of the home and into the hospital that it became synonymous with pain, suffering, and powerlessness? Now modern women want to escape from the experiences of labor, breastfeeding, and child care.

The denigration of everything female (except the capacity for nurturing) actually began long before the Christian Church and other patriarchal religions made it doctrine. Scholars continue to debate why the natural balance between male and female powers was disrupted. Few deny religion's numerous positive contributions to human civilization; however, religions have also institutionalized sexism and disempowered women, leading them to mistrust both themselves and the natural processes of birth, life, and death that flow through their bodies. Wherever women are not in control of their own lives, the effects will be felt by their children. When women are pathologically afraid of birth, view breastfeeding as an unnecessary inconvenience, and think of caring for young children as a curse, they will naturally want to distance themselves from these biological processes.

Society teaches that motherhood means giving up essential and innate needs, yet really the mother-baby unit is a symbiotic one, where each fullfills certain needs of the other. Child abuse and neglect, whether perpetrated by men or women, results from the devaluing and splitting of the mother-baby diad and from the attitude that considers children the possessions of parents and women the possessions of men.

It is human nature to seek direct experience with the force or entity many call God. People have been attempting to put into words, music, and art the awe and bliss of such experience since time immemorial. Before Christianity, no religion had attempted to deny the validity of individual mystical experience. But by doing so, the early church fathers laid the foundation for centuries of abuse. The murder of Joan of Arc at the hands of the Catholic Church was just one example of the devastating impact of this powerful institution, which regulated and judged individual spirituality. This point of church law, along with the Catholic Church's earlier splitting off of evil into a separate entity, resulted in the trial and death of thousands of creative, independent thinkers and scientists and led to the witch-hunts of the late Middle Ages.

Early fundamentalist sects often believed that the Bible was to be taken literally. Because the word of God said that Eve had tempted Adam to eat of the apple, which caused them to be expelled from the garden of Eden, all women had to suffer for their innate corruptibility. In addition, they would forever be dominated by men. This attitude continues to be part of many fundamentalist Christian, Jewish, and Islamic beliefs. They all come from the same roots.

A basic belief of seventeenth-century Calvinism, a Protestant sect that heavily influenced Northern Europe for many years, and Puritanism, another Protestant sect of the same period that heavily influenced both Britain and its

North American colonies, was that the female body was unclean and corrupt. The hallmark of Puritanism was its rigorous moral code, which emphasized strictness, austerity, and purity, and led directly to the suppression of all that was physical, including sex. Since it never has been possible to give birth without being both physical and sexual, women were seen as essentially unclean.

After Christianity became the dominant force in Europe, and later, after puritanical views predominated in America, how could any woman, whose body was considered inherently wicked, give birth in the same natural, accepting way as her ancient sister? The degraded view of the female body continued into Victorian times and continues in our culture—and our medical practices—today. It affects all women, whether or not they consider themselves to be religious.

THE VICTORIAN MIND
AND THE VICTORIAN BODY

Victorian attitudes toward the human body shaped Sarah Hanley's world, but this way of thinking had existed long before Queen Victoria came to the throne in England near the middle of the nineteenth century. The common thread of both Judaism and Christianity was a sense of shame and disgust toward all of the natural physical functions of the human body, especially sexuality. However, only in the second half of the 1800s, under the reign of Queen Victoria, did these attitudes dominate secular society.

During the mid-1850s there arose a movement to leash the passionate, animal nature of human beings. Rational thinking was elevated and the emotional and the physical were degraded. These Victorian attitudes toward the human body produced restrictive clothing styles that warped the female figure and made it difficult for women to expand their lungs fully or to digest food easily. (Curiously, it also produced the antecedent to modern-day Western-style vegetarianism. Eliminating meat from the adult diet and replacing it with grains in the form of cereals was believed to be a good way to curb passions and emotions in order to be more civilized.)

This elevation of thinking over feeling resulted from the desire of the middle class to live more "refined" lives, and to distance themselves from the land and the manual labor of the lower class. The impulse arose as a natural phase in human evolution. Europe had seen many kinds of excess and violence in the name of emotion and passion. But the pendulum swung too far. Victorian beliefs played right into the hands of those who viewed the suppression of feelings and sensations as the best way to discipline human nature. Childbirth suffered from this, just as did all normal bodily processes: breathing, digestion and elimination, sleep, and sexuality. The legacy of that time continues; adults today have lost the ability to breathe fully and are plagued with problems of digestion and elimination, insomnia, and sexual disorders—and birth, of course, has become an unnatural, complicated, and feared process.

WOMEN AND THE PROGRESSIVE MOVEMENT
FOR SOCIAL REFORM

It is important to understand just how physically unhealthy most men and women were in the mid- to late 1800s. In 1899, four out of every ten men who volunteered to fight in the Boer War were found to be too unhealthy to fight. The causes were numerous: inadequate housing, lack of sufficient fresh food, dirty water, poor sewage, poor hygiene, and miserable working conditions. In the cities the problem was compounded by smog and overcrowding. All across Western Europe and Great Britain there were epidemics of tuberculosis, typhus, typhoid, and cholera. Women often had deformed pelvises due to rickets.

The Industrial Revolution, which had begun with such promise, also had a harsh dark side. Automation did not necessarily improve people's lives. Children worked as day laborers in factories, and the practice of giving away children to be indentured servants was widespread in Britain and North America.

Against this background birth became unsafe and more dangerous for most women. Birth control was unknown. Poor women had a baby every year and often worked full time at menial, poorly paid jobs. They were malnourished and exhausted, and their husbands were often alcoholic. Upper-class women were also likely to be unhealthy, exercising too little and eating overly refined foods. Medical organizations and politicians moved childbirth into the hospital, believing that doctors could make it safer. What they did not understand was that health problems were social and economic.

There arose in Britain and the United States during the mid-1800s a strong social reform movement aimed at improving the lives of the masses. Britain took the lead. In the forefront were outspoken, educated, well-to-do women who believed it was morally wrong for a few to live in luxury while so many suffered. Women organized this grassroots movement, which grew until it became a political force in the first third of the twentieth century. Besides child labor laws, the focus was maternity care and the plight of mothers. In 1917 the Women's Cooperative of England demanded that the well-being of the mother be given as much attention as that of the baby. Until that time, when there was any question of the mother or baby dying in birth, attention was centered on saving the baby.

The first government report on maternal mortality in England was made in 1924 by Janet Campbell, a physician working for the Ministry of Health. She documented five major factors that could reduce the chronic ill-health of women and the high number of women dying during childbirth. Improving the quality of professional care women received before, during, and after birth was only one of the five. The rest were the need for sanitation, better housing, better wages and working conditions, and reducing rickets (which caused not only difficult births but also miscarriage and resulting infection). In 1930 Sylvia Pankhurst published *Save the Mothers,* which focused on the conditions in which working-class women were forced to live and work. She called for what she termed a National Maternity Service that not only would handle health care but also improve the overall condition of women. Her plea was heard. In 1932 a government report in England showed that almost 50 percent of maternal deaths were preventable!

It was women who introduced the concept of prenatal care to a modern culture that had long since forgotten what traditional and ancient cultures knew: How well a woman and a baby do in childbirth is primarily a result of how healthy the woman is when she becomes pregnant, not what is done to her in labor. The medical concept of prenatal care—weighing, measuring, doing tests—is an early twentieth-century notion. Early studies in the United States did not show that every woman benefits from prenatal care. What these and other, recent studies do show is that prenatal medical care is significant for a very small percentage of women, who can be easily identified. Most women do not need to see a physician or a nurse at any time in their pregnancy. What they do need is a skilled midwife.

The Traditional Role of the Midwife and Its Demise

Even while organized, patriarchal Western religion shaped and dominated Western culture and affected the way women viewed their sexuality, one constant helped maintain some semblance of normalcy in regard to childbirth: the midwife. All through the Middle Ages in Europe, midwives remained a soothing and supportive presence for women in labor. Most midwives were conservative in their approach to childbirth; they believed their role was to "be with the birthing woman," as the word *midwife* implies. From Middle English, the word *mid* means "with," and *wif* is another word for "woman," so the word *midwife* literally means "one who is with a woman," or assisting a woman in childbirth. As long as the midwife maintained her watchful, supportive vigil, the woman and the baby and the process itself would usually take care of the rest. For good midwives then and now, the formula for successful birth has been: (1) Keep a woman's spirits up; (2) Maintain her privacy and dignity; (3) Don't intervene in the process when it is working; (4) Do as little as is necessary to right things when they go wrong.

Eventually, however, midwives, too, were corrupted by the authority of the Catholic hierarchy. The church, which was the main civilizing and political force in Europe for centuries, held a paradoxical view of the midwife. On the one hand, she was seen as necessary and was therefore permitted to function. On the other hand, she was considered a threat, for her knowledge of herbs and abortifacients and for being the confidante of women. Although she was considered low class, the midwife had too much power. It was only a matter of time before midwives were labeled heretics and witches, simply because of their intimate involvement with female sexuality and reproduction, and then executed.

It is difficult to look back at the history of midwifery and the Catholic Church's role in the murder of thousands of women in the name of God without feeling a sense of outrage. The mass murder of women who were accused of witchcraft by their neighbors is one of the low points of human history. It arose from ignorance, which always feeds fear. The confusion of an earth-based, pagan religion called Wicca, or "witchcraft," with the practice of midwifery was simple enough. Pagans, like midwives, celebrated the human body and female sexuality, which they saw as connected to the earth, the source of all life. Like witches, midwives had special powers. Witchcraft was associated with magic, while the powers of midwives came from their special skills, including the use of herbs to heal and to end unwanted pregnancy. Pagans, witches, and midwives all regarded female sexuality as a healthy, vibrant part of life at a time when the Catholic Church considered sexuality shameful, albeit necessary for the perpetuation of the human race. The church saw women as empty vessels, to be filled with the seed of men, while "witches" and midwives regarded them as powerful humans because of their unique capacity to create life.

The Catholic Church attempted to eradicate pagan worship by incorporating major pagan holidays into Christian ones. When that didn't accomplish the goal of wiping out paganism, the church became more aggressive. It sanctioned the killing of those who refused to bow to the Christian God and the church itself. The one female Christian deity that remained, the Virgin Mary, was a mother, but she was supposedly nonsexual, so she bore no real resemblance to prior mother goddess figures or actual, living women. The witch was the Christian culture's projection of the female's dark, or destructive, side, the side the church wanted to control and suppress and which it considered evil. The Church's view of witchcraft was a clear distortion of a much older belief system.

Strongly independent individuals by nature, midwives never organized themselves into guilds for their own protection, as other professionals, including physicians, did. Nor did they engage in the politics of the times, which were closely linked to the church. Only in very recent years have midwives begun to organize on their own behalf.

Midwives traditionally did more than care for women who were bringing life into the world and practice herbal healing. They also prepared the dead for burial. During the Middle Ages, a time of plagues and epidemics, midwives were highly visible women who were identified with the great mysteries of birth and death. Thus they were easy targets during witch-hunts. Everyone knew who the midwives were, and they were particularly susceptible to criticism if a baby or mother died during birth, which must have happened often, since rickets and other diseases of malnutrition were also prevalent in cities and towns. In addition, midwives assisted women in aborting unwanted pregnancies, which was something the church had outlawed. Midwives were considered by women to be powerful resources and valuable helpers. By some women and many men, however, they were believed to be dangerous and evil.

In the period beginning in the fifteenth century and ending in the seventeenth, a time in which almost every woman who lived alone was suspect, thousands of women were convicted as witches and murdered throughout Europe and the American colonies. The women were usually drowned, or were tied to a stake in the center of town and set afire. Many of these women were midwives, and although the records that survive are far from complete, some names come down to us over the centuries. In 1591 a Scottish midwife, Agnes Sampson, was burned as a witch on a hill in Edinburgh for attempting to alleviate the pain of a woman she was attending in labor. In the early part of the seventeenth century, Anne Hutchinson, a midwife and religious dissident, was banished from her home in Massachusetts for supposedly being a witch. The witch-hunts of Europe and the American colonies helped take power away from midwives at the same time that power over women and childbirth was being coopted by the medical profession.

MEDICINE AND THE CONTINUING
DECLINE OF MIDWIFERY

When the first medical schools were established in Europe in the Middle Ages, midwives were excluded from the new profession of medicine. They could not enter the emerging sciences of anatomy and physiology (which had come about after physicians finally broke a long-standing cultural taboo about examining dead bodies by dissecting human cadavers stolen from graveyards). The results of this research were written up in medical books, none of which midwives could read because most women were intentionally kept illiterate at that time.

The exclusion of midwives from medical schools was part of a deliberate policy to take the control of childbirth away from women. At the same time, the prevailing cultural belief was that it was inappropriate for women to be taught to read. Thus medicine, along with all other forms of higher learning, was considered to be an exclusively male domain.

Midwives had always relied for their knowledge and skill on their practical experience with women's bodies, gained from apprenticeship and from sitting with women in labor. They did not have Latin or Greek names to describe what they knew. As the status of physicians slowly began to rise in European culture, the position of the midwife as wise woman/herbalist began to decline.

Over a period of a thousand years, the kind of woman who practiced midwifery changed as the culture changed and the status of women continued its downslide. Midwives had always been wives and mothers with experience in childbirth, a strong sense of practicality, and inquiring minds. Now, however, there was an almost universal disinclination to be so intimately involved with another woman's body. After the establishment of European medical schools, the age-old respected craft of midwifery declined to an all-time low. By the late Middle Ages and the Renaissance many midwives were not so skilled or so cautious in their practices.

MIDWIVES AND INFECTION

Traditionally, women had labored upright and delivered standing, squatting or sitting on the open lap of another person, sometimes the midwife herself. Because a midwife would not invade the woman's body in any way, she did not have the chance to pass along germs that could create serious infection. She did not need to be particularly careful about the cleanliness of her hands; they were usually in her lap until she extended them to catch the baby as it emerged from the mother.

For centuries women and their helpers had found objects near at hand to function as supports for an exhausted laboring woman. These evolved into simple horseshoe-shaped wooden stools, which by the late Middle Ages had become more elaborate when cloth skirts were added to them to hide the woman's buttocks from view. And with that they became carriers of disease, because the fabric trapped bacteria and was not washed between uses. Today we know the necessity of keeping all equipment and linens that come in contact with a birthing woman's vagina very clean to prevent infection. In the Middle Ages, the microscope had not yet been invented and there was no concept of microorganisms spreading disease.

PROFESSIONALIZING MIDWIFERY:
THE CONFUSION BETWEEN MIDWIFERY AND NURSING

At the beginning of the 1900s in England, a small number of physicians and some upper-class women began a grassroots movement to make midwifery a respected profession again. They wanted to elevate the status of midwifery and thereby make childbirth safer by giving back to birthing women the birth attendant they had always trusted. It was decided that the training of a midwife should no longer be permitted to occur through the age-old, time-honored tradition of apprenticeship. Because they followed their upper-class mores, the leaders of this movement to professionalize the midwife believed that midwifery would best be served by formal institutional education. So it was that one of the earliest and long-lived crafts and occupations in history became aligned with the new profession of nursing, which had been created to assist medicine and hospitals. People had always nursed the sick, and for many years it had been one of the roles of Christian nuns to do this. They largely ran the charity hospitals of the early Middle Ages, which were established for the poor. Originally, nursing, as they practiced it, was separate from herbal or other forms of healing, except for the more recent use of opiate drugs to obliterate consciousness and therefore pain. Nursing was for over a thousand years largely a matter of keeping the sick person clean and fed. The profession of nursing as it exists today really began at the end of the nineteenth century, but it did not develop fully until nurses began to be hired to staff hospitals. Now nurses provide 90 percent of all patient care.

In the name of making midwifery safer, in many countries nursing became a prerequisite course of study for anyone wanting to be a midwife. So began the twentieth-century confusion between midwifery and nursing, which are two distinctly different crafts. Except for the influence of the Catholic Church on midwifery, the practice had remained an independent profession. Suddenly it found itself an adjunct to, and finally under the control of, organized medicine. No longer were midwives able to make independent judgments about what to do for their clients in specific circumstances. Physicians had for several hundred years been attempting to influence the practice of midwifery, and had been writing books and designing courses to tell midwives how to practice, even though they never witnessed normal childbirths without intervention themselves.

Two countries that did not follow the trend toward making nursing training a prerequisite for midwifery—Denmark and the Netherlands—have for a period of years maintained the greatest amount of normalcy in childbirth and the lowest number of infant and maternal deaths, and were until very recently successful in keeping hospitalization, drugs, and other interventions to a minimum. Denmark went through some problems in the 1970s, when legislators put limits on the independent practice of midwifery. But the Netherlands have continued to be a model of what is best about traditional midwifery.

Dutch midwives are, by law, a distinct and separate profession from both nursing and medicine. They are a strong political force, organized and actively working to protect the right to a home birth. The government has granted them special privileges that enable them to retain authority over normal childbirth, and the independent practice of traditional midwifery is supported by the people and the culture, withstanding any outside political, religious, or financial pressures. Because normal childbirth has been maintained in the Netherlands, medical intervention is not seen to be always necessary.

Advancements in Obstetrics: Beneficial but Also Risky

Only a century ago, medicine relied solely on heroic human efforts to cure dreaded diseases, having very little in the way of tools to work with and no real

Childbirth in the Netherlands

In the Netherlands, 70 percent of all births occur under the guidance of midwives, and one out of three births is a home birth. Every mother and baby receives postpartum follow-up from her midwife. In addition, she is entitled to skilled postpartum support during the following weeks by a Home Health Aide.

Below, a Home Health Aide gives this new mother a bed bath after mother and baby have had some private time together. Called by the midwife at the second stage of labor, she was present for the birth as an extra pair of skilled hands. A midwife makes a number of home visits during the months following the birth and keeps careful records. Breast-feeding is standard in the Netherlands, and the midwife provides expert assistance. The only tools required in a normal birth—home or hospital—are something to listen to the baby's heart when the human ear is not sufficient (shown at right, a traditional wooden stethoscope); sterile cotton balls for wiping up; sterile clamp, scissors, and tie for tying and cutting off the umbilical cord. Above right, instructed by a midwife, a medical student learns how to conduct a normal birth.

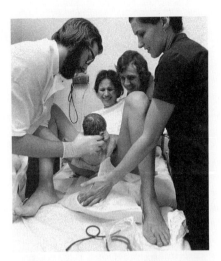

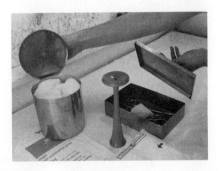

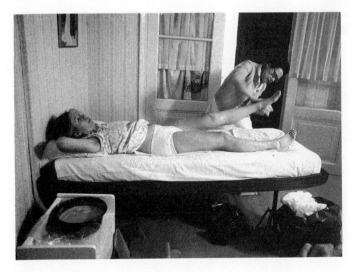

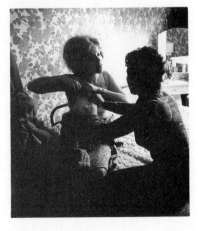

The Dutch Way of Birth

According to maternal and infant health indexes, the Netherlands consistently have the lowest percentage of babies or mothers who die or are injured during childbirth.

There seem to be two main reasons for these statistics. The Netherlands have the lowest rate of medical intervention during childbirth, lower even than Sweden and Japan, the other two nations that rank high in the indexes. The Dutch also use more midwives as primary birth attendants than are used in any other industrialized nation.

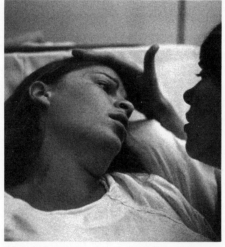

Women who give birth in the Netherlands— as well as their babies—experience less trauma as a result of excessive use of technology and fewer iatrogenic (physician-caused) problems than do their American counterparts.

Even the Netherlands, though, have been influenced by the American way of birth and its propensity for surgery. The cesarean rate has in the past few years crept above 5 percent. For decades it was a steady 2 to 4 percent, and many knowledgeable Dutch health workers and researchers feel it should not have risen above that. In the Netherlands, the rate of drugs and anesthesia used during vaginal births is extremely low among those who have home births (nearly a third of all women). The rate of episiotomies in the Netherlands is less than one in ten, compared with a nine-in-ten or higher rate in the United States.

It is unusual for a newborn in the Netherlands to spend time separated from its mother. There is really no such thing as a "well-baby nursery." When a mother asks to have some time apart from her baby, the infant is put in a room with a few baby cots just down the hall. The room is lit by the sun during the day and left dark at night so the babies are not overstimulated by bright artificial light.

Only a small number of babies spend time in intensive care nurseries. In the United States, even the most conservative estimates contrast sharply with this picture: one out of every five American newborns spends some time in an intensive care unit, where babies are routinely subjected to daily blood drawings and other painful "just-in-case" procedures.

In the Dutch health-care system, obstetricians, neonatologists, and perinatologists—the specialists skilled in treating complications of childbirth—see only those women and babies who need their care. The rest are cared for entirely by midwives: during pregnancy, birth, and postpartum.

Eight features of the Dutch maternity-care system stand out:

1. *A balance between physicians and midwives is maintained.* Because they are specialists in the treatment of disease, acute care, and surgery, physicians always have a special status in the public's eyes. To balance the tendency to grant them too much power, the Netherlands limit the numbers of specialist physicians. Obstetricians in private practice are required

to select a location where a need for their specialty has been demonstrated. This prevents a scenario commonly seen in the United States in which many obstetricians practice in wealthy urban and suburban areas, leaving rural areas without specialists.

2. *Midwives are the primary care providers for pregnant and birthing women.* They practice independently of physicians but do consult with them. Midwives examine women when they become pregnant and determine whether they should be transferred to an obstetrician's care. If the situation is uncomplicated, the midwife conducts the birth and is in charge of postpartum care, sometimes up to several months, of both mother and baby. Midwives can check women into any hospital in the Netherlands and automatically receive hospital privileges.

3. *Home birth is recognized as safe and is supported and encouraged.* The government recognizes that a reasonable percentage of home births is needed to maintain the high standard of childbirth practices and that hospital births tend to become complicated.

4. *The national health policy covers everyone. Every person receives the health care they need, no matter what their circumstances.* Health insurance is required, but people can choose to purchase insurance from either a private company or from the government. Maternity care and leave are fully covered.

5. *Maternity care policies are formulated by committees composed of lay people and health workers of all kinds.* Physicians do not dominate these committees, which review guidelines, such as the indicators that require a midwife to consult a specialist physician, and care limits, such as the amount of aggressive treatment that can be performed on babies born more than four months prematurely.

6. *Home Health Aides, who receive several years' training, care for postpartum women and newborns.* They provide daily postpartum home care for women in the first weeks after birth. Pregnant women must sign up for the service long before giving birth to be assured of having a helper, but it's well worth the trouble as they pay very little for the service and can have help for up to eight hours a day. Aides provide whatever the mother and family need—taking care of older children, doing laundry and shopping, even keeping records for the midwife.

7. *Physicians and midwives are paid a specific sum for each woman.* Because obstetricians are not paid extra for specialized medical procedures or cesareans, they have no financial incentive to order unnecessary tests or procedures. The health-care system covers the cost of hospital birth only if it is indicated as necessary. In most cases, it covers the cost of home birth with a midwife. Should a woman prefer to go to an obstetrician when there is no medical need, she must pay extra.

8. *In the Netherlands, true medical malpractice does not go unpunished, but malpractice lawsuits are not as common as they are in the United States.* Because the Dutch emphasize natural processes, they understand that accidents—welcome or not—are an integral element of nature; when something goes wrong in childbirth, no one is necessarily to blame. □

comprehension of how to prevent the diseases in the first place. Then, in the middle of the nineteenth century, Western medicine made a series of remarkable advances. Crucial scientific research and experimentation done at this time led to the development of a wide range of drugs for the treatment of myriad conditions, and other developments and techniques included antibiotics, blood transfusion and plasma expanders, microsurgery, laboratory medicine, and X-rays and other ways of imaging the inside of the human body.

From 1850 to the mid-1960s, childbirth was directly affected by the changing world of medicine. New techniques and medical equipment allowed doctors to intervene in the birth process, dramatically changing pregnancy, labor, birth, and, with the advent of the specialty of neonatology, the care of newborns. Many of these modern interventions in birth seemed to make childbirth safer and more predictable, but future generations may find them as barbaric as we view the earliest versions of forceps.

SOLUTIONS TO PROBLEMS AT BIRTH

Aggressive tactics to deal with difficult births have been attempted for centuries, with various success. Primitive methods for inducing or speeding up labor were apparently practiced by every society. When it was a matter of life and death, subtlety was not the priority. A woman might be laid on a blanket and shaken, or she might be suspended from a tree to encourage the baby out.

Until late in the Middle Ages, however, inserting hands or instruments into a laboring woman's vagina was avoided almost universally. Most cultures had virtual taboos on doing this, taboos probably reflecting an innate understanding of the possible serious harm that could be done to the mother and baby by such intervention. Today we can see clearly the kind of harm that was done when these taboos began to be violated by physicians.

Let us look for just a moment at early medical advances with regard to handling complications in birth. A small number of Bostonian women would have entered labor with the rare problem of their baby lying sidewise across the womb. Many traditional tribal cultures—and later the ancient Greeks—had discovered how to turn a baby in the womb who otherwise could not be born. This probably occurred even more rarely, since women in earlier cultures engaged in a high degree of physical activity while pregnant, so their babies were more likely to end up in the right position for birth.

According to the documentation of early anthropologists such as George

Engleman, in the late 1800s, many early tribal cultures apparently used massage throughout pregnancy as a way to keep the mother fit and the baby in a good position for birth. "External version," a means of turning a baby by placing hands on the outside of a woman's abdomen, is an extension of massage. It has to be done carefully, but it often succeeds in rotating the baby. Shepherds across the world have used this same technique when attending ewes in difficult births. "Internal version," or "podalic version," was a later, much more risky and painful procedure in which the baby's feet were grabbed and pulled down and out. It was rediscovered late in the Middle Ages, when ancient Latin and Greek obstetric texts were uncovered. A European-trained gentleman physician like Dr. Lewiston would have been knowledgeable in this skill, but he wouldn't have wanted to use it because it was so risky. By the 1850s, when Sarah Hanley was giving birth, obstetrics had developed other ways of intervening in childbirth. Most noteworthy was the invention of forceps, scissorslike metal blades with spoon-shaped ends that could be inserted into the birthing woman's vagina and clamped around the baby's head (assuming it was in the normal head-down position) in order to pull the baby out of the mother's body.

"Iron Hands" in the Hands of Male Midwives

In 1588, when forceps were first used, many women lived unhealthy, inactive lives in crowded and unsanitary cities. As a result, childbirth had become so complicated that even the calming and constant attention of a midwife was often not enough to help a woman give birth on her own. The men who first brought metal forceps into the rooms where women were giving birth were initially considered heretics by devout churchgoers for being present at a woman's labor. They were called "male midwives," because physicians did not normally attend births. Only midwives did that. They soon became known for "meddlesome midwifery," due to their habit of intervening even when things were going well. However, to the women who might otherwise have died from protracted labor, especially those with deformed pelvises through which a baby could not make its way, these early male midwives were a godsend.

Peter Chamberlen, who designed the first forceps, was an opportunist. He kept his invention secret within his family for three generations, each of which practiced the craft. A woman or midwife who could locate a Chamberlen and afford his fee would never see the contraption he carried in a locked box to a laboring woman's bedside. Working blind by touch only under the sheet that he extended, for propriety's sake, from the woman's neck to his own, the man would open the box discreetly and pull out and assemble the metal pieces, which came to be spoken of as "iron hands." The baby would be delivered and the man would be paid and walk out, leaving the rest to the midwife and the woman's relatives. The going price for the delivery, in today's terms, was approximately $7,500. This was an early instance of the practice of offering one kind of medical service to those who could pay a high price and denying it to those who could not.

After several generations, one of the later Chamberlens went public with the forceps. Soon they were produced in large numbers, and male physicians in eighteenth-century Europe who had them began to be sought after. Upper-class women, who had long since forgotten their connection to their bodies and whose lives were artificial in the extreme, wore tightly cinched corsets and restricted their diets to achieve wasplike waists. They found the raw physicality of birth shocking and repulsive. Even suckling a baby was considered repellent, giving rise to the prevalent use of lower-class mothers as wet nurses to breast-feed aristocrats' babies. Because midwives were now relegated to the lower classes, upper-class women had to depend on physicians, all of whom were male. No women had ever been permitted in European medical schools, nor would women be permitted to enter any medical schools in Europe or the Americas for another forty years.

In 1923, forceps were recommended as a routine part of birth. Dr. Joseph de Lee, an American obstetrician, said in the early 1920s that birth was by nature a pathological event and no more natural to a mother's perineum than "falling on a pitchfork." He further stated that the baby's head should be "saved from being used as a battering ram against its mother's iron perineum" by the prophylactic use of episiotomy (cutting the perineum to enlarge the vaginal outlet) together with forceps. Episiotomy and forceps went hand-in-hand from then on.

Today forceps are being phased out of use in favor of a suction device called vacuum extractor or, more commonly, cesarean surgery. Forceps are much more dangerous than vacuum extractors and are much more difficult to use. They have been misused horribly in midforceps and high-forceps deliveries, causing great trauma to both mother and fetus, and medical residency programs are currently dropping them from their obstetric curriculums.

THE INTRODUCTION OF DRUGS IN CHILDBIRTH

One pivotal and hotly debated medical issue during the second half of the nineteenth century had a broad impact on childbearing women and newborn babies. It was the use of drugs to diminish or obliterate the pain of labor. By early in the twentieth century the administration of drugs was a common practice in home births, and once birth was moved into the hospital it quickly became routine. Birthing women were given a combination of a powerful narcotic and a drug to eradicate their memory of the experience. Known as "twilight sleep," this was equally embraced by women and their physicians and continued to be in common use in the United States well into the 1970s (see pages 78–79).

At first, however, there was some debate over the "morality" of drug use. The question was: Should a "good Christian woman" take drugs or anesthesia in labor? The health and safety of birthing women and their babies was not the focus of this debate. Once the question of the morality of drug use was settled, it became a matter of what form of pharmaceutical was most convenient at any particular time, not what was truly safe or effective. Drugs proliferated rapidly, and their acceptance became so widespread that few births took place then—or take place today—without some kind of medication being given to the woman at some point during labor.

What's Good Enough for a Queen Is . . .

Queen Victoria holds a significant place in the history of childbirth for her role in popularizing the use of drugs in childbirth. In 1847, Sir James Young Simpson of Edinburgh discovered the anesthetic properties of chloroform. It was immediately considered a boon to surgery, since patients often died from physical shock when a surgeon cut deep into their flesh. It was also considered, but quickly rejected, as an aid to birthing women. Ministers, priests, philosophers, and politicians all took the podium to defend the belief that woman's God-given place was to suffer in childbirth. Anything that might prevent her feeling every sensation of labor was believed to be against biblical injunction. By the time Sarah Hanley, the fictional woman whose story began this chapter, went into labor, the idea that women had to suffer greatly to give birth was doctrine.

Sir James was not to be put off by religious injunction. He saw chloroform as a way to help women, and he apparently convinced the queen that there was nothing sacrilegious about taking it when giving birth. The queen took chloroform in 1853 for the birth of her eighth child. From that time on, the drug—called for many years Anesthésie à la Reine—was much sought-after by women who were terrified of the idea of pain in childbirth.

The use of chloroform allowed Victorian women to give birth—that primitive, elemental act—without having to deal with any of its raw elements such as emotions, physical sensations, bodily secretions, smells, or the sight of blood. Floating into euphoria as she reclined on her back on the doctor's table, a woman yielded everything—her attention, her effort, her responsibility, and her sense of protection toward her baby—to the authority of the physician.

Sarah Hanley's physician did not offer her chloroform because he was conservative in his approach to medicine, concerned that he should do no harm, and worried that this new drug had not been in use long enough to prove safe. However, because he had no knowledge of midwife practices, Dr. Lewiston did not know about any of the many natural aids that can be used to assist a laboring woman. Thus he did not suggest that Sarah take a hot bath, ask Mary to give her a vigorous leg massage, insist that Sarah eat and drink to keep her strength up, or instruct her to change positions and be active and upright. All of these things are part of traditional midwifery wisdom the world over. He also made no attempt to help Sarah to shift her attitude from one of helpless despair to one of confidence and trust.

THE LEGACY OF CHILDBED FEVER

The childbed fever so feared by Sarah Hanley was a virulent disease that caused perfectly healthy women to sicken and die within a matter of hours or days after giving birth. In some European hospitals in the sixteenth and seventeenth centuries, 50 percent of birthing women died of the disease. Although the Scottish physician Aberdeen in the late 1840s correctly guessed that childbed fever was an infectious disease that spread from one woman to another, news of medical advancements did not travel fast across great distances. Independently of Aberdeen, Oliver Wendell Holmes had the same insight at about the same time in Boston. So did Ignaz Semmelweis in Vienna. No one yet knew of the existence of microorganisms, particles so small that they could not be seen with the naked eye but which were the cause of infection. The prevailing belief was that childbed fever was due to a change in the weather.

Semmelweis observed that in his hospital the mortality rate for women in the division run by doctors and medical students was three times the mortality rate in the unit run exclusively by midwives and nuns. He also noted that there were no differences in the kinds of patients in either section, since women were simply assigned to one or the other section on alternate days. As a result, women in the physician-run unit were as frightened of the doctors there as they were of birth itself, and Semmelweis wrote that these women "believe the doctor's interference was the precursor of death."

The women were correct. Many of them did everything in their power to resist going into the hospital on the day when they would be placed in the physician unit. However, giving birth in a public hospital was the only choice many of them had if they were homeless, could not afford a midwife, or wanted the baby to be adopted by the state so that it would not be subjected to poverty. What Semmelweis first privately concluded, then publicly announced, was that the physicians must be doing something wrong. It was one thing for birthing women to complain—women were considered to be mentally inferior and to be ruled by their moods. But it was another thing altogether for a prestigious physician to declare that *physicians* were the cause of this scourge.

Childbed fever was in fact probably the first truly iatrogenic, or physician-caused, disease, a term that had not yet been coined. At that time it was unthinkable that a physician, whose oath of practice stated "above all do no harm," *could* cause disease, injury, or death. It would not be until the mid-twentieth century that iatrogenesis would be scientifically validated.

Semmelweis, Holmes, and Aberdeen all came to the same conclusion: that doctors should wash their hands thoroughly before and after vaginally examining any woman in labor. As a result of this recommendation, all three doctors were attacked and hounded by their physician peers. No one recognized that Semmelweis had inadvertently uncovered an equally important fact: that midwives not only did *no* vaginal examinations on the women in their care, they seemed to know the secrets for keeping birth normal and safe.

At the same time, a scientist named Joseph Lister theorized that it was microorganisms that were the cause of postsurgical and postbirth infections, and he discovered a way to keep microorganisms from infecting a wound or surgical incision: by spraying their hands with an antiseptic, physicians would not infect their patients. Establishing standards for antiseptic conditions made it possible for hospitals to change from being mere collection stations for dying people to places in which surgery could be done without automatically risking the patient's life from infection. Childbed fever, however, was not erased overnight. As late as 1920, 40 percent of all maternal deaths in the United States were attributed to "uterine fever," another name for childbed fever.

THE VALUE OF UPRIGHT POSTURE IN BIRTH

It is unfortunate that Sarah's Dr. Lewiston did not know of the benefits to a laboring woman of remaining upright and active for as long as possible. Many of the problems upper-class women experienced in childbirth at that time could have been prevented or treated by simple measures commonly used by midwives but unknown to doctors, including helping a woman labor with, rather than against, the downward pull of gravity.

Not only does an upright or squatting position actually shorten labor and make each contraction more efficient, but squatting causes the female pelvis to expand to its widest dimensions. Often when a woman has a mildly constricted or small pelvic outlet, her baby can still fit through if the woman is in a squatting position. The few extra centimeters created by squatting can mean the difference between a baby going through the pelvis or not. However, by Sarah's generation, women were being raised to accept second-class status and passivity and dependence on men. They had lost their connection to their bodies and lost their innate sense of power as human beings. All but women of the "lower" classes were by then laboring and delivering on their backs in bed, as if childbirth were a form of sickness. Sarah Hanley was a prisoner of her social class, and it would have been unthinkable for a gentlewoman to squat or get on her hands and knees. And so her labor was made longer and more difficult by the fashion of the day and might even have killed her, were it not for her doctor's heroic measures.

OBSTETRICS IN MODERN TIMES

Sarah Hanley came to adulthood at a time when, for the first time in history, men were the central figures in what had been an exclusively female domain: giving birth. Men had pieces of paper attesting to their formal training at prestigious medical schools; they had impressive mechanical tools; and they had drugs. The traditional birth attendants, midwives, had none of these. What midwives did have—and always have had—was an understanding of the women they served and an intimate knowledge of the birth process itself. They also shared their knowledge with the women they served, whereas physicians created a mystique, making themselves special by keeping their knowledge to themselves. The modern history of childbirth practices began with women abdicating responsibility for their bodies and their babies, and with physicians taking control. Today childbirth continues to be all too often a story of collusion, in which women agree with their physicians that they and their babies will be better off for having their births medically managed.

Why haven't women stood up for normalcy and defended their right to have successful childbirth without intervention? Remember, it was well into the twentieth century before a minority of outspoken and courageous women won the long battle for the right to vote. At about the same time, women finally won the right to enter universities and medical schools. The medical schools and training hospitals in which doctors do their obstetric residency have always been—and continue to be—dominated by the prevailing cultural belief that it is doctors who are the authorities in childbirth, not women, and that medicine functions best when physicians are in control. Even the strong entrance of women into the field of obstetrics has not changed that for the most part.

The issue is not just one of an imbalance of power between women and doctors in childbirth, but of laypeople and doctors in general. Obstetrics, after all, is a specialty of medicine and surgery. Its focus never has been normalcy. Only in a country like the Netherlands, where many obstetricians first learn about birth by assisting midwives, have physicians learned to respect the conservative approach of watching and waiting. The special domain of obstetrics is the use of tools, pharmaceutical drugs, and surgery to treat illness and cure disease.

Obstetrics today suffers as much from the lack of knowledge of how to maintain normalcy as it does from the overuse of medical intervention. This is understandable historically, since physicians never were trained in age-old herbal or hands-on forms of healing. However, there is no excuse for this lack of knowledge today, when there is widespread information about natural and noninterventive alternatives to most medical procedures and treatments used in birth.

When Women Don't Count

The rise in the power of men and the loss of the power of women in the Western world had begun thousands of years before Sarah Hanley was born. Women had long since placed all their trust in authorities outside themselves. With regard to childbirth this was a bizarre state of affairs, considering that birth is an arena alien to men. However, it is not strange when you consider that women like Sarah lived under the control of men all their lives.

By the nineteenth century, a middle-class woman in Europe, the British Empire, or the United States went directly from her father's home—for her mother could not by law own any property—into her husband's. To be single was to be a spinster, a term with a stigma that the word *bachelor* did not have. A man who was unmarried was free and independent and could be rakish as well; an unmarried woman was either suspect for unseemly sexual inclinations or pitied for her inability to find a husband. Middle- and upper-class women were unable to divorce their husbands for any reason, had no access to higher education, had even less access to paying jobs or careers, and were therefore dependent on men for everything. To be without one was a dangerous position.

Adult women had approximately the same rights as did children. They had no say in how government was run and little say in their own destinies. Women's work—and this has not changed much today—was ignored in the equation of a nation's wealth, because most of the work women did was unpaid, such as rearing children and running a household.

It is a small step from having no economic or political power to feeling and behaving like a victim. That is precisely what began to occur with women, and this of course affected childbirth. Women felt victimized by their body's natural functioning in the areas of sexuality and birth. They were alienated from their bodies just as they were alienated from the earth and the cycles of nature.

This lack of confidence and dissociation from the body continue today. Consider the fact that one out of every four births in the United States since 1988 has been a cesarean surgery. Moreover, consider that the overwhelming majority of cesarean births do not occur among those women who might be considered medically at high risk. Cesareans are much more often performed on healthy, well-educated, middle-class women who go to private physicians and give birth in private hospitals. Among the same population of women who have midwives at their births, the cesarean rate is well below 10 percent.

Noninterventive Aids to Birth

The healing arts, of which midwifery is one, have a long tradition in working with the human body's innate healing capacity rather than intervening in order to "fight" illness, and in doing simple things to correct serious problems. The list of effective aids to normal labor is long. It includes encouraging the mother to keep upright and move around as long as possible; having a calm person experienced in childbirth remain at her side continuously once labor becomes active; helping her maintain a positive attitude; giving her massage; helping her focus on her breathing and staying calm; feeding her and making sure she has enough fluids in her system to keep her strength up so the uterus can do its work; and helping her assume an upright position for delivery so her body can work with, rather than against, gravity.

The list of effective ways to initiate labor when a woman is more than two and a half weeks past her due date, or to make a sluggish labor more effective, is also long. It includes having the woman or her partner rub her nipples; having her engage in erotic play or intercourse (unless her bag of waters has broken, in which case clitoral stimulation is preferable in order to avoid infection); having her take a hot shower or bath; and giving her a vigorous massage, especially of her legs, to stimulate circulation and contractions. Each of these stimulates the body's production of the hormone oxytocin, which produces contractions.

Only in the last decade have such practices been seen in hospitals. Today in North America many hospitals now "permit" them, just as they permit a woman to have food and drink in labor instead of just ice chips. However, the activities tend to be accompanied with electronic monitoring, drugs, and anesthesia, rather than being done in lieu of these risky interventive procedures. Often the use of several traditional labor aids will be enough to get labor on course and no intervention will be needed. Where the practices listed above are now used, it has been the general public, midwives, and progressive nurses who have introduced them in hospitals, not physicians. Most physicians are resistant to learning them. They still don't know how to prevent a woman from tearing or needing an episiotomy. They do not learn in their training how to apply hot compresses to the woman's stretching perineum, how to do gentle perineal massage, or how squatting can prevent tears. These are just a few examples of the differences between normal childbirth and medical childbirth, between aggressive intervention that distorts the birth process and labor aids that support it. If they seem like two totally different approaches to childbirth, that is because they are.

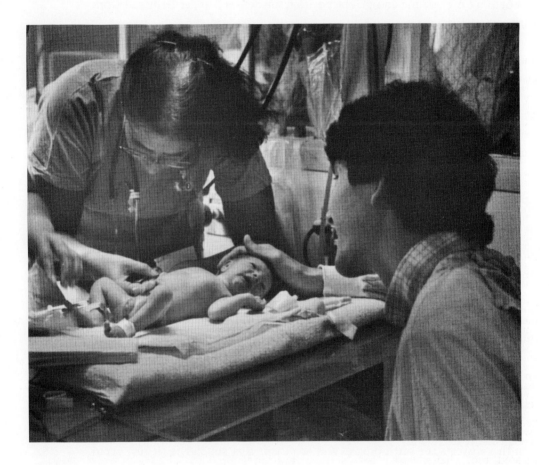

CHAPTER THREE

Hospitals and Birth

Your Mother's Two Childbirths

YOUR MOTHER HAS A SON: 1963

"Honey, guess what! The rabbit died!" Marion whispered excitedly into her husband's ear as she gave him a hug on his return home from work. Marion and Mark's marriage of two years was mutually supportive and they considered themselves a "progressive" couple. Having children had always been in their picture of their future, but they hadn't planned for Marion to get pregnant just yet.

Marion tried the pill, but it contained very high amounts of synthetic hormones and she had negative side effects. When she gained a lot of weight and couldn't lose it, she stopped taking the pill. She didn't want an IUD because she didn't like the idea of having an object in her uterus. Several of her friends were using them, but they were having very heavy periods. Mark hated condoms, so they finally settled on Marion using a diaphragm with spermicidal jelly. She found it messy and forgot to use it on more than one occasion. The most recent time had resulted in this pregnancy. However, she found herself unexpectedly excited at the prospect of motherhood, and Mark was rather pleased, too. That was fortunate, because abortion was not a legal option in the United States in 1963.

At her first prenatal visit, Marion was introduced to the doctor who would deliver her baby. He took down her medical history, did a routine physical exam, and had a nurse take several blood samples to send to the lab for tests. Then he did a vaginal exam to ascertain how far along the pregnancy was.

Marion was brimming with questions, but she felt suddenly tongue-tied and foolish, and didn't ask any of them. The doctor didn't volunteer any information about prenatal care or procedures during labor and delivery.

"I'll see you in four weeks, and once a month after that, until the last two months when you'll be coming in every week," the doctor said. "You'll get to be a regular around here. Just remember to watch what you eat. I don't want my mothers using pregnancy as an excuse to eat like pigs and gain lots of weight." He laughed jovially. "That would just make my job a lot harder." He noticed Marion's flush and wasn't sure whether she was sensitive about her weight or anxious about the birth, so he added, "You have nothing at all to worry about. Everything will be fine. Just leave it all to me."

"How much weight should I gain?" Marion asked the nurse on the way out.

"Twelve to fourteen pounds. That's all the doctor likes. It's the total of the average newborn plus the weight of the average placenta. It's all you need."

Marion was a sophisticated and well-read young woman and didn't feel completely comfortable putting everything in the hands of a stranger. She left the doctor's office with a vague sense of unease, but decided to pay it no attention. "After all," she told herself, "this man went to medical school and had a four-year residency in obstetrics. He should know what he's doing. He's delivered hundreds of babies, and I've never even had one before!"

Marion had grown up in a world in which men were the authorities on virtually everything except housework and rearing children. All of her professors at college had been men; all of the business owners she had contact with were men; all but a few of the authors she read were men. So she never thought about the appropriateness of a man acting as the authority on the workings of her female body.

At the library Marion found only one book on childbirth. Its author, Nicholson Eastman, seemed to be quite an expert. He was chief of obstetrics at a medical school Marion had heard was top-notch. On the cover of the book was printed: "If you are going to have a baby, you will, of course, visit your doctor regularly and listen carefully to his advice. Between visits you will find this book a convenient reference book to remind you of what he said . . ." Marion was not offended by the paternalistic tone, for this was something she had heard every day of her life. She checked the book out.

On the way home Marion stopped by a used bookstore. There she found a well-worn copy of a small book whose author, Grantly Dick-Read, was a British physician. The book was copyrighted 1944 and titled *Childbirth Without Fear*. The subtitle, *The Principles and Practice of Natural Childbirth,* piqued her curiosity. She had never heard of anything called "natural childbirth." It seemed different from the book she got at the library, which had chapter titles like "Weight Control" and "Danger Signals." Marion stood and read the first pages. The opening chapter was entitled "Childbirth as a Natural Process" and was the story of a home delivery the doctor had attended in a very poor section of a city in England.

"In due course, the baby was born. There was no fuss or noise." The author went on to describe his surprise when the laboring woman refused his offer of chloroform as the baby's head appears. When he asked her why afterward, she said, "It didn't hurt. It wasn't meant to, was it, doctor?" That, according to the author, began his investigation into the reasons for pain in childbirth.

Amazed, Marion read further. Apparently, in his travels to other parts of the world, areas not considered modern, this physician had witnessed many births in which women did not appear to suffer, although he had seen others in which the women were in horrible pain. "Unbelievable," Marion told herself. She closed the book and paid for it.

That afternoon, Marion curled up on the couch with a cigarette and read the British doctor's book, cover to cover. She hadn't recognized all the anxiety she'd been feeling over her pregnancy as fear, but after reading the stories of some of the women in the book she realized that she *was* actually afraid of the process of birth and doubted her own ability to have a baby. Dick-Read was reassuring, but then so was the doctor she had just seen. There was a difference, however. She was moved by Dick-Read's enthusiasm over what he called "natural childbirth," and his conviction that women had an innate ability to give birth successfully without needing any drugs. Marion was particularly intrigued with all the chapters related to fear, and she read the one on relaxation with close attention.

Still, nothing in this book related to what she had heard about birth, from her mother or any other woman. No one, including her doctor, had discussed the idea of fear and its negative impact on the process of labor. While this made a good deal of sense to her, the idea of not taking drugs during childbirth seemed like a very radical and risky thing to do.

Now she picked up the American obstetrician's book and turned to the chapter entitled "Painless Childbirth." It described the three phases of giving birth. First were the pains of early labor, which served the useful purpose of warning a woman that labor was starting. The woman would know it was time to go to a place that would be safe for her and for her baby. The second phase was marked by "more severe pains," when the cervix dilated. The third phase was again characterized by pain, caused by the "expulsion" of the baby.

After reading the description of a potent combination of drugs called "twilight sleep," used for the second stage, Marion stopped for a moment. Her mother had told her that she had had it for all four of her births. She remembered that her younger brother had needed resuscitation when he was born and had been kept in the nursery for several weeks. "Nicholas had a hard time as a baby. Could twilight sleep have caused his problems?" she wondered.

She returned to the book. Barbiturates, she read, induce a sleep state, and are used in combination with other drugs that reduce pain. "The results are usually very satisfactory, the patient knowing nothing about her labor and awakening in her own room several hours after the baby has been born." The description of natural childbirth was brief, stating that few women can get by without the benefit of drugs. These words satisfied Marion and calmed her anxieties. She closed the book and put them both aside.

In the course of her pregnancy, Marion found abundant reinforcement, both from her physician and various women friends, that birth was far too painful a process for a woman to try to go without modern medication. That is, they said, "unless you're crazy or want to be some kind of martyr!" Everyone seemed to have at least one horror story they were eager to relate about a friend or relative who, for one reason or another, was not able to have drugs and found the experience a nightmare.

At the seven-month visit, Marion's doctor spent twenty minutes with her, instead of his usual five, in order to discuss his plans for her delivery. "When you think you are in labor, you'll come to the hospital. A nurse will check you to see if you are in fact in labor, and if you are you'll be admitted. Then I'll see that you have sedation to relax you and make you sleep, as well as something to make you forget all about the pain afterward. When the baby's head is coming you'll be given gas to breathe. And when you come to, you will have your baby!"

Her doctor's plan sounded fine, until Marion suddenly recalled a section in the Eastman book that said that doctors generally withhold medication for premature births, because of the risks to the baby's respiratory system. She asked her doctor, "Are the drugs safe for my baby?" He immediately assured her. "Do you think we'd even consider giving you something that might harm you or your baby? Young women today just don't know how lucky they are." And he gave her a reassuring pat on the back.

Marion's husband, Mark, grew more and more anxious as the baby's due date approached. He and Marion had not talked about the anxiety they each harbored about the birth or their ambivalent feelings about all the changes the new baby would bring about in their lives. He was relieved when Marion finally packed her hospital bag, because it signaled to him that the most worrisome part—the birth—would soon be over. He told a friend, "I'm sure glad I don't have to go through it!"

OCTOBER 24, 1963: The great day had arrived. Marion woke up with more energy than she'd had in a month. She cleaned the entire house and set about preparing dinner. In the early afternoon she lay down for a few minutes and noticed a sharp tugging sensation deep inside her groin. It was a little different from the sensations she'd been feeling on and off the past few weeks. An hour later they were coming more regularly. She thought that this might be labor, but she decided not to phone Mark at the office, thinking, "He'll be home in a little while." In the meantime, she took a long hot shower, which felt very good, since she now had an aching sensation all across her lower abdomen along with the sharp twinges. She focused her attention on washing and setting her hair and sat down to have a cigarette.

When she went to the bathroom and discovered bloody mucus on the toilet paper, she was immediately anxious. No one had mentioned this. She phoned the doctor's office and, with embarrassment, described it to the nurse. She was told, "It's probably early labor. The mucus plug must have come loose from your cervix." Marion felt somehow ashamed that she needed to be told this but was glad to know it was normal. The nurse told her to wait until the pains were coming five minutes apart and lasting a minute or longer, and then to go to the hospital. "Don't worry about a thing," she said.

Marion went through her packed bag one more time, and then placed it by the front door. She considered calling her mother, whom she knew would be at her home in Virginia, but she decided to wait a bit to make sure it really *was* labor. "I don't want to make her worry any longer than necessary," she thought. She finished the preparations for dinner and smoked another cigarette.

Mark came home from work and became agitated at finding his wife in labor. Neither of them could eat. It took hours for Marion's contractions to become five minutes apart so they could finally go to the hospital. They arrived at the emergency room entrance at 1:00 A.M. Mark was asked to wait and sign Marion in while Marion was guided to a wheelchair and wheeled to a labor and delivery unit. Marion was embarrassed when she had a contraction while a strange man was pushing her wheelchair. When Mark found his way up to the unit and knocked on the door, he was handed a paper sack containing Marion's clothes. The nurse told him, "Go home and get some sleep. We'll call you when the baby's come. There's nothing you can do here."

Marion was taken into a tiny white room that smelled of antiseptic. The nurse told her to undress and handed her a pale green hospital gown. Marion noted with alarm that it was open all the way down the back, revealing her buttocks.

She was excited and anxious; the contractions were now definitely harder to cope with. Left alone, she began, unconsciously, to hold her breath and tense her entire body during each contraction in an attempt to control it. The nurse returned to "prep" her. Marion had never heard of this, but she found that it meant she must lie down on her back so that the nurse could shave off her pubic hair and administer an enema. "We've got to make sure you are clean, inside and out, before we take you into delivery," the nurse said cheerily. After that she did a vaginal exam, then she inserted two fingers into Marion's rectum. Marion found the rectal probe humiliating and painful, but the nurse told her she was checking the position of the baby.

"Well, you're two centimeters, but the baby is not well down in the pelvis, and I'm not certain about its position. Maybe it's breech," the nurse said. She left to phone Marion's doctor, who prescribed an X-ray, and Marion soon found herself being wheeled downstairs to the X-ray room. Afterward, she was brought back to her room. Two centimeters, she knew, means she was only in the early stage of labor. She felt discouraged. The contractions were coming four minutes apart now and felt quite strong. "How will I ever get through hours of this?" she asked herself again and again.

For the first time she wished that her mother were there with her. As soon as the nurse left the room, she turned her face to the wall and began to cry. The contractions grew stronger and closer together over the next hour. Marion rolled from side to side during each contraction and talked to herself to control her urge to moan or shout. A different nurse came and examined her, wheeling a cart with bottles and tubes and needles. Marion was given a shot in her buttocks. She soon lost all track of time and place, and for the next five hours she experienced a swirling series of unpleasant dreams. When a nurse came in to do another vaginal exam, Marion was well under the effects of the drugs, unaware that she was making wild animal noises and thrashing about in the bed. So that Marion could not hurt herself, the nurse had tied Marion's wrists to the bed rails and placed some thick leather cushioning all around her. She checked to make sure the side rails were secure and then wrote in the chart that Marion was dilated six centimeters and that the labor was progressing normally.

Marion's baby was born at five-thirty in the afternoon. He was pulled from her inert body with forceps, for she was fully unconscious from the effects of anesthesia given through a face mask at the end of pushing and could not participate at all. It was a boy, and he was pale bluish-white in color, and limp, and needed minutes of resuscitation before he was able to breathe on his own. Then he was taken to the nursery. It was almost eight hours after delivery before Marion was alert enough to hold her son. He was groggy and unresponsive for most of the following seven days in the hospital. Marion felt frustrated that she had so little time with him when he was awake. He spent most of the time in the nursery, only being brought to Marion during the day, once every four hours, so she could feed him formula out of a bottle.

Meanwhile, Marion was preoccupied with the immediate concerns of her own convalescence. The entire area between her vaginal outlet and her rectum ached and burned whenever she urinated. Her bowel movements were difficult because of large hemorrhoids. Her breasts had become swollen with milk, despite the medication she was given to stop them from producing and the tight binding cloth the nurse wrapped around her. She felt depressed and bored and there was a sour taste in her mouth. There was nothing to do when her baby wasn't there, and she was too uncomfortable to walk or move around very much.

Mark listened sympathetically to Marion's complaints when he came to the hospital each day during visiting hours. He felt helpless. What could he do to make Marion feel better? He was secretly glad that he didn't have to go through all that misery, but he worried whether his wife would ever be the same.

Marion's recuperation was slow. Her episiotomy stitches continued to cause her discomfort for months after she returned home. Mark did his best to help out whenever he was not at work and got up in the night to give baby William his bottle. Marion did not breast-feed him; he was fed skim milk at the suggestion of her doctor. Marion was so depressed for the first three months as her body continued to slowly recover from the birth that she had barely enough interest or energy to care for her new child. The women in the neighborhood helped her out, bringing food in the first weeks, then dropping by unannounced over the next months to see how she was getting along. They insisted that she get out of the house, and they took her shopping and invited her to their homes for coffee and conversation. When they talked about their childbirth experiences, the conversation usually turned into a recounting of war stories of who had had the hardest time and the most complications. The litany of complaints always included how horribly painful it was—although most of them had been heavily sedated or anesthetized for much of active labor—and usually how unpleasant the recovery was as well. None of them seemed to find it unusual that they could not look back on their childbirth experience with any warmth or joy.

Slowly, Marion's depression lifted and her life began to look a little brighter. She took more interest in her baby, she began going out more on her own, and she and Mark resumed their sex life, although this time she was extra careful to use her diaphragm consistently, as she dreaded becoming pregnant again.

YOUR MOTHER HAS A DAUGHTER: 1968

The family had moved to the Northeast, and Marion was pregnant for a second time. She was initially excited at the prospect of another baby in the house. She chose an obstetrician named Dr. Alan Dickerson on a neighbor's recommendation that he was "the best in town," because "he does four hundred births a year. He should know what he is doing!" Dr. Dickerson delivered all the babies at a large teaching hospital affiliated with a major medical school that prided itself on its progressive birth practices.

The doctor's waiting room was full of pregnant women and decorated to resemble a large living room, with toys for the children and current magazines on housekeeping and child rearing. Marion's first visit lasted twenty minutes, and she surprised herself when her first question was, "What can I have for pain?" The doctor looked at the records sent to him from her other doctor and noted that she had had "twilight sleep" and inhalation anesthesia when her first child was born. He told her that he preferred not to use either one because there were much safer medications today. Marion was surprised to learn that what her other doctor gave her might have been unsafe. The doctor then told her about a new form of spinal anesthesia called a "caudal block." "I'll give you a tranquilizer and a little bit of Demerol to get you through early labor, then you'll get your spinal," he explained to her.

"As long as it doesn't hurt," Marion said. "I can't stand pain." After the doctor did an exam, he handed her his instructions for pregnancy, which included "no smoking." Marion was a little upset about this, but noted gratefully that she was allowed to gain a little more weight than she had been with William. She'd had to go on a rice and Jello diet prescribed for her by her other doctor during the last three weeks of her pregnancy with William, and a lot of her other women friends had had to do the same thing. She was glad that that thinking had changed; it wasn't easy to stay on a diet when your body was constantly hungry. Marion left the doctor's office feeling very good.

On succeeding visits she had her "fundal height"—the distance from her pubic bone to the top of her uterus—measured, her blood pressure taken, her weight recorded, and a urine sample analyzed. The doctor always asked her how things were going, but she had the impression from his manner, and from the number of women always waiting in the waiting room, that he didn't really want her to say more than "I'm fine," unless something was *really* wrong.

This pregnancy was more uncomfortable than her first. Marion had morning sickness almost all day long for the first three months. "I don't know why anyone calls it *morning* sickness!" she complained. This was made worse by the nicotine withdrawal she suffered—and she couldn't even have a cigarette to calm her stomach!

Marion never did get the surge of energy she had had with William in the middle months, and felt increasingly tired as her due date approached. The neighborhood women gave her a baby shower. While they sat around talking, drinking coffee, and eating little sandwiches, a few of them began to reminisce about their childbirths, but, once again, they were tales of suffering told with pride.

One night Marion had a nightmare about falling into a black hole. She woke in a sweat, vividly recalling the awful months of depression after William's birth. "I can't face another time like that. What will I do if it happens again?" she asked herself. She didn't wake Mark, but she did decide to talk to the doctor.

At her next visit the doctor explained to her about postpartum depression. He tried to comfort her by telling her that some women had it so bad they needed to be hospitalized for months. He assured her that he would prescribe a tranquilizer for her if it happened to her again. "I'll see to it that you won't have to suffer," he said. He didn't tell her that some of his patients had been given shock treatment for it.

*   *   *

Toward the end of her pregnancy Marion began having dreams about giving birth. Mostly it was to baby animals, and in every dream there were problems. In one particularly vivid dream there was a drawbridge over a wide river separating her from the hospital on the other side, and she could not find anyone to let the bridge down so she could get across. Every time she had these dreams Marion woke up tense and unsettled, and the feeling lasted well into the day. She didn't mention the dreams to Mark. "He wouldn't understand," Marion told herself. She did tell her mother about them during a phone conversation, but her mother only said she thought it was very strange and advised her to talk to the doctor. Marion didn't feel comfortable doing that, though. She preferred to show him how well she was doing.

At the end of her final prenatal visit before her due date, Marion's doctor dropped the news that he would be out of town the next week at a medical convention in Hawaii. "I don't feel good about leaving you. Why don't you come into the hospital on Wednesday morning and we'll induce you?" he said. Marion had read an article in a women's magazine entitled "Baby by Appointment," in which the woman reporter wrote glowingly about how it was now possible to plan the very day of your baby's birth. The idea appealed to Marion, who was very tired of pregnancy, but she hesitated. Her doctor said, "This is your second baby, after all. Second babies are often troublesome. Lots of women end up going weeks beyond their due dates and having labor start and stop for days. Think of it this way; you won't have to worry about making it to the hospital in time. Second babies sometimes come very quickly!" Marion agreed and went home to tell Mark, who was relieved.

On Wednesday Mark drove Marion to the hospital after he got home from work. Marion was once again put into a wheelchair and rolled down the hall to her room by an attendant. Mark was once again told to wait in the fathers' waiting room while the nurse examined Marion and "made her comfortable." Then he was permitted to go in and see her for a few minutes before leaving to pick up William from the babysitter's. He had heard from Marion that a few hospitals were now allowing fathers to be present for the birth. He was glad this hospital wasn't one of them. The whole idea made him anxious; he imagined fainting in front of the doctor.

Once again Marion was put into a small, windowless room with nothing to look at but a clock on the wall, to labor alone. This time the nurse did what she jokingly called "a poodle cut," which was a partial pubic shave. Apparently Marion was not the only woman to have complained of the weeks of itching while her pubic hair grew back; or maybe the change was due to recent studies showing that shaving a woman's pubic hair in labor actually increased the risk of infection. A needle was inserted in the back of her hand and attached to a long plastic tube connected to a bottle of clear fluid hanging alongside her bed. Marion was given several wafers to put between her gum and her lip. She asked what the wafers were for and was told they contained an artificial hormone that would speed up labor. She was given more wafers as soon as the last ones dissolved, every half hour or so, until her contractions were strong and regular.

Marion didn't have to ask for medication; the nurse told her that her doctor had prescribed something called Demerol. Marion was given a shot and felt a comforting dizziness, and the pain of each contraction grew duller. Her contractions seemed to go on forever. Another nurse came and gave her more wafers, then another shot, then helped her up onto a bedpan to urinate; finally she slipped into another dimension, where everything was a blur.

On his lunch hour Dr. Dickerson came in to check on Marion and told the nurse to start the spinal anesthesia. Then he went back to his office. A little while later, an anesthesiologist came into Marion's room and instructed her to curl up on her side and remain very still so that he could inject anesthesia through a long needle alongside her spine. It was very difficult for her to keep still, as it was more painful having contractions in that position. But a little while later Marion began to feel numbness spread down her body from her navel.

The clock was watched closely by the staff because they didn't want Marion's baby to start coming before her doctor could get back to the hospital. Finally Marion was moved onto a gurney and wheeled into the delivery room, then rolled onto a high, narrow table. Her hands were strapped down at her sides with leather handcuffs, and her feet were placed in metal stirrups. Her doctor was called. Marion was waking up; she had not been given sedatives for some time, because that was the policy in this hospital. Current studies showed that the sedatives commonly used for labor inhibited a newborn baby's ability to breathe and to breast-feed. Marion felt very cold. A team had assembled, dressed in gowns and hats and face masks. Suddenly her doctor entered, holding his hands up and out in front of him. A nurse unwrapped a pair of sterile rubber gloves and helped him into them. "You'll be fully awake, but you won't feel any pain," he told Marion as he sat down on a stool between her outstretched legs.

Marion felt her hospital gown lifted up around her breasts. She could not feel the cold wetness as a nurse liberally swabbed her pubic area, upper thighs, and lower buttocks with a bright orange antiseptic solution.

"Well, it's time for this baby to be born," the doctor said. After cutting an episiotomy and carefully inserting the blades of his forceps, the doctor clamped them together and began to slowly and firmly pull the baby down the birth canal. "Give me some fundal pressure," he called out. Because of the spinal anesthesia, Marion had no urge to push to help the baby be born. A nurse reached across Marion's abdomen and took hold of a metal hand grip across the table. She then straightened her elbow, put her other hand on top of her outstretched forearm, and began leaning her weight onto Marion, pressing down against Marion's abdomen and downward toward her feet. "More pressure!" the doctor called out from his seat at the bottom of the table. Marion could not see what was going on at the other end of her body, which was draped with blue sterile sheeting, but she did feel a heavy pressure inside, despite the numbness. With the doctor pulling and the nurse pushing, it was all over in a matter of minutes. "You've got a girl!" he said.

Her daughter was briefly held up for Marion to see. Then she was carried across the room. Marion could see a bit of her between the backs of the nurses.

Jessica, as she and Mark had decided to name a girl, had arrived pink, with good respiration and good muscle tone. The nurse said she had an 8 out of a possible 10 Apgar score.* Despite her visible good health, she was held down while her mouth and throat were deeply suctioned, the bottoms of her feet were flicked repeatedly until she began to scream, and she was vigorously rubbed, then wiped dry with a towel. She was wrapped tightly and was still screaming when she was brought to Marion's side for her first good look.

Marion tried to reach out to her daughter, but her hands were still strapped down. Meanwhile, the doctor sat down between Marion's legs and began to stitch up her deep incision. The combination of the fundal pressure, the forceps, and the scar tissue from her previous episiotomy had caused Marion to tear beyond the initial incision into her rectal sphincter muscle—"a fourth-degree tear," she was told later. Her doctor had to be particularly careful in his repair work, lest his patient end up with a hole between her vagina and her rectum. He didn't like this kind of repair, but he found himself doing it fairly often. He took the opportunity to tell Marion he was making her "as tight as a virgin," saying, "Your husband will appreciate this." Marion thought that the remark was crude, but she laughed politely just the same.

In the nursery, Jessica had drops of silver nitrate solution put into her eyes. Since it caused her to cry loudly, she was laid down in a bassinet and fed her first food, a bottle of sugar water, to quiet her. Six hours later, her mother got to hold her for the first time; the nurses had been too busy to bring the baby to her earlier.

Mark came to visit Marion during visiting hours each day. He had to scrub up and put on a gown to be allowed to see his daughter in the nursery, as fathers weren't allowed into the mother's room when the baby was there, in order to prevent the possible spread of infection. Marion thought it strange that the TV repairman and the person who delivered her meals were allowed to come into her room without gowns even when Jessica was there, but her husband was not.

Marion only suffered a mild postpartum depression this time and her stitches healed without complication after a few weeks. It was a good thing,

*Apgar is the basic score used to judge the immediate well-being of a newborn. It evaluates the heart rate, skin color, muscle tone, reflexes, and respiration at one minute and five minutes after birth. A baby with an Apgar score of 7 or more at five minutes is statistically shown to be in good shape. A low one-minute score is not significant if the five-minute score is good.

because Jessica was not a quiet baby; she fussed almost all the time and Marion found herself placing Jessica's crib in her and Mark's room and taking her into her bed many nights to feed her. Fortunately, the new pediatrician told her that was just fine, because newborn babies cannot be spoiled. "Newborns need all the cuddling and attention they can get," he said. As with their firstborn, Mark helped out with the bottle-feeding when he was at home, since Marion did not want to breast-feed. Per the doctor's suggestion, Jessica was fed a manufactured formula rather than skim milk.

Marion was constantly grateful for not being depressed after Jessica's birth. Jessica grew steadily, and the doctor said she was in fine health, but at nine months she was still quite fussy and became upset whenever she was separated from her mother. Her difficult behavior continued through kindergarten and was a marked contrast to William's. A passive baby, William had grown into a quiet and submissive child. In the first grade Jessica was diagnosed as having learning disabilities, including difficulty concentrating. It was recommended that she be placed on a drug called Ritalin to calm her.

Birth and Drugs

DESPITE ALL OF THE technical advances in medicine, virtually every one of which is quickly being applied to childbearing, the predominant technology in childbirth from the beginning of the 1850s right up until today in North America has been the routine use of drugs. The history of twentieth-century childbirth practices can be told in terms of drugs: drugs to stop excessive bleeding, drugs to reduce or numb the body to pain, drugs to treat mothers or babies with infections or disease, drugs to start labor, drugs to stop it or speed it up, drugs to maintain pregnancy, drugs to force fertility, drugs to force fetal development. Every one of these pharmaceutical products has some useful function, even though negative side effects sometimes make it questionable whether a particular drug is really of value. The issue is not whether we should stop all drugs, but how and when drugs ought to be used.

The most important thing to remember about all drugs used in pregnancy and birth—and while a mother is breast-feeding—is that whatever is given to the mother is also given to the baby. Second, we must realize that a baby's system is not mature enough to metabolize and throw off the residual effects of drugs the way an adult body can. This makes *all* drugs suspect in terms of the risks they present to fetuses and newborns. A third consideration is the effect of drugs on the baby during the birth process. The act of being squeezed and pushed down the birth canal is the first journey in life. The baby has an active part to play in this journey in the way it positions itself to be born. The baby's whole body is massaged by this process, which serves to stimulate its entire nervous system. This is the preparation for breathing. It also readies the baby's brain for a huge learning spurt, in which it takes in all the new sensory information from the world it enters the moment it is born, and begins to make the complex series of adjustments that will enable it to survive.

For the mother, the physical sensations of labor create a shift in her consciousness, from an ordinary to a heightened state. Naturally produced hormones dull the pain that comes from muscles and tissues expanding. The process of labor is an important passage to prepare the mother emotionally to receive and bond with her child. After birth, such hormones as prolactin, aptly called the "falling-in-love hormone," are produced and course through her body in profusion, triggered by the mere presence of her baby. Labor creates a set of naturally produced hormones in the baby too. Thus the body's own natural hormonal orchestration works to support a mother and baby through their birth and bonding processes. Artificially dulling the sensations of labor alters the mother and the baby physiologically, alters their relationship, and alters the way in which the baby perceives its new world.

DOUBLE-TALK ABOUT DRUGS

Despite all the talk about the joys of living sober, drug-free lives, modern culture, especially in the United States, continues to be a culture of widespread drug use. We promote the use of drugs in every aspect of life, from allergy aids and laxatives to personality changers such as Prozac. Our medicine cabinets are more full of drugs than they were fifty years ago and so are our childbirths. We are terrified of our children using marijuana, yet we continue to take drugs such as caffeine, alcohol, and nicotine to cope with the stress of our overly busy and fragmented lives.

We are bombarded with warnings about the dangers of alcohol, cigarettes, and street drugs like crack cocaine and their harmful long-term effects on babies whose mothers have used them in pregnancy. Yet we naively exempt the drugs prescribed by doctors to women during pregnancy and labor. We continue to ignore the fact that drugs given to a mother pass quickly from her body directly to the baby through the blood via the umbilical cord that binds them together. The baby gets the same dosage the mother gets, yet the baby is only one-twentieth the size of the mother and in a much lower state of physical development.

In rare cases, a small amount of drugs can be worth the risk in picking up a very slow labor or to calm a woman in difficult moments in labor. Even epidural anesthesia can sometimes be used effectively to facilitate an obstructed labor. It can relax a woman's tissues so that she goes to full dilation, thus preventing the need for a cesarean, which is major surgery and always poses potentially greater risks to the mother and baby. But for the most part, drugs simply are used as they have been ever since women were brought into modern hospitals for childbirth: they are used to replace human caring and support. They make it possible for administrators to staff maternity units so that nurses can care for three or four patients at a time, and for physicians to continue on with their office hours or their nighttime sleep while their patients labor somewhere else.

FROM TWILIGHT SLEEP TO EPIDURALS

The 1970 edition of the Nicholson Eastman book on childbirth, a later edition of the book that Marion read in the last chapter, gave a good layperson's description of the various forms of medication and anesthesia used for childbirth. Little with regard to those drugs has changed today.

Twilight sleep was the most popular form of anesthesia in the United States for nearly half a century. Why was it so popular? It allowed women to go through childbirth without recalling any of the effort or pain associated with it, and it allowed nurses and physicians to be fully in control. Twilight sleep was a combination of morphine and scopolamine devised in Germany early in the twentieth century and used in the United States as late as 1980 in some hospitals, despite the mass of evidence that accumulated over the years showing the harmful physical and psychological effects on babies and on mothers.

Eastman's description was honest: "A woman under twilight sleep may shriek, make grimaces and show other evidence of pain, but upon awakening from the drug will remember nothing about her labor and will vow that she experienced no pain whatsoever." He did not, however, mention that the drugs actually induced a kind of wild psychosis in many women, who fought nurses, scratched themselves, or tried to throw themselves out of the bed. For this reason, the side rails of hospital beds were kept up, heavy leather pads were put inside to protect women from bruising themselves on the metal rails, and women were physically tied down. Many women were shocked to find themselves covered with bruises when they awoke after the birth, with no memory of the cause.

Others found themselves completely hoarse, having no recall that they had lost their voice from screaming. Many harbored doubts that the baby they were shown was really theirs. This is the way many of our mothers, grandmothers, and great-grandmothers gave birth.

Barbiturates, such as Seconal or Nembutal, are sleep-inducing drugs that went into common use in childbirth later than twilight sleep, but they also continued to be popular in many hospitals into the 1980s. Given in combination with other drugs, their effects, Eastman wrote, were similar to twilight sleep. "The results are usually very satisfactory, the patient knowing nothing about her labor and awakening several hours after the baby has been born."

Demerol, which in Britain was called pethidine, was extremely popular in North America and Britain for decades and still is. It is a derivative of morphine, and in 1970 was by far the most popular drug used in labor. It was often given to a woman as soon as she entered the hospital and given repeatedly, in the form of shots, to sustain its effects all the way through labor. Eastman wrote that this drug, like barbiturates, while very likely to impair the functioning of a premature infant, had "little or no effect on the normal, full-term infant." That is what they believed in 1970, but as we shall see later, nothing could have been further from the truth, and today the use of Demerol in labor is controlled and somewhat discouraged.

Tranquilizers, not considered a wise choice today because of their negative side effects, were still being given during the 1970s and were thought quite safe. They were commonly used along with a barbiturate and/or Demerol. For many years the drug diazepam, known in the United States by the brand name Valium, was the most commonly prescribed drug in the nation. Today Valium is known to be extremely addictive, and is difficult and dangerous to kick if someone has been taking it for a long time. Even in just a few hours of labor, Valium can be hazardous to the progress of labor and dangerous for the baby.

Spinal and caudal anesthesia are methods of numbing the nerves that convey sensation to the brain. They are given by injection to the area around the spinal cord. Eastman did not include in his description what anesthesiologists today are taught, that *all* forms of anesthesia injected into the body are poisons. They must be used under extremely controlled conditions and given in just the right doses and in just the right part of the body or they can paralyze or kill. Both spinal and caudal drugs are injected into the interior spaces of the vertebral column. They bathe all the nerves in that area and temporarily deaden them to all sensation—pleasure as well as pain. The differences between spinal and caudal anesthetics result from where they are given along the spine and therefore how much of the area is deadened.

The most popular form of conduction anesthesia for the past twenty-five years has been what is known as "epidural anesthesia." Epidural is anesthetic injected into space inside the spine, blocking nerve transmission. Epidurals were first touted by doctors and nurses because they made for quieter labor wards than did twilight sleep. Today in some hospitals, 80 percent of laboring women are given epidural anesthesia. They can often be seen chatting with relatives, watching television, or playing cards in the midst of contractions, showing no sign whatsoever that they are part of the process because they feel nothing from the waist down. Epidurals have been a boon to cesarean surgery because they make it possible for women to undergo a cesarean, yet be awake to see their baby born, and to be able to hold it in the first minutes of life. When a cesarean is done under general anesthesia, the mother is completely unconscious, and it takes quite awhile for her to become fully aware of her surroundings and her baby. Unfortunately, women have the impression today that a cesarean surgery is not a serious or risky procedure, and that is partly due to epidural anesthesia.

Epidurals today can be given continuously, making it possible for a woman to have anesthesia from early labor right through delivery. Because epidurals can cause a lowering of the woman's blood pressure and make for problems in her pushing during the second stage of labor, most doctors and nurses try to let it wear off at this stage. However, so prevalent is the use of epidurals, and so widespread is the belief in the United States that epidural anesthesia is the greatest boon to childbirth that in many hospitals an epidural is given as soon as the woman arrives. Women come into hospitals demanding "my epidural." Yet, as you will read in the interview with two obstetric nurses, epidurals have their risks and not all nurses support their use (see pages 261–262).

Many women decide to have epidural anesthesia early in their pregnancy, thinking that an epidural will make it possible for them to avoid the pain of labor. The risks of epidural anesthesia are now well understood, even though the public has not been made aware of them. They fall into three categories: effects on the mother; effects on the baby; and increased need for other interventions in the birth, each of which carries additional risk.

A randomized controlled trial reported in the *American Journal of Obstetrics and Gynecology* in 1993 compared the use of epidural anesthesia (which is now being called "epidural analgesia," presumably because it sounds less serious) to analgesia for pain relief and showed an alarming 1200 percent increase

Active Management

In the 1970s, Kieran O'Driscoll, the chief obstetrician at the National Maternity Hospital in Dublin, Ireland, developed a set of standard practices for his unit that became popular in hospitals across North America. O'Driscoll's two goals: Providing optimum safety for mothers and babies, and guaranteeing women and staff that all births would occur within a specific time limit. His need: An orderly system to deliver babies—"military efficiency with a human face."

The name for the set of policies O'Driscoll instituted is "active management." Similar to the 1970s policy in British hospitals of "9-to-5 obstetrics," the intent is to manage birth so that staff (and laboring women) don't have to wait out long labors. Under active management, birthing women are expected to produce a baby in a given number of hours, that number set by doctors. The underlying assumption of this was—and still is—that both staff and mothers benefit when birth is made to conform to a standard. O'Driscoll also hoped that mothers who could be guaranteed a twelve-hour labor would be willing to forgo pain medication (which is both costly and carries risks to mother and baby).

As a result of his active management policies, O'Driscoll achieved good outcomes in terms of the immediate physical health of the mothers and babies in his unit. Relatively few births required the use of forceps or vacuum extractor, and the cesarean rate was kept to 5 percent (although those figures are rising in the hospital now that women can have epidural anesthesia on demand).

O'Driscoll had correctly observed that many women are admitted to a hospital before they are in active labor and that when a woman is admitted too soon, the chance of medical intervention rises, increasing both cost and risks. His policy: No woman to be admitted until dilated to five centimeters. Once in, she would receive one-to-one attention and care from a staff midwife, who acts like a doula or midwife at a home birth—staying with the woman for each contraction and giving comfort and encouragement.

This use of midwife support in combination with limiting the number of hours a woman would be in labor to twelve (ten for dilating and two for pushing) did not increase hospital costs because there was a lower rate of costly intervention and fewer babies ended up in intensive care.

On the negative side, to guarantee that every woman dilated according to the clock, laboring women's membranes were routinely ruptured. If a woman did not dilate at least one centimeter every two hours, oxytocin IV drips were used (resulting in a 40 percent oxytocin use rate). Studies show that women whose membranes are ruptured find labor hurts more and is more difficult to handle. Women also dislike the frequent vaginal exams to check dilation.

In the United States, "active management" has meant the aggressive use of intervention to keep labor to a schedule but unfortunately *without* the one-to-one attention from a nurse or midwife. This has been routine in most U.S. hospitals for years. It fits neatly into cultural attitudes that view labor as without value and sees the best labor as the shortest with the least pain.

But we must ask ourselves, is the best labor really the shortest or the most painless? What is the real value of labor and birth? Are they not important rites of passage for the woman and the baby? Don't women in early as well as active labor need and deserve the attention of one-to-one care, support, and encouragement? Who should be in charge of managing this important time? □

in cesareans among women who had epidurals early in labor. The risk of cesarean was found to be 50 percent when a woman had an epidural put in at two centimeters, 33 percent at three centimeters, and 26 percent at four centimeters.

For the mother the most common direct complications resulting from epidural anesthesia, other than an increased risk of cesarean, are the lowering of her blood pressure, an increase in her temperature, and the inability to push her baby out. In addition, there are rare but life-threatening complications that include convulsions, breathing paralysis, cardiac problems, allergic shock reaction, nerve injury, and spinal headache.

For the baby there are two direct risks. The first occurs when the mother's blood pressure drops, reducing the amount of blood—and therefore oxygen—to the baby through the placenta. The second is the tendency for the baby's heart rate to change. In one recent study 11 percent of all the babies whose mothers had epidurals showed "profound" and "prolonged" heart rate changes.

Increased intervention that often results from epidurals includes the need to artificially stimulate contractions, because they are now ineffective, placing the baby under greater stress; catheterizing the woman's bladder because it becomes paralyzed and the woman is unable to urinate (a full bladder lies in front of the uterus and can actually prevent delivery); instrumental delivery because the baby gets stuck in a position where it cannot come down the birth canal on its own; and cesarean surgery, which can result from fetal distress or any of the other problems caused by the epidural.

In addition, epidural anesthesia given to the mother results in an indirect but serious complication for some infants. These are babies whose mothers get a fever as a side effect of the epidural. Because infection is a serious threat to a newborn, it is generally hospital policy to put these babies in a high-risk nursery for three days. During this time they undergo painful procedures and are put on strong antibiotics.

I recall visiting one large, well-regarded hospital in Florida in 1980 in which every woman was given an epidural anesthesia as soon as she reached three centimeters—despite the fact that at three centimeters a woman may not be in active labor. Each laboring woman was in bed, hooked to her anesthesia, an IV, and an electronic monitor. In a different part of the hospital was the newborn intensive care nursery, jammed full of isolettes. There were five rows of them and so little room to walk in between that the cords to all the equipment hooked up to each baby went overhead and plugged into a strip on the ceiling alongside the fluorescent lights. Walking through the hospital, I was able to make a clear connection between the numbers of mothers who had epidural anesthesia throughout labor and the number of babies who ended up in intensive care.

MEDICAL FADS

This history of drugs for pain relief in labor is the story of one drug after another becoming popular and then being phased out altogether with no explanation or apology to those women who were subjected to them. The rate at which drugs are phased out once they are proven to be more risky or less effective than was originally believed varies from region to region and hospital to hospital. It is not uncommon for a drug or a form of anesthesia that is considered at one hospital to be too risky to be used—except in very rare circumstances—to continue to be in common use or given routinely at another hospital just across town. They can be directly attributed to what physicians are taught at their particular medical school, and which they tend to continue doing forever.

Some drugs and anesthesia had very brief popularity in the United States, yet they were used on millions of women—and therefore millions of babies—over a period of just a few years. An example of this was an anesthetic known as the paracervical block. A long needle was inserted up into the vagina, and an anesthetic was placed directly into the nerves alongside the cervix and the lower part of the uterus.

Paracervical blocks were very common in some hospitals in the late 1960s and early 1970s, because they did not require putting a needle near the spinal cord and the woman was not totally numbed from the waist down. However, injection at the cervix itself proved to be more dangerous than injection to the spine, because it was not possible to control the amount that went into the local area. As a result, with a paracervical block contractions often slowed or became ineffective, the cervix sometimes swelled and went backward in dilation, and babies sometimes ended up with heavy amounts of anesthesia in their system. Paracervical blocks also caused babies' heart rates to slow down for prolonged periods and could easily get into the baby's bloodstream.

For the actual delivery, inhalation anesthesia was very popular in North America and Britain well into the 1980s, but is no longer popular in most hospitals. It is oxygen combined with an anesthetic gas that a woman breathes through a mask. Women liked it because they could hold the mask in their hand and decide how much they wanted to inhale. Spinal anesthesia—which eliminates all sensation in the pelvic region—never caught on in Britain, whereas an inhalation anesthesia called Trilene was commonly used in Britain even by midwives at home births.

Eastman mentioned the now-well-known fact that any anesthesia given too early or too late in labor can have the nasty side effect of slowing the progress of labor or of obstructing labor altogether. As a result, the mother's contractions are not as effective in moving the baby into the best position for the delivery, and the baby gets stuck in the outlet of the pelvis, as in the case of epidural anesthesia. However, he endorsed a variety of drugs that could be given by mouth, inhalation, or injection during the dilation phase of labor and pronounced them to have "little or no effect" on most babies.

Physicians in Marion's decade of childbearing were as dependent on drugs as were their counterparts in the 1920s. Drugs were—and usually still are—the first choice when a doctor wants to get labor going or give support to a laboring woman. Nicholson Eastman and his 1970 coauthor, obstetrician Keith Russell, who was at one time president of the American College of Obstetricians and Gynecologists, represented most obstetricians when they gave full support to the notion that all women should be able to have drugs for birth. They wrote that women should not only look forward to birth with "equanimity," but with "nonchalance." Nonchalance is a strange choice of word with which to describe one of the most significant experiences of a woman's life.

The physicians and nurses who prescribed and administered all the drugs given to Marion and to countless other birthing women all across the modern world considered what they were doing to be both humane and safe practice. It took many years, numerous studies, and—most important—vocal public protest before medical professionals become more cautious about drugs. Even midwives in countries like Britain, where they staffed maternity units, routinely administered drugs in labor and gave anesthesia at delivery without questioning their safety or real benefits. When it was finally publicized in the mid-1970s in Britain that almost 90 percent of births were being induced as a way of streamlining obstetrics and having all births occur between the standard working hours of nine to five, the outcry was slow to come. Everyone assumed there was nothing wrong with the idea of forcing nature.

Research eventually proved what a few pediatricians and nursery nurses—

and mothers themselves—had been observing for decades: any drug given to a woman in labor and at delivery usually affects the baby. The placenta is not the barrier it was once thought to be; indeed, drugs pass through it as if it were a sieve. Drugs reach the baby in higher dosage and settle in the liver and the brain. It is often weeks or months before all traces of drugs given during birth pass out of a baby's system, because human infants are born physiologically immature and vulnerable to foreign substances in their bodies. One classic series of studies can serve as a reminder to us about the serious problem of drugs and childbirth.

The Lessons of Drugs and Babies

Martin Richards, a scientist in Cambridge, England, conducted several studies during the 1970s and 1980s on the most popular drug then being used to control pain in labor, Demerol/pethidine. Although no other studies have been done that back up Richards's findings, his studies have some basic warnings to give us. He found evidence that babies whose mothers were given just one 50-milligram shot of the drug often showed negative neurological effects for up to several years! At that time, most mothers who received this narcotic were getting not one, but two, three, or more doses. The problem with Demerol/pethidine is the way in which such opiates suppress basic physiological functions crucial to the ability of a baby to breathe on its own and to suckle. These two functions— breathing and suckling—are obviously vital to a baby's survival, and they in turn affect subtle functions related to speech and other behavior, such as how calm or irritable a baby is. Physicians have long been extremely cautious in giving opiates to an adult who has sustained a serious, painful injury whenever there is any possibility of affecting the brain and respiratory system, because the person's breathing may be impaired. We should be at least that cautious with an unborn baby.

Newborn examinations at the time did not show any of these effects. It was too soon in the baby's life for the full spectrum of side effects to have been seen, and the techniques for examining a newborn were not refined enough. Teachers of learning-disabled kids often had a hunch that what they were seeing in those children was in some way related to what happened to them at the time of birth. But no one was listening. There is an intimate relationship between what goes on during pregnancy and childbirth and in how a child develops, but in the United States there is still no long-term follow-up on babies and young children, except for immunizations. Furthermore, the professionals who see the babies at birth are not the same ones who see them at six months or at six years.

Today, newborn exams are much more precise, but they still do not catch the long-term neurological problems associated with drugs and other interventions in birth. In the United States there's the additional problem that mothers and their babies who are not considered at risk or are not in an ICU leave the hospital just one or two days after birth, and all care is suspended. Parents could be taught simple ways of observing their child's development, but we are not yet doing that. We do not even try to see that every baby is breast-fed for at least six months, though we already know the long-term hazardous effects of bottle-feeding: increased incidence of allergies, dental caries, hospital emergency room visits for infections, and chronic conditions such as asthma and heart disease.

Parents do not need to be made any more anxious about the state of their baby's health than modern culture and medicine have already made them. But they do need to be made aware of the implications of the kind of gestation or birth their baby has had. Most of them already sense there is a connection. Parents' instincts and observational skills are quite good, but the medical system does nothing to help parents feel more confident about their own judgment. It's important to understand that when you are the parent of a child with a feeding or sleeping problem, a learning disability, or what's known as attention-deficit disorder, the effects are in no way minimal. Parents have to cope with them on a daily basis, and they know how it increases the normal frustrations of parenting to have a child who is difficult to work with and has a very hard time controlling his or her moods or behavior. Imagine the frustration of being that child and continually getting the message at home and at school that you are difficult or a problem.

We have to take the message about drugs and childbirth seriously. Regarding the use of all drugs, Nicholson Eastman cautiously admitted in his 1970 edition, "None is without its drawbacks . . . none is without some slight risk to the mother or child under certain circumstances." The risk, it turns out, is more than slight for a significant number of mothers and babies, and that risk continues today.

Long-term studies of children show the dramatic increase in all kinds of learning disabilities associated with both complicated delivery and the use of drugs in pregnancy and birth, yet the practice continues of resorting to drugs without first exhausting every other alternative. Drugs should not be used instead of one-to-one human support for a woman in labor. The most effective and safest support for a birthing woman is the continuous presence and reassurance of another person.

It is safest to follow this principle: no drug given to a woman who is carrying a baby inside her can be considered safe for her baby, no matter what the reason for its use. After birth, for women who breast-feed, the same rule should be followed. Whatever the drug, whatever the reason for taking it, we must consider the possible effects on the natural process and on the baby. It is worth investigating any possible alternative before resorting to drugs, including homeopathic remedies or acupuncture, for giving drugs to a birthing woman is always a gamble: you never know in advance which drug will cause problems for which mother or baby, or for how long.

Regarding drugs for pain relief, nothing will change until we stop associating the pain of childbirth with abnormality. Most physicians make the erroneous association between the pain occurring in labor and the pain and suffering from physical injury or disease. Eastman in 1970 linked childbirth to having a cavity drilled in a decayed tooth. "Indeed, you need have no more fear of labor pains than of those of the dentist's chair and should follow a similar policy in dealing with both of these situations."

Regarding other drugs—including fertility drugs and drugs to stop premature labor and force fetal growth—we will continue to use these drugs widely until we begin to examine their long-term effects on babies. Most people do not even believe that what happens to a fetus in the womb or a baby at the time of birth matters very much. We are still focused on very general measurements of physical health. We aren't looking at the subtler, but equally important, aspects of life, such as patterns of behavior, especially under stress, that may be initiated in the pre- and perinatal period and may last for years, or for an entire lifetime. We have, as a culture, only begun to acknowledge the importance of psychological and spiritual development. The field of prenatal and perinatal psychology, which is only a few decades old and has not yet earned the respect of most health workers or scientists, has something to teach all of us. The dangerous and lasting effects of drugs on mothers and babies are just the tip of the iceberg; what makes the issue of drugs so central is the fact that they alter the normal environment of childbearing and affect the relationship between a child and its mother in so many different ways.

Cesarean Birth

In the United States most cesareans are now performed under epidural anesthesia, but in other parts of the world (top photograph shows a cesarean in Mexico), general anesthesia remains the norm.

The woman's abdomen is shaved and scrubbed. Her arm is taped to a board for the IV and blood pressure. With general anesthesia, an endotracheal tube is inserted, then taped onto her cheek. A screen is put up to separate the mother's eyes from the operating team. Numerous metal clamps (hemostats) tie off bleeding blood vessels cut during surgery. A metal retractor holds the incision back to keep the abdominal wall out of the way. Once the baby and placenta have been removed, the uterus is lifted out through the same opening, laid on the mother's abdomen, and sutured.

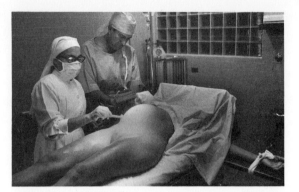

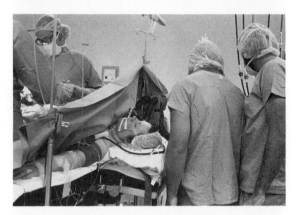

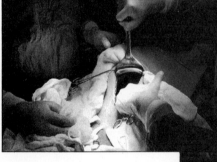

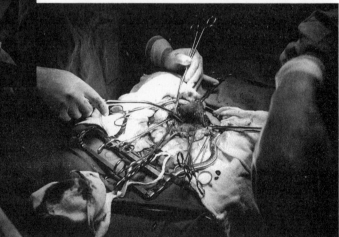

The Cesarean Epidemic

Cesareans—removing a baby through an incision in the mother's abdomen and another in her uterine wall—were uncommon before 1850. That was because there was no known scientific technique for keeping a patient undergoing major surgery such as this from going into shock from the pain. Even if a woman survived the cutting of her body, she was likely to die of blood loss (uncontrollable hemorrhage) or to develop infection in the wound, which would rapidly spread through her bloodstream. Cesareans were resorted to primarily when the mother was expected to die but there was some hope that her baby could be brought out alive. It then required a full-time wet-nurse and a mother substitute to survive.

With the advent of opiate drugs, ether, and chloroform in the mid-1800s one hurdle was removed. However, without any knowledge of how to calibrate the proper dosage of a drug so as not to kill the patient with it, and without a way to handle hemorrhage or infection, physicians were very reluctant to attempt cesareans.

Today the main risks of cesarean for a mother are much smaller than they were fifty years ago. However, the risks are the same as those of any major surgery: unexpected adverse reaction to the anesthesia or other drugs used, uncontrollable hemorrhage (which can happen even today), or infection that does not respond to treatment. There is also the risk of an injury to other organs such as the bladder, which lies right against the uterus. The long-term dangers of cesarean are adhesions in the scar tissue that can cause chronic pain, bowel obstruction, infertility, or miscarriage; and placenta acreta (where the placenta grows into or through the wall of the uterus) in the next pregnancy. The psychological hazards of cesarean are now known to include the mother's having to start motherhood while recovering from major surgery and having to deal with self-esteem and other issues that result from major surgery or missing vaginal birth.

For the baby the primary risks continue to be side effects of the drugs given to the mother, which pass quickly into its bloodstream, and breathing problems, which primarily stem from having missed out on the natural stimulation to the lungs and central nervous system that occurs in the birth canal. If the cesarean is performed before labor has naturally begun, there is the additional risk that the baby will be delivered prematurely. Prematurity carries its own risks because the baby may be born before its body is sufficiently mature.

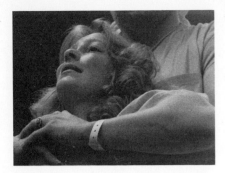

Vaginal Birth After Cesarean (VBAC)

A vaginal birth after cesarean (VBAC) is possible for as many as nine out of ten women, and is often a healing and empowering experience for a woman who felt cesarean was traumatic. The woman above gave birth vaginally to an 8-pound boy after previously having a cesarean birth.

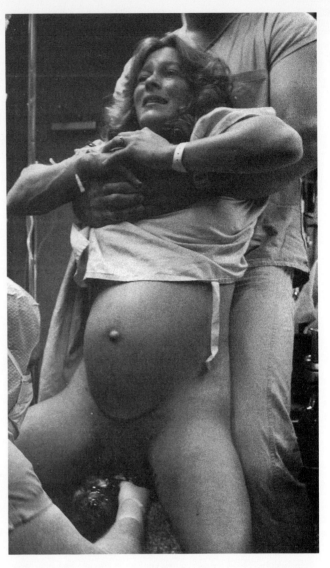

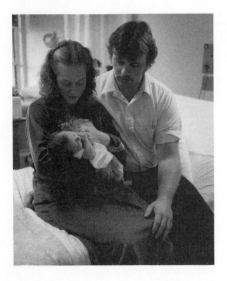

For more information on cesareans, cesarean prevention, and VBAC, contact the International Cesarean Awareness Network (see Resources).

Up until the early 1970s cesarean was considered so risky that hospitals were routinely monitored to make sure they did not have an unduly high rate of cesarean births. The rate considered reasonable was 6 to 10 percent of all births. This changed dramatically when cesarean began to be considered by physicians, and judges and juries, to represent the best possible care. Almost overnight in the United States, as the public began to sue physicians more frequently, the cesarean rate began to skyrocket.

The public soon came to believe that cesarean is a quick, relatively easy, and risk-free solution to any problem that occurs in birth. By 1980 women in the United States were beginning to accept cesarean birth without question. By the mid-1980s a growing percentage of pregnant women could be overheard telling friends they were planning to have a "scheduled" cesarean—one done before the onset of labor—because they wished to avoid the pain of birth. By 1985 U.S. hospitals and obstetricians were freely doing cesareans at rates of 20 percent or more. The cesarean rate in the United States reached an all-time high of 25 percent in 1990. We are usually alarmed when we hear of any disease or problem increasing by 40 or 60 percent. Yet the above statistics mean that in a twenty-year period, cesarean surgery increased in this country by 400 percent with only passing public and professional outcry.

Along with the increased rate of cesareans came the belief that a woman's subsequent birth would also have to be cesarean. Research on the subject was slow in coming, but what it clearly showed is that each subsequent cesarean is more dangerous than the last. By the 1970s obstetricians switched from doing vertical incisions on the uterus to much safer horizontal incisions on the lower part of the uterus. The new cut was called the "bikini incision" (named because most women could hide the scar with a modest bikini). Research from 1960 to 1985 showed that it is safe for a woman to have a vaginal birth after cesarean, with a success rate of 75 percent of hospital VBACs. In fact, it is almost as safe as if she never had a cesarean at all. The term vaginal birth after cesarean (VBAC) was coined and with it a consumer movement to give every woman the chance of a VBAC. Consumer organizations such as the Cesarean Prevention Movement (which recently changed its name to International Cesarean Awareness Network—ICAN) took the lead in raising public awareness and putting pressure on obstetricians to stop performing unnecessary cesareans.

The complication rate due to cesarean can be five to ten times the rate for vaginal birth. Cesarean surgery continues to be two to five times more likely to result in the death of a mother than vaginal birth. Not only is each subsequent cesarean more risky than the last, each subsequent pregnancy is as well.

Cesareans have raised the cost of birth by hundreds of millions of dollars and have subjected millions of babies to the risks of anesthesia and of breathing problems caused by not going through the birth canal. We do not yet know the subtle but long-term effects of depriving a baby of the full process of labor. One of the risks of scheduling cesarean surgery before the onset of labor is that some babies are delivered prematurely and are then placed in intensive care for the problems of prematurity as well. A high proportion of non-premature cesarean-born babies are also sent to the ICU as a precautionary measure, "just to be observed." However, once inside they are usually subjected to the many painful intensive care procedures done routinely "just in case" they turn up a problem. This is only one example of how our culture takes newborn babies who, because of the kind of birth they've had, need the comforting presence of their mothers and time to recover, and instead punishes them by subjecting them to invasive tests and procedures.

WHO IS HAVING CESAREANS?

In most countries, the healthier a woman is when she enters labor, the lower the chance of all kinds of medical intervention, including intensive care for her baby after birth. The opposite, however, is true in the United States. Most of the women who take drugs or have epidural anesthesia in labor and who undergo cesarean surgery in the United States are healthy, well-educated, well-fed middle-class women. These women tend to go to private doctors and private hospitals.

The United States has the highest cesarean rate in the developed world today, as well as the highest percentage of epidural anesthesia. The overall cesarean rate remains at approximately one in every four birthing women, despite the fact that even the American College of Obstetricians and Gynecologists has come out against the overuse of cesarean surgery. Yet there are hospitals where the cesarean rate is less than 15 percent and epidurals are hardly ever done. These are primarily either small rural hospitals that cannot afford a staff of specialists twenty-four hours a day or hospitals that belong to a health maintenance organization (HMO), such as Kaiser of California, which realizes that cesareans and drugs cost too much.

The rate of cesareans among the population of women in the United States who are healthy, middle-class, and having their first baby in their mid- to late thirties or early forties is 50 percent or higher in a number of private hospitals, whereas for low-income women of the same age in public hospitals the rate is commonly 10 to 15 percent. Among the former, the rate of epidural anesthesia for labor runs as high as 75 or 80 percent. Clearly, cesarean birth and epidural anesthesia for labor are a class issue. If we weigh the risks against the benefits of epidural anesthesia and cesarean surgery and compare this to doing everything we can to keep labor normal through noninterventive aids, we find that we all pay a high price for the unnecessary cesarean surgery being done on close to a million women and a million babies each year in the United States.

The cesarean epidemic is the result of a combination of factors, not the least of which are that private obstetricians, who do the most cesareans, get paid more for cesareans than for vaginal births, and because middle- and upper-class women can afford to have cesareans done. But the increased use of this procedure is primarily due to two things. The first is the routine use of the electronic fetal monitor, a device that is attached to a woman and baby in labor and prints out a continual strip showing the baby's heart rate and the mother's contractions. The second is the rising incidence of malpractice suits against hospitals and physicians, which began increasing in the late 1970s.

The Electronic Fetal Monitor

For several hundred years, people have checked a baby's heart rate during labor by placing an ear or a simple wooden or metal stethoscope against the woman's abdomen. In 1968 the first electronic fetal monitor (EFM) was introduced to hospitals. Hewlett-Packard quickly became the world leader in sales, with sales on every continent and in extremely poor countries. Hewlett-Packard estimates that in its first twenty-five years one of its monitors had been used in 45 million births worldwide and 25 million pregnancies. The design was changed so that a smaller version could be sold to doctors for use in their offices. In 1990, 73 percent of labors in the United States were electronically monitored.

The monitor has several parts: an external sensor that, when taped or strapped around a laboring woman's abdomen, gives a readout of the frequency, length, and intensity of contractions; an external auditory ultrasound component; a sensor on the end of a wire that is screwed into the baby's scalp in the uterus and transmits its heart rate; and a machine that displays a continuous reading of the information. In addition, there is an audible beep that sounds the baby's heartbeat throughout the room, and a paper printout, or "tracing."

Many routine procedures are not harmful in themselves, yet they can cause harm because they can alter the attitude of the care providers. The anxiety or impatience of care providers directly alters the course of pregnancy, labor, and postpartum for mother and baby. Therefore, a procedure can be "invasive" even if it doesn't fall into the traditional definition of entering an orifice or going beneath the skin. Obstetrics and newborn care today are full of such procedures. The question always needs to be asked, "Will the information we get from this procedure cause us to do anything different in the care of this woman or baby?" If not, it is useless information. It does nothing but make everyone expect problems, and that is a sure way to create problems.

—FAMILY-PRACTICE PHYSICIAN

Some hospitals are beginning to use new high-tech devices that nurses and physicians can carry in their pockets and record data on (blood pressure, temperature, fetal monitor results). The data are then entered directly into the central hospital computer of patient records, and displayed on banks of EFM screens showing the information from each laboring woman's EFM. These screens, which can be located anywhere in the hospital, even in the doctors' lounge, allow those responsible for a laboring woman to process data and issue orders far from her side.

EFMs, which in the early 1970s cost five or six thousand dollars each, were highly promoted at obstetrical and nursing conferences and marketed aggressively to every hospital in the United States. The marketing premise was—and is—that the electronic monitor is necessary to accurately tell how a baby is doing during labor. Prominent U.S. obstetricians contributed to EFM promotion by doing research on how to interpret the readings and then speaking glowingly about it. Nurses were hired by these same companies to enthusiastically show other nurses and doctors how to use the devices. Many medical conferences were underwritten by monitoring companies. (This is not an unusual practice; infant formula manufacturers have for years been the sponsors of major maternity conferences.) It was a masterful marketing job.

Within a decade virtually every hospital in the United States had been sold several of these expensive machines, and many had one for each labor room. It's astonishing that EFMs had not yet been studied sufficiently to prove whether they were safe or effective.

Because EFMs are mechanical devices, they are subject to malfunction at any time. They require regular maintenance to transmit an accurate reading of heart tones. Even early studies showed that external monitoring (the belt around the woman's abdomen) was inaccurate as much as 40 to 60 percent of the time.

Randomized trials (which are considered the most accurate way to conduct a study) of EFMs have now shown no benefit in fetal outcome, and use of these devices results in a significant increase in instrumental deliveries (forceps and vacuum extraction) and cesarean. The research has now proved that EFMs are not reliable predictors of a baby's well-being at birth. Yet that is what the monitors were designed to do. Another important point to consider is that of those babies who do show signs of distress in the uterus in labor through an EFM, only a few will end up with any long-term physical disability. Most babies recover fully on their own from the physical stress of birth.

A major survey of ten studies that appeared in the *American Journal of Obstetrics and Gynecology* in 1993 failed to show that any particular fetal heart pattern (fast or slow) is predictive of how a baby is doing. Nowhere have EFMs accurately predicted brain damage in babies, even high-risk ones. Despite the use of EFMs there has been no decrease in the incidence of cerebral palsy in full-term infants.

In addition to their unreliability and ineffectiveness, EFMs present other problems. Nurses, already in short supply on hospital obstetrical units, are pulled away from giving direct patient care by having to spend their time going from room to room reading monitor printouts and keeping the machines in order. Women may feel they are getting more attention when there is a monitor in the room, but in fact they are getting less. Hospital administrators have been sold on the idea that EFMs cut down on the nursing staff and can be used in lawsuits to support the hospital's side.

Another problem is that hospital staff tend to focus on the monitor and the limited amount of data it provides, and not on the woman herself. Cesareans have occurred when physicians, who haven't analyzed monitor readings accurately, have become nervous about a slow or fast fetal heart rate and rushed in to do a cesarean before getting a complete picture of what was really going on.

With electronic monitoring devices dominating the labor rooms of U.S. hospitals and cesarean surgery suddenly popular, an alternative birth movement began in reaction in the early 1970s (see pages 151–154). The emphasis on high-tech equipment and medical specialists made birth in hospitals seem very risky. Women who had hospital births usually were not told they had any options. Even today, most birthing women do not know that they can refuse to be electronically monitored and insist that a nurse or midwife listen regularly to the baby's heart rate during labor. They are told during hospital tours that it is hospital policy, and their physicians tell them the same thing. They are never told about any of the possible disadvantages of the fetal monitor.

The results of fetal monitor studies done over the past two decades are now clear: electronic fetal monitoring has no significant value when used on normal, healthy women. It also has no significant value when used on women who are considered "at high risk" for developing problems in birth. Fetal monitoring may save one baby in ten thousand when the machinery is functioning correctly and the monitor printouts of the fetal heart rate are interpreted properly, but in exchange it increases the danger to many mothers and babies, many of whom end up in a cesarean surgery as a result. Electronic monitoring results in more babies being separated from their mothers and put in intensive care nurseries, where they are subjected to routine ICU procedures and tests.

As a result of having the fetal monitor wire screwed into their scalp, babies often develop a bruise or sore at the site, and it is not uncommon for them to develop an infection in the sore, which is treated with antibiotic drugs. Nurses have their time taken up with reading tracings on a piece of paper or a screen instead of looking at and talking with the laboring woman. But perhaps the most hazardous side effect of the electronic monitor is that it takes the control of the birth process away from the birthing mother and sends out the message that expensive machines are essential to deliver babies.

Konrad Hammacher, primary inventor of the Hewlett-Packard monitor, stated in a 1993 company publication that obstetricians shouldn't use the machine to create an alibi for engaging in particular practices, nor allow it to form the focus of care or be the basis of diagnosis. Yet this is precisely what happens the world over. For over two decades the misinterpretation of information from fetal monitors has led physicians to do hundreds of thousands of unnecessary cesarean surgeries. This is common knowledge among physicians; even their medical associations admit to this.

Why, then, do doctors continue to insist that their patients be hooked up to these monitors throughout labor? Because in malpractice cases, judges and juries can be swayed into thinking that the use of continuous electronic monitoring in labor represents the best of care. Meanwhile, hospitals continue to use monitors because they have them.

Ultrasound

Electronic monitoring is only one flagrant example of unnecessary, costly, and risky technology that quickly became a routine part of medical care without careful study. Another is ultrasound. Handheld ultrasound devices have been used for a number of years to listen to the baby's heart during pregnancy or labor, and are a component of the electronic monitor. Some researchers and clinicians have questioned the use of these handheld devices (doptones or ultrasonic fetuscopes), which look harmless enough, and their effects on the ova of female fetuses. (It is important to note that the entire supply of eggs a woman will have during her life is present when the female fetus is in the womb; therefore any concern is a serious one.) It will take several generations of women to see the possible long-term consequences of ultrasound in pregnancy, particularly if it is used in the first three months, when the fetus is forming and at greatest risk.

Many practitioners today use ultrasound machines in the first weeks of pregnancy to view the baby and reassure themselves and their pregnant patients that all is well with the fetus. A randomized trial of fifteen thousand women at low risk for problems in birth, which was conducted at forty-eight different sites in six states in the United States (published in the *New England Journal of Medicine* in 1993, volume 329), reported that there was no significant decrease in fetal deaths as a result of routine ultrasound use for screening in pregnancy. Moreover, at an average cost of $200 per scan (1993 figures), if diagnostic ultrasound is used on the four million women who give birth in the United States each year the total cost is more than a billion dollars! This study did not recommend that ultrasound never be used, only that it be used sparingly, for specific medical indications.

It was awful being at odds with my physician. By the end of the pregnancy I allowed him to do a test that I was opposed to—that I didn't feel was safe for the baby or would give us any information we didn't already have—just because I felt I had to let him do something. It was easier than to do battle.

—PHYSICIAN AND MOTHER

Today, virtually every pregnant woman seeing a private obstetrician in the United States has at least one, and often a number of, ultrasound scans done of her uterus. The newest technique involves going in through the vagina, which many women feel is more physically invasive, but which also results in even less protection for the fetus from anything harmful in ultrasound. Parents-to-be have been led to believe that the scan is necessary to tell whether the placenta is functioning well and the fetus is healthy and growing. Today hospitals and physicians use ultrasound scanning as one way to promote their business. Physicians use scans regularly because they can charge extra for each one and thereby pay for the expensive machine and make a profit.

Physicians claim that their patients are demanding ultrasound to hear the fetal heart amplified, to determine the baby's sex, and to see a picture of the baby. Consumer demand is there, but it has been created by physicians, hospitals, and media who have failed to talk about any possible risks of this new piece of machinery and to question its value. This raises the deeper, philosophical question of whether it serves our interests to take away the mystery of life with machinery.

Intensive Care Baby Units

Today various studies show that between 15 and 25 percent of full-term, healthy babies born to healthy mothers are spending days or weeks in intensive care units (ICUs), known in Europe as "special-care baby units." Why are they there? Mostly as a result of the interventions done on their mothers in labor, which create symptoms in either the mother or the baby that lead health workers to believe the baby might have a medical problem. Many more cesarean-born babies have difficulties after birth than do vaginally delivered babies. Most of their difficulties are associated with breathing, and are caused by the lack of the central nervous system stimulation they would get if they were squeezed and pushed through the mother's birth canal, by drugs and anesthesia given to the mother, or by a combination of these two factors.

Epidural anesthesia, especially when given to a mother for a number of hours in labor, tends to cause a slight rise in the mother's temperature. Because any rise in the mother's temperature can be a sign of infection in the baby, many doctors routinely put these mothers' babies in intensive care, believing they may be suffering from infection picked up in the womb during labor. Infection in newborns is quite serious, so these babies are given aggressive medical treatment, even before results have come back from blood tests to show whether any infection is indeed present.

The "septic workup" done on such newborns is not only quite painful but also risky. First, blood is drawn as often as every few hours, which stresses the newborn's body just reproducing its blood supply. Second, one or more spinal taps are done on the baby. In this procedure, a needle is inserted between two of the baby's vertebrae and into the outer covering of the spinal cord in order to remove some of the fluid that bathes the spinal cord. That fluid is then "cultured" in a lab to see whether it is growing anything dangerous. The practice of doing spinal taps on babies is now so common that parents are led to believe it is nothing more than another blood test. It is, however, a far more painful and risky procedure than a blood test, and most parents are not even told it is being done, much less given a choice.

These kinds of unnecessary and aggressive interventions on healthy newborns have serious ramifications. Not only does placing a baby in an ICU strain the beginning parent-child bond, it also results in fewer mothers choosing to breast-feed and in more of those who do breast-feed having problems and giving up early.

The Drive Toward Physician Specialization

In tribal societies, the needs of the group took precedence over those of the individual; otherwise, the group would not survive. Over eons, the drive toward individualism has led us away from cooperative tribal living. The history of Western civilization is the story of this drive, and technology has been both a cause and a result of specialization.

This drive toward specialization, in combination with a dualistic and mechanistic view of the universe, has had a disastrous effect on childbirth. Today the human body is seen as the sum of many separate parts, with each one having a specialist physician to attend to its needs but no one attending to the whole person.

Modern physics has shown us the fallacy of this way of thinking and approaching life, yet medicine continues to follow the old Newtonian model. Women are cared for by obstetrician-gynecologists, with gynecologists functioning as if they were specialists in women's health care when they are only specialists in the physical aspects of reproduction, focusing on pathology and surgery rather than wellness. In large hospitals, the physician in charge of obstetrics is a subspecialist known as a perinatologist, and newborn babies are the proprietary domain of neonatal pediatricians called neonatologists.

Seeing human beings as a conglomeration of separate parts began during the

Renaissance and became entrenched during the Enlightenment. The scientific method was developed to explain the workings of nature, which was followed by the Industrial Revolution, during which people were seen as serving the needs of machines and factories. Eventually people came to be seen as a kind of machine themselves. This very limited and inaccurate view of ourselves, our world, and our place in it has resulted in massive destruction of the environment in the name of progress and a mechanistic view of the human body that prevails in medicine even today.

Medicine in the Far East has always been based on the holistic principle that the human body/mind cannot be understood by breaking it down into separate parts, and that a person can only be understood within the context of their family and physical-social environment. In Asian or ayurvedic medicine, when a person becomes sick the physician first attempts to find whether the cause lies in the person's diet, personal habits, or relationships. The basic assumption is that all illness results from an imbalance deep within the person. Correct the imbalance, and the body will do its best to heal itself.

Until the eighteenth century, there were two groups of orthodox medical practitioners in Western Europe and North America: physicians, whose tradition came from the gentleman observer-scholar, and surgeons, whose tradition came from barbers and hog gelders, men who were skillful in the use of metal tools. Physicians practiced in people's homes, much as midwives did, bringing their bag of simple tools and drugs (mostly opiates for pain) and working humbly at the patient's bedside. Over the course of the eighteenth and nineteenth centuries, physicians began to practice surgery, and the hog gelder–barber–surgeon disappeared altogether. In the middle of the twentieth century, general practitioners began to be replaced by specialists, who combined medicine and surgery and focused on one part of the patient's body. These, in turn, are being replaced by an ever-growing variety of subspecialists, who base their practice on tests and procedures rather than on patient observation.

But the care of mothers and infants does not lend itself to specialization. Why not? First of all, because birth is a normal, healthy process, not a disorder or disease. Second, because it's impossible to clearly separate a mother and her baby: they are a symbiotic pair, two separate organisms living together as one in a mutually beneficial relationship. Even in terms of basic physiology, it is not easy to say when a mother and baby truly are "separate." Breast-feeding mothers and their babies, for example, have been found to have the same REM patterns, while mothers and babies who are formula-feeding do not.

Even before the birth of a baby, most doctors regard the mother and fetus as separate entities requiring separate attention, and at birth the obstetrician is not allowed to care for the baby any more than the pediatrician may assist the mother in delivery. From the moment of birth, a baby is considered to be a totally separate being that is supposed to tolerate separation from its mother for any reason: weighing, measuring, examination, observation, testing. Yet for weeks after birth a baby remains directly connected to its mother in a symbiotic relationship in which each is dependent upon the other. Modern postindustrialized people are the only ones who believe that a baby should sleep apart from its mother, and that a baby does not need to spend much time in direct physical contact with its mother or other primary caretaker.

Midwives and Doulas in Hospitals

It has been amply documented that midwife care for women during labor and before and after childbirth in hospitals dramatically lowers the incidence of all kinds of intervention in birth and recovery and results in women being more satisfied with their experiences. Even when the population of birthing women in a particular hospital is at much higher risk for developing problems in labor, the presence of midwives dramatically reduces the number of problems that do occur and keeps many babies out of intensive care who would otherwise have been sent there. The rate of drugs and anesthesia in labor in hospitals with midwives has been found to drop to 10 percent or less, and the rate of cesarean surgery has been documented at close to 5 percent, rather than the 25 percent we have come to believe is normal.

Not only that, hospitals using midwives do not have to make any other changes in routine practices before showing these positive results. In countries where midwives are the backbone of the maternity care system, the number of routine medical procedures done in birth and on babies is kept to a minimum. The number of mothers and babies requiring special, intensive medical care is far fewer. And the cost of birth is dramatically lower. There is also much less dependency on doctors, drugs, emergency rooms, and surgery in the years after birth and a greater reliance on self-care and maintaining wellness.

In cases where midwives are not permitted to do much labor support, because of hospital staffing policies, a doula—a female labor companion—can make all the difference between having a normal, uncomplicated birth and one with medical intervention. Many communities are starting their own doula programs, training women to provide continuous emotional and physical—but nonmedical—support before, during, and after childbirth. (For more information on midwives, see pages 156–161; for more information on doulas, see pages 161–163.)

The advantages of both midwives and doulas underscore the importance of a community of women in supporting normal birth. Perhaps more than anything, education and group support are the antidote to the fear of birth. Mothers who have had positive birth experiences are more confident in their own judgment and in their ability to care for their babies. And those who feel they have the support of a group of knowledgeable, experienced women are far less likely to feel isolated and overwhelmed by child care.

The Hallmarks of Hospital Birth

Despite the proven long-term benefits of midwives and the more recent proven benefits of doulas, in the United States we continue to train more specialist physicians, to build larger hospitals and bigger intensive care nurseries, and to buy more equipment rather than invest in more hands-on nursing care. Only since the mid-1970s has consumer pressure on hospitals brought about any changes. Today more and more hospitals are redesigning their maternity units so that a woman can labor, deliver, and recover in the same room and with her family—even children—present. Unfortunately, in most North American hospitals the emphasis continues to be on buying more machinery and paying for more tests rather than hiring more nurses and midwives so that laboring women can have constant care. And the care that is given in hospitals continues to be regimented by changing shifts of nurses and other staff, keeping elaborate hospital records to prevent lawsuits, managing birth according to the clock, and fragmenting care so that many people are involved in any one birth, but no one person is responsible to the birthing woman.

The "team" approach at hospitals is valuable in many acute-care settings. In childbirth, however, it is usually a disadvantage in the care of a mother and baby, who need quiet and privacy to bond and breast-feed. The team approach involves a dozen or more people attending a birthing woman in the course of a twenty-four- to forty-eight-hour hospital stay. Most of these people are strangers who do not know anything about the woman before she entered the hospital. They include an admitting nurse, an initial-labor nurse, a change-of-shift nurse, often an extra nurse during delivery, various postpartum nurses, a dietician, and the nursery staff. This is not even counting the physician, who may be someone the birthing woman has never met, or additional medical students or residents if the birth is in a teaching hospital.

"AVERAGE" IS NOT "NORMAL"

One hallmark of hospital birth is the supposition that every woman's labor must conform to a standard. That standard is not based on the idea of normal birth, but on a mathematical average. What is considered a "normal" first labor in the United States, for example, is very different from what is considered "normal" in the Netherlands or Denmark. As a result, any variation from the *average* birth experience is considered to be a complication.

Many hospitals in North America still follow a standard set up in the late 1970s called the Friedman curve, despite the fact that it has proven to be unreliable. It is named for Dr. Emmanuel Friedman, the obstetrician who developed it. According to the Friedman standard, every woman should be expected to dilate one centimeter during each hour of labor. Studies show that the Friedman standard fits less than half of all women in labor. It is normal for many women to reach a certain point in dilation and plateau for a period of time. Even Dr. Friedman is distressed that his curve has become doctrine. Consider the wisdom of holding a woman to a standard that does not take into account her body structure, her state of mind, her genetic inheritance, her mother's birth history, the position of her body during labor, what she has eaten during the past twenty-four hours, her stress level, or the kind of emotional support she has.

Modern obstetrics, and more recently modern neonatal care, is run by the standards of big business: control and management. But normal childbirth encompasses a wide range of variations in the length and pace of labor. The principles of control and management don't give women and the process of labor a chance. At the first sign of any variation from the norm, intervention is used. And, unfortunately, one intervention tends to lead to another.

For one woman, a normal labor can be three hours from start to finish; for another, it may be three days of uncomfortable contractions before true labor sets in and another ten hours before her baby is born. Yet both babies are likely to be healthy. A third woman can hover at three centimeters for a day, then suddenly dilate to ten in a matter of minutes, have no urge to push for twenty minutes, then push out a baby in half an hour. Although a first birth is most often the

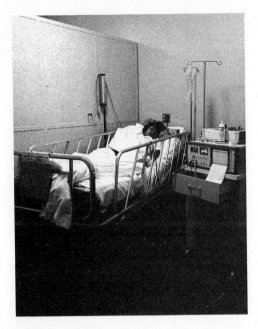

Hospital Birth in the 1970s

These pictures show some of the disturbing routine practices I observed in hospitals across the United States while I researched the original *Immaculate Deception* in the early 1970s. Most went unquestioned well into the 1980s; some continue today in many hospitals.

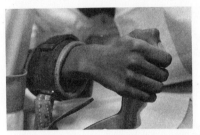

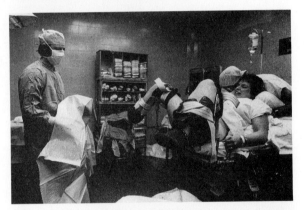

Above: This laboring woman is confined—the bed rails are up, the needle in her hand hooks her to an IV solution, and a belt wraps tightly around her abdomen.

Top right: Women who were awake presented a problem, as they might reach down and contaminate the doctor's "sterile field," so some women were handcuffed to the delivery table.

Middle right: The standard position for women who insisted on "natural childbirth" was supine, legs stretched wide apart in stirrups, allowing the physician easy approach for an episiotomy.

Below right: If a woman insisted on no episiotomy, the physician expected her to tear, a common result of this position.

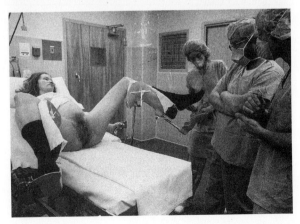

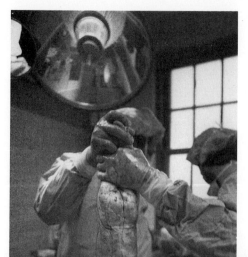

Many newborns, held by the heels, were hung upside down, even into the early 1970s. After being curled in the womb for nine months the spine was suddenly pulled straight by the head's weight. All babies were put on a warming table as soon as the cord was cut. Any resuscitation efforts would be done here. When deemed warm enough, a baby was weighed, measured, footprinted, and wrist-tagged. Here (below right), mother and baby are left alone for a few minutes in the delivery room, but on opposite sides of the room. The few women who succeeded in giving birth without medication or an episiotomy were still subjected to routine separation from their babies (for four to twelve hours) as the babies were "observed" in the nursery.

hardest, that isn't always true. So much depends on the size of the baby, how it is lying in the uterus, how well its head is applied to the cervix, whether its face is toward the front or the rear of the woman's body, the woman's body type, and what the woman is doing and how she is feeling.

A very short labor is not necessarily one that is either normal or easy on the mother or baby, and a long labor is not necessarily either complicated or traumatic. Besides that, what is traumatic for one person might not be so for another. And each mother and baby, although connected and affected by each other throughout pregnancy and birth, can experience pregnancy and delivery very differently. The range of normalcy in labor is wide enough to include one or more unusual factors. When labor is not going well, and the problem does not correct itself, it is necessary to try a series of procedures to see what will work. It is always safest to try doing the most good with the least intervention. Without taking part in a wide variety of normal births in which intervention was not used, it is difficult to trust in the inherent normalcy of the birth process. That is why, for decades, nurses and physicians have applied one intervention after another without considering them to be interventions. Thus they will routinely write in a chart that labor was "unremarkable," or "normal," to indicate that it did not include any major medical complication. It is also why, with aggressive management of labor, physicians and nurses view every birth as a potential complication and treat every mother and baby as potentially at risk. And this is why women today are labeled "high-risk" or "low-risk," but never "normal."

THE DECEPTION OF
THE HOSPITAL ENVIRONMENT

Despite the results of studies showing the greater value in putting more money into staff, not equipment, hospital administrators still prefer to pay for expensive electronic monitoring equipment or to buy expensive "borning beds" rather than to assign one nurse to each laboring woman. There will always be a limited amount of money to spend on medical care, and whenever the priority is placed on equipment, there is that much less to spend on human beings. Furthermore, when equipment is available, it is used even when it is not needed, simply because it is there. Private hospitals are for the most part no more receptive to the individual voices of the people they serve or the staff who provides the majority of care than public hospitals, HMO hospitals, or military hospitals, who tend to only make changes that reduce their costs.

Today, most hospitals have begun to make some changes in the physical environment of maternity wards to make it more inviting. But making substantial changes, such as providing one nurse or midwife for each laboring woman and using high-tech equipment only when it is clearly indicated, is not a priority.

Many hospitals in the United States have recently purchased birthing beds that can be moved into various positions and permit a woman to sit or half-squat for delivery. Some have bars across the foot of the bed to help women get into a squatting position. These beds also convert, at the push of a button, into a traditional delivery table complete with stirrups. These new beds cost thousands of dollars. It needn't cost this much, however, to fully equip a birthing room. A low padded platform big enough for the birthing woman and her partner, perhaps a low chair her partner can sit in while supporting the birthing woman in a squatting position, an inexpensive U-shaped birthing stool, plus a light switch to darken the room for privacy are all that is needed. Birthing women would also benefit from having a shower or a tub that can be filled with warm water, large enough for the woman to completely immerse herself in, as this helps her to relax. Many women find being immersed in warm water toward the end of labor makes them more comfortable, and studies have shown that it prevents edema, or swelling. Environments that are conducive to privacy, informality, making noise, and freedom of movement result in more normal births.

HOSPITALS: BIG VERSUS SMALL

In comparison to the several hundred small birth centers currently operating in the United States, in which birthing women are guaranteed a large measure of privacy and support, there are many hospitals where six thousand births or more occur every year. When ten or twenty women are in labor at the same time, there is little privacy and little individualized care, but a great number of routine procedures are done in order to keep the system working smoothly. The policies and practices of large hospitals are designed for efficiency, not for normalcy or to meet the needs of the individual birthing woman, her baby, and her family.

The trend toward building larger and larger hospitals and closing small hospitals across the United States and Canada was a part of a national public health policy to consolidate medical facilities, technology, and specialists in big hospitals in order to give better care for less money. It may have worked in areas of medicine such as organ transplants, but it has not served childbirth at all. Bringing large numbers of birthing women together into big maternity units has not resulted in making birth safer or in making it more satisfying for mothers and babies. It has increased the number of routine procedures, the incidence of surgery, the use of intensive care, and therefore the cost.

Who Cares About Normal Birth?

For the most part, hospital nurses and physicians in the United States continue to view natural childbirth as a foolish and impossible goal for most women. They endorse the idea of childbirth classes, but see Lamaze and other childbirth-preparation programs as a way to make women feel better about standard hospital routine and accept whatever is done to them and their babies. Many nurses and physicians can be hostile to women who write up a "birth plan" and want it attached to their hospital chart. A birth plan is a list of the important features the parents want protected, such as having the baby remain with them after birth. The plan also lists what parents want to avoid if at all possible, such as having an IV, electronic monitor, or episiotomy, being separated from their baby, or giving the baby sugar water or eye drops. Pregnant women and their partners learn about their rights and options, and how to write a birth plan, from reading various books and articles or in birth preparation classes. People who bring birth plans to the hospital make most nurses and physicians uncomfortable. Yet it is normal for mothers of any species to be aggressive in the face of any possible threat to themselves during labor or to their newborn babies. Such actions are the mark of a responsible parent, not a difficult patient.

Few nurses or obstetricians in North America have ever witnessed a woman conducting her own labor and giving birth on her own two feet. Today, a nurse's time is increasingly taken up with handling and maintaining equipment and recording data in charts. It's no wonder that so few obstetrical or neonatal nurses are excited today about the work they do; they've been turned into technicians.

Obstetricians, at least in the United States, have to pay more and more money for the privilege of being insured against malpractice suits. They find themselves increasingly restricted by unreasonable hospital policies, and often view every pregnant patient as a potential adversary in a lawsuit. More and more obstetricians, in fact, are giving up attending births altogether. The system is now set up to make normal birth as unlikely as possible, and no one, neither mother nor medical staff, finds birth a positive, life-affirming experience.

The good news is that cost containment is likely to eventually lead hospitals back toward normal birth and the use of midwives, because in the long run it will be necessary to cut costs for hospitals to survive. Midwifery care results in less intervention and fewer malpractice suits. Midwifery training costs less than physician training, so eventually we will probably see midwives as the standard attendants at births in North America. Hiring midwives in hospitals will also solve the problem of who will care for low-income women.

The root of the problem with childbirth in the United States, however, remains the modern hospital itself. Women who go to a hospital to give birth simply do not retain control of their bodies once they are there. They often have to fight the system and the medical staff and stay vigilant every step of the way, or the birth and care of their baby is taken from them. Parents need to know that legally they do not have control over the decisions made regarding what is done to their baby once the baby is out of the mother's body and out of her arms. And there is an increasing tendency to view even the baby in the womb as the property of the hospital and its health workers. Studies show that the larger the hospital and the more births at that hospital per year, the greater the risk of unnecessary intervention and the greater the risks to the mother and the baby. In fact, a Cambridge University study done in England in the early 1980s revealed that the most important factor determining whether a baby ends up in an ICU unit is how many feet from the ICU the mother is when giving birth.

Placing midwives in charge of all hospital birthing units, including high-risk or intensive care, and having a midwife present at every birth, even when an obstetrician or neonatal physician is required, would make a dramatic difference in hospital childbirth.

Today midwives have organized, they know their own worth, they are setting standards to bring normalcy back to childbirth, they are fighting for hospital privileges and medical backup, and they are eager for their chance to change the face of maternity care. Their numbers are increasing every year, and more and more women are requesting their services. The rising costs of birth created by specialist physicians, high-tech medicine, and hospital stays will eventually work in favor of midwives and greatly increase a woman's chances of having a normal birth in a hospital. Within the decade we may see a nationwide effort to move childbirth out of large hospitals and into small community hospitals, birth centers, and women's homes, with midwives at the heart of the system and physicians providing special expertise for rare but serious complications.

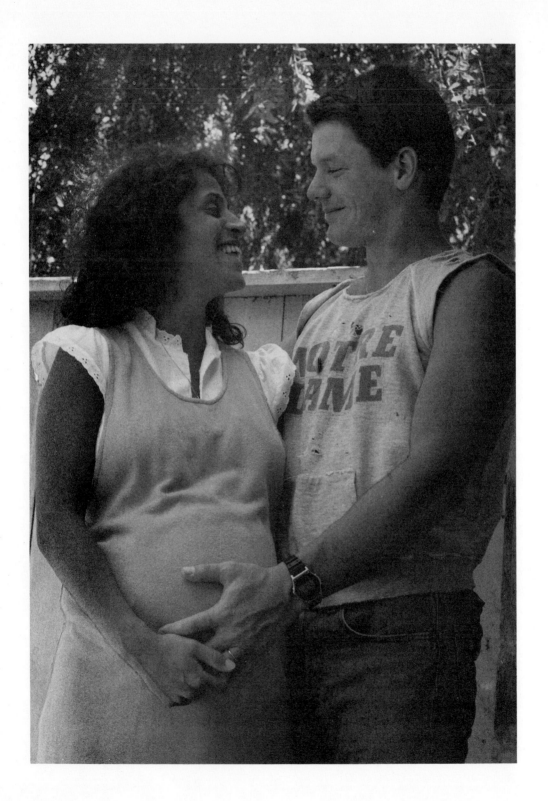

CHAPTER FOUR

Easing the Fear of Childbirth

I N THE VAST MAJORITY of U.S. hospitals epidural anesthesia is used routinely in labor. Women demand it. Fifty percent of American mothers do not breast-feed at all or quit within the first six weeks. Professional women don't want to be "tied down" to a breast-feeding infant. It's fashionable to believe that neither mothers nor fathers are needed to provide most of the baby's care, and society does not support parents and babies being together.

Today, when the needs of babies come in conflict with the needs and desires of their parents, people say "babies are flexible," and "babies learn best when they are in day care." Babies are expected to yield, or at least meet their parents halfway. Our culture supports all of this by making it difficult for women and men to stay at home when their babies are young, and by making it virtually impossible for any parent—male or female—to bring a baby to the workplace. Who suffers from all of this? We do—so do our children and so does society.

How is it that we humans are so susceptible to fashion and fads when it comes to something as fundamental as the way we give birth, and the way we care for our young? The answer lies in the nature of fear and how fear shapes our lives.

Fear in Birth

A doe moving through the forest suddenly catches an unfamiliar scent as the wind shifts in her direction. She stops and stands as still as a statue. To an observer she seems frozen, but inside her body she is anything but still. Within milliseconds of her sense of smell being aroused, her brain has received a message, translated it, and sent it out to all parts of her body: Be on guard! In the blink of an eye her entire body has become organized for flight or fight from the effects of the adrenaline and other hormones now flooding her body, causing her breath to come quickly and her heart to pump fast.

She does not break into a run yet. She stands still a few seconds longer as her primitive brain runs a rapid check on this scent she has smelled to see if there is any record of a similar scent having meant danger in the past. It comes up with nothing; there is no past danger with which to associate this present scent. It is merely unfamiliar. The doe looks cautiously around her, still poised for flight, should it prove necessary. Slowly and gracefully she begins to move through the trees, still alert, her body no longer tensed for action.

In those few last seconds her brain has initiated the release of other powerful hormones to counteract the effects of the first. These rebalance her system so that her body uses no more energy than necessary in a state of alert.

For humans, fear is equally compelling and equally vital to our survival. Its function is to alert an organism to the possibility of danger—especially imminent danger—and initiates preparation for self-defense. In humans, like most other animals, the body has two instinctual ways of responding to a threat: fight or flight. In humans, fear produces strong, urgent, and painful emotions along with the powerful physical reactions that are triggered. Although today we have no natural predators to fear, we still have an innate fear of death and a strong tendency to fear the unknown. We have all felt many forms of fear in our lives: from concern, worry, or anxiety on the mild end of the spectrum, to dread, panic, or even terror on the other end. Fear is both mental and physical agitation in the presence, or anticipation, of danger.

In terms of childbirth, we humans have always had some things to fear. In the course of history, however, our fears regarding this normal human process have greatly increased. Many of them are based on the high rate of death caused by childbirth during periods of history when women lived physically limited and unhealthy lives that affected their ability to give birth. Yet knowing this does not necessarily alleviate our fear of childbirth. So it is worth taking a good look at fear itself, how it affects us physically and mentally, and what kinds of things are likely to trigger it. Then we can discover how to deal with it more effectively.

One immediate problem is that fear can be mild enough that we do not even identify it as fear. Some people live for years in a state of chronic fear, called anxiety, without ever knowing it. Their bodies are constantly being bathed internally with adrenaline-like hormones, so that true relaxation, normal digestion and elimination, and deep sleep are not possible. Outwardly, these people might look as if they are functioning normally, but they are not; their higher brain is simply blocking awareness of the fear and they are living in a state of denial and psychological numbness.

People who live in a state of chronic fear live in a state of constant tension. They spend much of their energy trying to gain a sense of control over their environment. Fear often disguises itself as a need to control everything within and around us. In a culture such as ours that values control so highly, we forget that it is likely to be fear, not pleasure or love, that drives us. The more we strive for control, the less at ease we are in our lives and also in childbirth.

Birthing women and their partners, as well as medical professionals, are in the grip of fear but usually don't know it. What it translates into is a constant mental state of "What if?" "What if?" childbirth practices create a mindset that views everything and everyone as at risk—either high-risk or low-risk, but never healthy or normal. What plagues childbirth today is a constant free-floating anxiety that is not attached to any particular event or situation, but that becomes fixated on first one thing and then another and is never resolved.

Fear has always been women's Achilles' heel when it comes to childbirth, the place where they are most vulnerable. Childbearing women are particularly subject to fear because they have an innate sense of the responsibility they bear for the life they carry. Most women would sacrifice themselves if it meant the survival of their child, and most will agree to any procedure or test if they are told it will result in better chances for the baby. This natural vulnerability to fear makes a birthing woman easy prey for anyone who, consciously or unconsciously, tries to control her through fear. That is precisely what happens in childbirth all too often, and it happens very easily because our doctors and nurses are filled with fear regarding birth, partly from the way they were trained and partly from their hospital experiences. As a result, they are hypervigilant for any sign of something going wrong, and their medical procedures are governed by the constant expectation of danger.

This kind of fear, and the view of childbirth as a disaster waiting to happen, is catching. Here's an all-too-typical scenario. A woman is told when she enters a maternity unit that she has to have an electronic fetal monitor, that it is part of hospital policy for every birth. She usually gives in, either because she has confused the words "hospital policy" with the idea that it is some law she cannot break, or because she likes the idea of having her baby's heart rate continuously monitored since it makes her think the baby will be safer, or because she doesn't want to make a fuss. A nurse periodically comes in to read the printout and record it on her chart, or she simply watches a screen at the nursing station.

Usually at some point in labor, the monitor shows some slowing down or speeding up of the baby's heart rate during contractions. Studies have shown that it is common and normal for a baby's heart rate to have variations in the course of labor, and during pregnancy as well. Research also has shown that electronic monitors, like all machinery, often malfunction and give inaccurate readouts. Nevertheless, a nurse reads the monitor tracing and grows anxious. "What if?" immediately comes to her mind. She consults the doctor and a procedure is usually suggested and a warning is given to the woman. "If this doesn't improve in the next few contractions, we're going to need to . . ." Perhaps the nurse first tries to get the woman to change position. This can be difficult, as usually the woman is in bed, and often she is hooked to an intravenous drip and also has a catheter in her spine with anesthesia flowing through it. If changing the mother's position doesn't immediately change the heart rate of the baby, the nurse will usually talk to a doctor about what to do next.

A physician—perhaps the woman's own doctor, but sometimes someone else who happens to be on the floor, perhaps a resident in training—comes into the room. The woman and her partner are told what the procedure is that the hospital staff want to do. Often today it's cesarean surgery, because doctors and nurses have been trained to be so afraid of something going wrong and of being blamed in a malpractice suit that they do not feel secure in spending any time watching to see if the problem will correct itself or in trying some less-invasive technique before turning to major intervention.

Let's assume the woman is told she needs a cesarean to make sure the baby will be all right, since that is what happens most often today when there is thought to be any possibility that a baby might be in distress. If she hesitates at all, what happens next is one of two things, depending on whether the particular doctor prides himself or herself on being progressive or not. The couple may be told in graphic terms all the terrible things that could result from a slow or fast fetal heart rate and how quickly things can get worse if they wait. Or, the partner is taken outside the room. The doctor places an arm around the partner's shoulder and, in a conspiratorial tone, explains how serious the situation is. "We don't want anything bad to happen to the mother or the baby, do we?" Thus fear spreads as easily as an infection from health worker to parent.

THE PHYSICAL NATURE OF FEAR

Even mild fear can be compelling enough to obliterate all other physical sensations but those associated with the fear: a tightening deep in the gut; shallow breathing or a stoppage of breath; constriction in the throat; tension in the muscles of the face, hands, arms, buttocks, and legs that causes blood to drain from the digestive system and flood the large muscle groups that would be used in fight or flight. In the grip of strong fear, we become pale as the blood drains from our face, and our stomach literally feels hollow.

Fear is such a powerful reaction that it can be triggered by the merest hint of surprise, if the primitive brain believes that surprise might mean danger. This is especially true if what surprises us bears some similarity to the memory trace of an early experience stored deep within the brain, and if that earlier experience once posed a possible threat to our survival. It is important to remember that the primitive brain—the brain stem and lower regions, which developed long before the neocortex—treats similar situations as if they are the same. Any thing or event that resembles something that caused us to panic in the distant past, especially when we were very young and very vulnerable, is likely to produce the same reaction of fear. That is just the way our nervous system and brain are organized, in order to sense situations in which we need to protect ourselves. The most recently developed part of the brain, located near the top of the forehead, allows rational thinking. Our higher intellect, however, is not always able to override our more primitive reactions. But it has serious implications for childbirth today.

Some of us may have had traumatic births or other early experiences that were traumatic. We can be easily frightened by anything that seems to threaten us or our baby just because it is reminiscent of an earlier fearful or traumatic situation. Health workers too have had traumatic events occur to them early in life. They too are likely to have free-floating anxiety about birth, even more so because they have seen many problematic births, and because they are expected to be able to correct all problems connected with birth. Few of the doctors and nurses we count on to help us are able to make decisions based simply on good judgment rather than "What if?" fears.

THE MENTAL ASPECT OF FEAR

Think of a time when you stepped off a stair or a curb, expecting your foot to touch down on something solid, but found only air. This can happen when the height of the stair or curb is only an inch more than your body expected it to be. Suddenly your breath caught, your arms shot out to protect you from falling, your leg jerked as the muscles tightened. All this happened within the milliseconds it took for your foot to come to rest on something solid. Then, again within seconds, your body had to completely reorganize itself to adjust to the fact that the danger had passed.

Fear can be triggered by a mere thought. In fact, fear *arises* as a mere thought. Therefore, we know that the brain is the key to fear. The most effective way to stop our body from reacting fearfully is to prove to it that there is no basis for fear at that moment and then to calm the ancient brain that governs our autonomic nervous system. This primitive brain is our protector, and it must be reassured that all is well.

WHEN FEAR CAN BE OUR ALLY

In general, we need not fear childbirth today; we have the means to solve almost any of the rare serious problems that can occur.

All too often physicians fail to understand what women really need when they express the fear of giving birth. Because women today doubt their natural capacity to have a normal birth and a healthy baby, what they need most is reassurance—not reassurance that everything can be done will be done for her and the baby, but reassurance that her body and her baby know what to do during a process that nature has designed for success.

Still, fear does have its place. As one physician aptly puts it, "I don't think women are as ignorant of their bodies as we doctors make them out to be. They can, however, be scared out of perceiving what's going on inside. But I don't know of one instance in my practice where the need to do something wasn't clear to the woman long before it became clear to me."

When a woman who otherwise has trust in the birth process suddenly has a strong sense that something is wrong, at any time during pregnancy, labor, or afterward, she should be taken seriously. There are too many instances in which health workers magnify unwarranted fears but fail to listen to a woman when she is convinced something is wrong.

FEAR OR TRUST?

For centuries women have given birth in all manner of circumstances from deprivation to danger, and survived. It has only been in relatively recent history that birth has been made dangerous because of cultural conditions and conditioning, and only in the past century that women have been routinely drugged or anesthetized when giving birth. That has been long enough for us to pass along the belief that every birth requires hospitalization, obstetricians, drugs or surgery, and all sorts of other procedures when in fact, for healthy women, only one birth in ten requires special caution. Among that 10 percent of women and babies, the vast majority needs only a little help at some point in the process of gestation, birth, or afterward.

Many traditional societies understood that labor itself produces an altered state of consciousness. This altered state is created by the endocrine system. Certain hormones released into the bloodstream not only raise a woman's pain threshold and therefore naturally dull the perception of pain during contractions, they also make it possible for virtually any woman to birth her baby unassisted if she has to, even when she is alone and would otherwise be afraid. There are millions of examples of women giving birth successfully without any assistance at all, even in bomb shelters during war, and during natural disasters.

This natural altered state of consciousness produces a feeling of trust and acceptance during labor and a sense of euphoria with the appearance of the baby. From that state of consciousness the body shifts into another altered state, one of calm and well-being, once the baby is suckling at the breast. This is a state that occurs each time a woman breast-feeds and that helps her focus on the baby and shut out all distraction. Of course there are things that can inhibit these altered states of consciousness. Pain is one. For example, if the baby is not suckling well because it is not properly on the breast, this can be painful to the mother, and the sensation of pain can override the sense of pleasure breast-feeding normally produces. A feeling of disgust or anger can inhibit a sense of well-being, and so can fear. Nevertheless, the body is designed for pleasure as well as pain, and it is designed so that a birthing woman can sense when all is well, as this furthers survival.

Fear is an intrinsic part of human existence and is vital to our survival, catalyzing us into action in our own defense. But the kind of fear that is unhelpful and that inhibits the birth process is the kind that so many childbearing women and health workers today possess: the ever-present expectation of something going wrong. *There must be a dynamic balance between trust and fear if we are to live with an appropriate sense of awe and reverence for those forces beyond our control.* Without fear, there can be no appropriate sense of caution, and without trust we are always imagining the worst. It doesn't take a lot of fear to produce caution; it's trust that we need more of. Too much focusing on possible problems actually creates problems physiologically by triggering a whole series of reactions within the body to the state of anxiety.

No one should ever be belittled or patronized for fearing childbirth. Every person's fears are real and legitimate and therefore deserve compassion. We come by our fears honestly, even though they are often unfounded. The fears of many women today are based on what their mothers experienced in childbearing and in caring for a baby. We hear of horrible labors, in which a woman who was totally ignorant about the process going on inside her was left alone for much of her labor, was frightened by the pain, and had no emotional support. Many of us had traumatic births and we carry this primal fear without having any conscious memory or awareness of it. These personal experiences with fear only add to a cultural legacy of fear.

In a healthy woman there is little to fear and much to trust in birth, especially now that modern society has adequate—and sometimes superb—first-aid care, emergency transport to hospitals, and specialized hospital care. Yet most womens' fears today center around the mistaken belief that they cannot successfully give birth to a healthy baby without outside intervention and the aid of a hospital and a specialist physician-surgeon. Most doctors' fears have to do with the birth process somehow being faulty and with women not being capable of taking responsibility for their pregnancy and labor.

Physicians and nurses tend to fear the kinds of situations in which they have felt helpless in the past, and this differs from person to person. One doctor might fear premature rupture of membranes, because he or she has encountered several situations of an umbilical cord prolapsing and the baby dying. Another might fear hemorrhage, because that is where he or she has encountered the most problems. It helps for birthing women to know that their care providers are only human and capable of irrational but understandable fears.

Dealing with Fear

The danger of focusing on any fear is that by doing so we perpetuate it and increase its strength. A Buddhist saying can teach us how to deal with fear that has no basis in present reality:

Be hospitable to an unwelcome emotion, as if it were an unexpected guest. Offer it a cup of tea. Greet it kindly and see if you can learn something from the message it brings. If it does not bring you something useful, say "thank you" and send it on its way. Above all, do not invite it to share your supper and offer it a bed in your house for the night, or you will have a difficult time getting it to leave.

Fear can show up at our door at any time. It may sometimes bring a gift. We can learn something from any emotion, including fear. Resisting an unwelcome emotion only makes it bigger, and it then takes up a lot of attention and energy. But we shouldn't make too big a fuss over it, either, for it might take up permanent residence inside us!

Unfortunately, much of what passes for childbirth education and preparation today actually increases women's fears by giving them too much concrete information to hang their anxiety on, and too many names for all the bad things they already fear will happen. In the course of trying to calm the higher brain by giving it lots of data, we can end up defeating our purpose by feeding our fears. It's a tricky business, a little like telling a child who wakes in the night with a nightmare about a boogeyman that there is no such thing as a boogeyman, then going on to name all the things he *should* be afraid of.

USING OUR MINDS TO CREATE INNER BALANCE

The best antidote—and prevention for that matter—for unwarranted fear is to place a little space between ourself and the fear. It helps to realize that we are not synonymous with fear; it is simply an emotion that arises within us and can be let go of. One antidote to unreasonable fear is to become an observer of it, to see how it is affecting our body and mind. Another is to do something that puts us into a state of peacefulness by shifting our attention to a mental or physical activity that is pleasurable, like taking a long walk to some place beautiful or taking a journey in our mind to some place we love.

Learning how not to be afraid, especially when we've spent a lifetime becoming quite good at it, takes practice, just as learning to be good at anything does. It's important, when learning this skill, to be kind to ourselves and not judge ourselves for having fear. We need to be as gentle with our minds as we would be with a new kitten or puppy. If, when practicing the technique of shifting our attention to something pleasurable, our thoughts wander back to whatever makes us anxious and we find ourselves swept away by obsessive thoughts, we just turn our minds back to what we want to focus on, as if it were an impish pet.

The paradox is that it doesn't work to pretend fear isn't there when it is. Denying fears, like dwelling on them, can cause them to become pervasive and exaggerated. Whatever we try to push away takes a lot of effort. It's easier to allow it to be there and then direct our attention toward something better.

Many a birthing woman has found it especially helpful to remember that she is connected to all women who have birthed successfully before her. These are her ancestors and they live in her. Others have found it helps to remember they are connected to all living things and to the earth itself.

It is a subtle process, learning to create a sense of inner calm and spaciousness. But with it comes a sense of well-being. Perhaps the very easiest way to do this is to think of anchoring yourself to the most stable yet fluid part of you, your breath.

RECONNECTING WITH OUR
NATURAL ANCHOR: THE BREATH

Our breath is always there, one thing we never have to force. Most forms of relaxation, contemplation, or meditation are based on learning how to breathe the way a child does, naturally and fully. Rediscovering our natural way of breathing in and out, which is a matter of allowing it to happen, is central to finding an inner sense of balance and calm. The simple act of shifting your attention to observing your breath as it is—shallow or deep, rapid or slow—and allowing it to go on just that way works wonders.

The best analogy I know for what happens when we turn our full attention to our breathing, without trying to change it in any way, was given by the Vietnamese Buddhist monk Thich Nhat Hahn. He tells a wonderful story about a little girl he served a glass of apple juice to who refused to drink it because it was unfiltered and did not look "clean." A few minutes later he offered the same glass of juice to her and she took it and drank it. He then told her it was the same juice. "How could that be?" she asked. He explained that in the process of sitting the sediment had fallen to the bottom of the glass, leaving the clear juice on top. In the same way, by simply allowing ourselves to sit, while giving quiet attention to our breath, we find that our emotions settle and our minds are clearer. This same technique works as well to calm our fears before going into labor as it does in the midst of a contraction during active labor.

THE POWER OF MENTAL IMAGERY
AND VISUALIZATION

A number of years ago, a series of landmark studies were undertaken in several European countries of athletes preparing for the Olympic games. The purpose was to examine the value of combining mental, or psychic, training with physical training. The athletes were divided into different groups. One group went through only physical training, which was the standard approach at the time. Another spent half of the training time physically going through their paces and the other half doing a form of visualization. One of the most interesting studies was done on weight lifters. The form of mental training used was to have the athlete close his or her eyes and form a vivid image of lifting a weight of a particular size. The weight was one size heavier than the athlete had ever successfully lifted. The study showed—and this was later replicated with tennis pros, golfers, and others, including nonathletes—that the athletes who scored highest in subsequent trials were those who did the least amount of physical training and the greatest proportion of visualization.

The kind of visualization used in this study employed as many of the senses as possible. So the weight lifters had to literally feel, smell, taste, and hear themselves lifting the weight, sensing the pressure of the metal against their hands, and so forth. This study led to further research on the nature of the brain, which showed that when visualization calls up specific physical sensations, the physiological changes in the body are the same as if the body had actually been through the physical experience. The athletes who did the least physical training might have done the best in competition because of the fact that muscles can get overly

> *You can have book knowledge, and that's important, but when it comes to your baby and what you do, it gets down to your body and your baby. You must consider your own rhythms and what you want and how you can work it out.*
>
> —OBSTETRIC NURSE AND MOTHER

fatigued during physical training, but not during psychic training. Cancer treatments involving visualization also have been used with success for a number of years now.

Using visualization in preparation for birth and during labor to remain calm during contractions and to assist the body in opening the cervix and bringing the baby down the birth canal can be very effective as well. Labor can be so demanding that many women forget that the point of the whole process is the delivery of a baby. It's easy to forget that the natural rhythm of labor—except sometimes at the very end of the dilation phase—provides for regular rests between contractions for the baby as well as the mother. Caught up in thinking about the next contraction, it's all too easy to forget to stay in the moment. We get ahead of ourselves, lose our balance and lose perspective. The next moment we find ourselves feeling hopeless and like a victim of our own body.

It is important to help a laboring woman remember that her body is not trying to hurt her but simply doing what it needs to do to deliver the baby. We should not feel betrayed by our bodies when contractions hurt, any more than people should feel betrayed by their bodies during the effort of going on a long hike. We need to remain present in order to do what most helps our body do its work. This means adopting physical positions—such as squatting or standing or sitting on someone's lap—that will allow gravity to help draw the baby down, and perhaps immersing ourselves in a tub of warm water to allow the body to feel weightless and relaxed. Labor is not an athletic event, and many women who have easy labors are not athletes. There is much we can learn, however, about how to approach labor from those who do sports or other strenuous physical activities for recreation. It is a matter of mind more than body, of the mind either getting out of the body's way, or actively assisting it.

We should keep in mind that just as breathing, falling asleep, digesting food, eliminating waste, and becoming sexually aroused are meant to occur without our consciously willing them to happen and without our trying to control them, so birth is meant to occur spontaneously. Occasionally something will go wrong. In some situations—such as the extremely rare instance of the placenta beginning to separate from the uterus before the baby is born—there is nothing else to do but to remove the baby surgically. But in many other situations—such as a very slow labor without much progress, or a woman bleeding heavily after the birth—visualization can be used to change the physical conditions. Not only can women speed up their labors by using mental imagery, a woman can stop her bleeding simply by being told, or by telling herself, "You're bleeding too much. I want you to stop! Now!" In normal circumstances, however, there is no need for the intellect to do anything in childbirth, as it usually cannot improve on the natural process when all is going well.

Labor and Birth Without Drugs

Those who have lived among primitive tribes report that they tend not to respond as we do to the physical discomfort and pain of life. This may be due in part to a worldview, shared by everyone in the tribe, that does not see nature as separate from people, the mind as separate from the body, or pain as separate from pleasure. We pay the price for our addiction to personal comfort. In tribal societies, people accept unpleasant experiences and discomfort as part of life. Instead of responding to the pain of childbirth with fear and denial, women are raised to accept it as an integral and essential part of the birth experience.

For most women, giving birth to a child requires a steep descent into a place they have never been before within their conscious memory. Today this journey is often done unwillingly, with little or no vision of what is taking place and with little real preparation or guidance. Few women find labor to be what they expected. One part or another, and sometimes the whole of it, feels overwhelming. Many women in modern societies are shocked by the pain of labor. Past generations pronounced that women need to feel the pain of childbirth. It was said that only through this pain would a woman learn to love her child and be a good mother. Considering the source of such pronouncements—male clergy, male philosophers and physicians, and male legislators, all of whom allied against the right of women to receive anesthesia for birth in the late nineteenth century—it is no wonder that women have in ensuing years had scorn for such beliefs. Yet many women who have gone through labor without drugs but with the benefit of loving support claim that the experience changed them forever, for the good.

WHY WOMEN CHOOSE TO HAVE DRUGS IN LABOR

For as far back as we have information, humans have birthed without the use of *any* external substances for relief from the intensity and pain of labor. Except in rare and extreme circumstances, common sense dictated that anything the mother took might harm her or the baby, or inhibit the birthing process. It is

Early Labor

Paradoxically, normal birth usually demands that a woman's inner reserves of strength and confidence be used to allow her to yield to the forces of labor. Some women find that allowing the body to do and feel what it must as the cervix opens is when they work most easily with the birthing process. Others have a hard time waiting through the dilation stage and much prefer actively pushing.

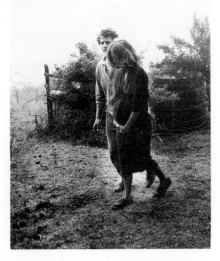

First-stage labor, or dilation, is a matter of settling into the sensations, which can be difficult to do because of their surprising intensity. Envision this stage as being like settling into an uncomfortable armchair: you must find a way to make yourself most comfortable. It may mean tucking your legs under you, throwing them over the arm of the chair, or cushioning your lower back with a firm pillow. The secret is turning your attention inward, getting your mind and your body settled.

Early first-stage labor can be challenging, because although contractions can be frequent, there's no obvious sign of progress. You may think: If it hurts this much and it's only the beginning, I'll never make it without drugs. Ride it out! As labor gets harder, your body's reserves will rise to meet the challenge.

You may feel you need help from others early in labor. However, during this time, actively continuing with your normal day and taking care of yourself allows the right hormones to kick in, making labor stronger while taking the edge off the pain. Do what you can to avoid the three perils of dehydration, exhaustion, and depression. Eat and drink, luxuriate in a warm shower or long bath, rest and sleep as much as possible. Most of all, don't resist your contractions. Find your body's rhythm and get in sync with it. Contractions, like a swell in a vast ocean, arise, build to a crest, then dissolve into calm.

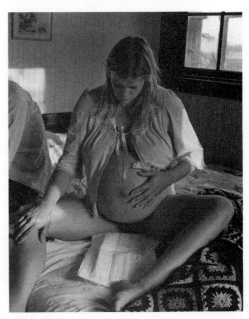

Active Labor

Once labor becomes really active—and the contractions are strong enough to open the cervix—your greatest challenge is maintaining your confidence. You literally cannot afford the energy it takes to be doubtful or hesitant. Most women find contractions are more

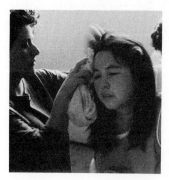

effective and less painful if they remain upright (standing or sitting) or get on their hands and knees. Let your body go. Use what—and who—is nearby to lean on. Deep moaning helps many women.

Think of sinking into, or riding over the top of, each contraction. If the contraction is strong, it's good. Change positions. Keep drinking lots of fluids. Above all, focus on only the present moment, only that contraction.

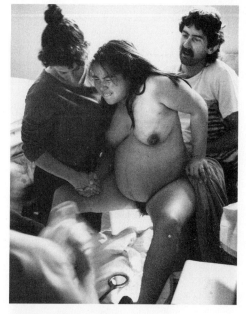

At the end of dilation, contractions can come one right after another, and there's no time to catch your breath or rest. Don't panic. All is well. Your baby will be in your arms soon!

You may not feel the overwhelming pushing urge for a while. If you don't, take a well-earned rest. Some women fall asleep at this point; others sleep between pushes. Once pushing urges begin—a few women never do have them—they build in intensity. Breathing is the key. You might feel your body will split wide open. It won't. Your uterus is propelling your baby down the birth canal. Being upright, in a well-supported squat, or sitting on a low, U-shaped stool or toilet really helps now. Lean back against someone you love.

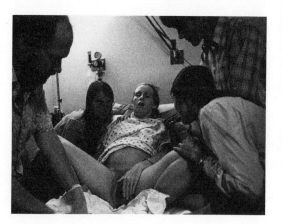

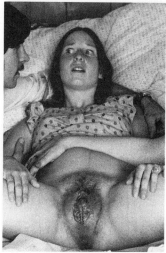

Delivery

The goal of pushing is not to give birth in the next push but to bring your baby down slowly. You may find that reaching your fingers inside to touch your baby's head makes you connect better with pushing.

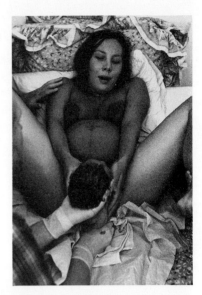

When your baby's head no longer disappears back inside you after a contraction, it is about to slip out. At this point, not pushing can allow you to stretch without tearing. You may feel pressure, heat, or burning. This too shall pass! If you open your eyes now, you will see your baby emerge and you may even want to reach down and bring your baby up to your chest. Ask that the umbilical cord not be cut until it has stopped pulsating so your baby has a backup supply of oxygen while it starts to breathe.

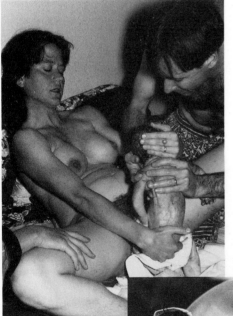

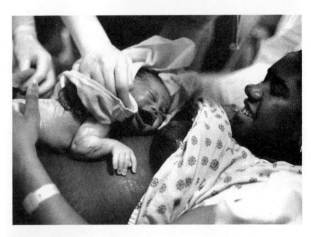

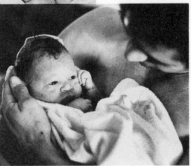

After your baby is in your arms, it will be time to expel your placenta, the nourishing source on which your baby has thrived. Soft and warm, the placenta will often slide right out with a contraction.

only in the past seventy-five years that women have been routinely drugged or anesthetized for birth. That is a very short period of time, but long enough to have imprinted on our culture the belief that birth requires the use of drugs.

Most traditional societies have understood that labor produces an altered state of consciousness that brings a woman extra strength and endurance and makes it possible for even a rather frail woman to deliver her baby unassisted and without any drugs stronger than herbs. Most cultures found ways to help a woman keep up her confidence and strength in labor and cope with the pain of contractions. Only modern Western culture has built an entire system of care around the patriarchal belief that women are not able to birth successfully on their own and that the human female body is not designed to cope with the pain of birth.

The primary reason for routinely hospitalizing women for childbirth, which began early in this century, was to provide a more controlled environment in which physicians could administer drugs to laboring women. Today the vast majority of pregnant women expect that they will need drugs in labor and believe they should be able to have them on demand. Physicians and nurses, for the most part, agree with them and encourage the use of drugs. The main difference between women giving birth today and their grandmothers is that their grandmothers found the whole process of birth so disturbing that they did not even want to be awake for it, whereas today women want to be awake. They just don't want to feel pain.

Traditionally women have sung, chanted, or repeated prayers to take their mind off the pain of contractions or to change their state of consciousness so that the pain becomes only one element of the experience. Often, women today do the opposite: they focus so much attention on pain, from early in pregnancy and during birth classes right into labor, that they end up priming themselves for unendurable pain. There is an entire culture around the avoidance of pain, not only in labor, but in all aspects of modern life. And many people single out the pain associated with giving birth as being somehow different and particularly unbearable. They have lost sight of the whole picture and focus compulsively on only one aspect: how much labor hurts. Anyone who engages in aerobic exercise or enjoys taking long hikes or jogging knows how easy it is to become a victim of the body's sensations, all the aches and pains that come with doing things that push physical limits. If we are climbing a hill and focus on how hard the ascent is, on how tired we are, on how strained our muscles feel, on how fast our heart is beating, and on the shortness of our breath, we can make ourselves miserable the entire trip. But keeping a cheerful attitude and focusing our attention on the pleasure of being in good health and out in nature make the effort worthwhile. It helps to admit that the discomfort is there but not to feel a victim of it. And the purpose of labor, after all, is the birth of a child.

THE PARADOX OF PLEASURE AND PAIN

The area in the brain that receives sensations of pleasure is the same area that receives sensations of pain. The brain cannot respond to sensations of pain and pleasure simultaneously; when one is predominant, the other is shut down. Thus anything that heightens our fear automatically raises our sense of pain and diminishes our sense of pleasure. This is why at some times our threshold of, or tolerance for, pain is greater or lesser than at other times. If a state of fear or anxiety can increase pain in labor and actually alter the course of labor, it is equally true that anything that heightens a birthing woman's sense of well-being lessens her perception of pain. And therein lies the key to preparation for birth and for how to keep birth both normal and within a woman's tolerance for pain without drugs.

It may seem like a cruel hoax evolution has played upon humans that, in the course of developing our neocortex, or thinking brain, we have had to cope with some difficult side effects. In the first place, our neocortical brain is quite capable, and often succeeds in, getting in the way of the more primitive parts of our brain, which govern such basic aspects of our body as breathing, digesting food, sleeping, and giving birth. Merely believing that you will suffer greatly during labor makes it likely to happen. Second, along with the refinement of our intellect has come an increased awareness of both pleasure and pain.

Alan Watts, the late Anglican cleric and philosopher who brought an awareness of Zen Buddhism to an entire generation of Westerners early in the second half of this century, wrote and spoke eloquently on the subject of pain: "Unquestionably, the sensitive human brain adds immeasurably to the richness of life. Yet for this we pay dearly, because the increase in overall sensitivity makes us peculiarly vulnerable." He went on to state that it is our very vulnerability that makes it possible for us to experience the deliciousness of earthly existence: "Sensitivity requires a high degree of softness and fragility—eyeballs, eardrums, taste buds, and nerve ends culminating in the highly delicate organism of the brain. These are not only soft and fragile, but also perishable."

The paradox exists: To be sensitive to pleasure we must be equally sensitive to pain. This is why any attempt to cultivate comfort to the exclusion of discomfort or pain always backfires. We live by the myth that we can control and suppress whatever we don't want to feel—such as the pain and discomfort of normal life—and that there will be no consequences of our actions. We have forgotten a simple truth: Joy or suffering is only a state of mind and separate from physical sensations or emotions.

DOING WITHOUT DRUGS

It's awe-inspiring to be with a woman in labor who is up on her feet, or on her hands and knees, rhythmically swaying, making low moans with each contraction. Unfortunately what you usually see in hospitals today—since sedative and analgesic drugs are out of fashion and the epidural is all the rage—are tense, frantic women lying in bed watching the clock, making high tight noises or crying out in hopelessness and pain, until the anesthesiologist arrives. After the anesthesia has taken over you see a very strange sight—strange at least for anyone who knows what labor is about: a woman lying or sitting up in bed, casually chatting with the people around her or watching television, as if nothing at all were going on inside her body.

Labor pain should not be treated as if it were a sign of illness or injury. The best form of pain relief—and the only form we know of that has no side effects—is the kind of emotional support that encourages an optimistic, calm attitude in the laboring woman.

The last contractions of the dilation phase of labor are often very hard, and, when a woman is not medicated or anesthetized, they may seem to come nonstop, peak after peak. The woman often looks around frantically, sensing that a change is coming and needing reassurance that all will be well. The primitive parts of her brain have taken over and are looking out for her safety. This is the moment, as French obstetrician-author Michel Odent states, when a woman is showing how near she is to delivery and when she really needs close support. That moment of panic triggers, or perhaps is triggered by, a release of a set of different hormones that pick up the pace of the labor and prepare the woman for the final pushing phase.

From his decades of observing women cared for by midwives in his hospital unit, Michel Odent observed a commonality among women having normal childbirths. At this point of momentary panic, something occurs that actually triggers the delivery. Odent named this "the fetal ejection reflex." And the lack of it, in his eyes, is a sign that the woman's natural hormonal mechanism has been thrown off, either by drugs or by too much interference, including too much fussing over the woman early in the labor, when she needs to settle into the contractions.

The problem is not that modern woman cannot tolerate the sensations of labor, but that the sensations become intolerable when she is in a state of fear and living in the expectation that labor will never end. The mind's conception of a repetition of a single painful moment over and over and over again is enough to frighten it, and this brings real suffering in its wake.

Fear is completely intertwined with what we experience as labor pain. If there is a single barrier separating modern woman from her ancient sister and preventing her from experiencing what it is like to give birth under her own power, it is not woman's weakened physical condition, nor the overly refined nervous system of our bodies. It is fear. And it is the fear in our physicians and nurses as much as the fear within ourselves. This is one negative aspect of putting many laboring women together in one place. In a hospital, whenever there is a serious problem the staff tends to respond in panic—because their own fears are stimulated—and they pass along this sense of danger to every patient they see.

The subconscious responds better to a hand calmly stroking the back of the neck than to verbal assurances that all is well. This is why the traditional practice of midwifery, which depends on careful but calm observation done while sitting or walking with a woman and giving her encouragement, works so well. Being present continuously makes it possible to spot a deviation from what is normal long before it becomes serious. And being present while giving continuous encouragement—especially nonverbally, through touch, or humming a tune, or sitting in a rocking chair and knitting—tells a woman that all is well. "All is well" is the message every woman in labor needs to get.

Some midwives make it a practice of telling each client after the first vaginal exam, "You have a beautiful pelvis. It's so roomy, just made to give birth." They have observed that the planting of this message actually aids labor, especially since the configuration of a baby's head and a mother's pelvis are almost always compatible. What is the alternative? Certainly not to do what some obstetricians have done for years: at a teenager's first vaginal exam, when there is any dimension of the pelvis that is smaller than average, to declare: "Your pelvis is rather small. You are probably going to need a cesarean when you have a baby."

A second alternative is more commonly used today, especially by physicians who are consciously trying to make women more comfortable by means of giving them lots of data to chew on. "Well, Michelle, your pelvis is not gynecoid in shape. It is flatter than the typical woman's pelvis. Here, let me draw it for you. You see, it's the shape that most men's pelvises are. I think we may be able to have a vaginal birth, but you should be prepared for the possibility of a cesarean."

The subconscious messages we give a woman begin long before we ask her to remove her own familiar clothes and put on an impersonal-looking hospital gown. It begins when she leaves her home and enters an institution. For years, many hospitals have had—and some still have—the practice of making women in labor come through the emergency room entrance. What message does this give? "If I don't have an emergency now, it's likely I will soon."

Labor makes one essential demand on the woman's mind. It asks that she give up intellectual thought and drop into an altered state of consciousness in which she can allow her body to take over. Her entire hormonal system is geared to create this altered state. What confuses the hormonal system and causes it to switch to a physical state of fight or flight is fear. Any interruption from the outside environment can be especially disruptive during early labor, before the woman is in the altered state in which her body has taken over. On the other hand, anything in the outside environment that encourages the shift into the altered state will be likely to help keep labor moving along normally and keep the fetus doing well, too.

What are some environmental aids to normal childbirth? A place to labor that is familiar and comfortable to the woman, especially a place where she can see the moon or sun, can smell fresh air, can see or sit outdoors beneath a tree, can watch water flowing. It could be an artificially created interior garden, or the out-of-doors, which she can walk into. Some sounds are conducive to focusing inwardly, such as certain kinds of music on a tape or someone playing an instrument in a soothing fashion or singing a comforting tune. The feel of warm water playing over the woman's body in a shower or a tub, especially one large enough to let her feel weightless and to take the pressure of gravity off her during contractions, is a natural labor aid. The touch of a calm person can aid labor, whether it is brushing the woman's hair or placing the palms of his or her hands against her feet, or deeply massaging her buttocks, especially if she is experiencing labor in her back. A pervasive sense of calm and quiet are the important aids to normal childbirth, as are surroundings in which the woman and her companions feel comfortable and free to move around and act as they would at home. Wearing her own clothes, rather than a hospital gown, reminds a laboring woman that she is an individual, not a "patient."

Today, drugs and other interventions in birth still symbolize freedom to many women. But ask women who have had cesareans in which there was no prior labor and you will find that they often express sadness at what they sense they have missed. If you show a woman you are truly interested in hearing the entire story of her birth, you are likely to hear a lot of unfulfillment today. The drugged mother has missed out on discovering that her body works. She has been denied the actual experience of giving birth naturally. She needs to mourn that loss in order to fully heal, but she is expected to put on a smiling face to friends and relatives.

The process of having completed something difficult, of allowing ourselves to be pushed beyond what we think is our limit and finding ourselves to be more capable than we ever dreamed possible, is where much of the joy in childbirth lies.

Failure to Progress?

We modern people are obsessed with the concept of progress and of having to outdo nature with human invention. We've taken that obsession into maternity and newborn care. We insist on measuring progress in pregnancy and birth in linear ways—measuring weight and length and levels of pH—and in believing that these measurements tell us what we need to know about how healthy someone is and how pregnancy and birth, or a newborn baby, are progressing. We then hold everyone to a single standard. Long early labors that do not lead to a specific amount of progress in dilation of the cervix are classified by the phrase "failure to progress."

Sometimes there is a true problem and intervention is necessary. From recent research on the impact on babies of overly long second stages in labor, it appears to be true that babies should not remain in the birth canal for longer than a few hours or they show signs of trauma. The second stage of labor, also known as the pushing phase, begins with the efforts of the uterus to propel the baby down the birth canal. In cases in which the second stage is not progressing, it's important to get the woman to focus on getting the baby born and to be in a position physically conducive to bringing the baby down and out, and it may be time to ask everyone to leave the room so she can concentrate on the task at hand.

Much more commonly, however, the problem of failure to progress lies in the standards we have set for laboring women, which are unreasonable and do not take into account the individuality of each mother-baby pair. This, combined with the extreme lack of privacy and the lack of sufficient emotional support for mothers going through labor, often results in women needing medical intervention and believing that they or their baby would surely have been injured or have died without it.

Failure to progress has in recent years become commonplace in the labor wards of modern hospitals around the world, wherever physicians attempt to hold women's labors to an unrealistic standard and to control and manage the process of birth. "Failure to progress" is more frequently listed on birthing women's charts as the cause for a cesarean surgery than any other.

Most of the causes for failure to progress in labor today come down to environmental factors: a lack of adequate emotional support, a lack of privacy, and the hospital environment itself, in which paraphernalia and procedures such as electronic fetal monitors and IVs dominate the scene. A woman's subconscious identifies any procedure done to her body or attached to her body as sign that something is wrong or is likely to go wrong. Even a woman who trusts her body and has confidence in her own ability and in the process of labor can lose faith. She stops listening to herself and her baby and turns to outside authorities to tell her what is going on and what to do.

> *The worst intervention in childbirth today is the clock.*
>
> —MIDWIFE, MOTHER, AND GRANDMOTHER

Facing Risk: Possible Problems in Birth

We cannot talk about the unwarranted fear of childbirth without acknowledging the problems that can arise in pregnancy or at birth, however uncommon they might be. Sometimes things go wrong and require quick thinking and medical intervention. This happens much more rarely than you have been led to believe. At those times, we are grateful for doctors, for medicine and technology, for well-equipped and well-staffed hospitals. Medical intervention can save lives and prevent injury; that is the appropriate use of doctors and modern medicine in childbirth.

None of us want to go back to a time when crisis intervention was unavailable, when there was no anesthesia, no antibiotics, no aseptic conditions for doing surgery. Mothers who choose to give birth at home or in a birth center, as well as their midwives and physicians, are thankful when they have a good hospital to go to if the need arises. They are appreciative when the hospital staff is welcoming and does not judge them for having planned a birth outside the hospital. Having a backup plan for an out-of-hospital birth is crucial to the safety of that birth. But all too often birthing women and expectant fathers believe that simply by being in a hospital the mother and baby will have a safer birth and a better experience. This isn't true, and studies show that planned out-of-hospital births where there is a skilled attendant present and a hospital within a half hour's drive are as safe as those in any hospital. Not only that, the mother and baby avoid unnecessary medical intervention by staying out of a hospital if they don't need anything a hospital can provide.

The truth is, however, that when a woman is healthy going into her pregnancy, it is very unusual for her or her baby to require a hospital and a team of medical specialists. Even if she has had problems getting pregnant or problems during pregnancy, if the woman is healthy and problem-free when she enters labor, it is rare that she or her baby needs to be in a hospital. What modern medicine has done is to give women who are particularly frail or ill a better chance of giving birth safely and having a healthy child.

Often even a woman who is in poor health or has a chronic disease can give birth without the need for any medical intervention. She needs to be watched more closely, of course, and a few extra precautions might need to be taken. Such a pregnancy is correctly called "high-risk," a term that frightens women and their families and makes physicians and nurses more anxious too. All it means is that special attention needs to be paid to a mother and baby pair.

Approximately one mother and baby in every ten will have some complication arise during pregnancy, birth, or immediately afterward. The majority of these complications can be anticipated. Problems that complicate the normal process usually fall into one of two categories. The first is those that are self-correcting, that run a natural course and then disappear spontaneously, without any intervention. The second is those that, if spotted early, can be handled simply and effectively with only minimal assistance or intervention.

Let's look at the first group of problems, those that are self-correcting. Physicians and nurses are trained to know that the majority of illnesses and diseases

Normalizing "At-Risk" Birth

1975: This first-time mother had preeclampsia, a serious condition in which a woman, at the onset of labor, suffers high blood pressure that can result in seizures. Magnesium sulfate was administered to reduce the risk of convulsions. Standard care usually meant spending one's entire labor period lying in a hospital bed, with no visitors allowed, taking barbiturates.

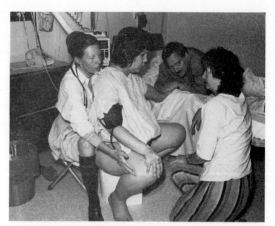

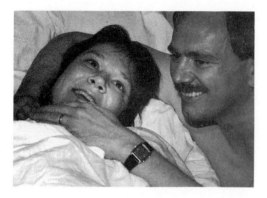

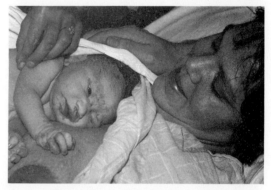

This woman chose a holistic alternative to this approach: to give birth in a hospital and to take the necessary drugs, but also to have friends and family by her side for support. A shorter labor was facilitated by walking and by squatting upright and pushing on a birthing stool. With continuous emotional support and careful medical observation, a safe and optimum birth was the result despite the complications of preeclampsia. She and her baby went home in good health the next day.

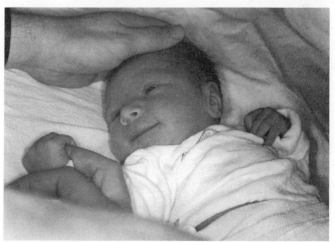

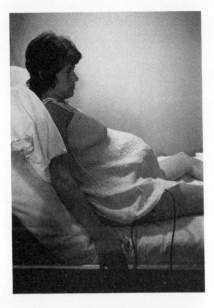

Twins

Many hospitals consider the delivery of twins a high-risk birth, because of the complications that can occur. Despite the high-risk label, this mother fought to keep her childbirth normal. She wore her own clothes for labor, and when her overdistended uterus required the use of an artificial hormone to stimulate contractions, she insisted on controlling the amount herself. Though there was a crowd at the delivery, she made sure she had the space she needed; she even had the bottom half of the delivery table lowered so she could half-squat, making the birthing process easier. After the birth, she refused to let the babies be taken away.

If you are carrying twins, consider choosing a hospital that has experience with twins and that can provide adequate neonatal care. For more information, contact the National Organization of Mothers of Twins Clubs or Twin Services (see Resources).

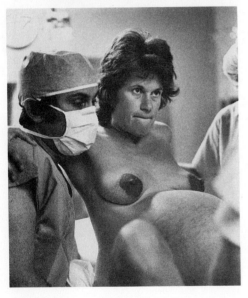

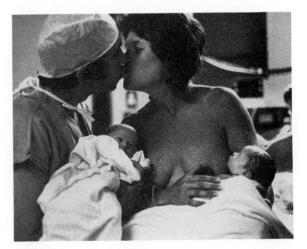

are self-limiting and that most problems will correct themselves given time. Their job with regard to these kinds of problems is just to help the person be more comfortable and wait it out. That is why it is so important during labor and childbirth to have a skilled person present to continually observe how you are doing. When someone is with you every minute, he or she can identify anything that might become a problem and assess whether it is likely to be self-correcting or not.

Two good examples of conditions that can occur early in pregnancy but are usually self-correcting are nausea (morning sickness) or spotting blood from the vagina. Once in a while, in each case, these conditions continue past early pregnancy or become so severe that they pose a real threat. But the rest of the time they go away on their own. An example of a self-correcting problem in labor is when the cervix dilates to six centimeters and then stops dilating for several hours, until the woman is either able to rest or sleep for a while or to otherwise relieve some of her stress. Then the contractions suddenly become more effective and the cervix continues to reopen.

Let's look at the second category of problems, those that, if spotted early, can usually be handled simply and effectively by doing something that changes the environment. There are many situations during labor that fall into this category. Since they are usually given as the reason for major intervention but seldom truly require intervention, you should be aware of them.

A baby's heart tones suddenly speed up or slow down markedly to where they are outside the range of normal. Although this may be self-correcting, it is potentially too serious to wait very long to see if it changes on its own. The usual and probable cause of a sudden, dramatic change in a baby's heart tones is that the baby's umbilical cord (through which it receives the blood carrying its oxygen) is being compressed. Usually the cause of cord compression is that the baby is lying on it. The first course of action should be the least interventive: simply have the woman change her position. She may need to try several different positions such as getting on her hands and knees, with her buttocks higher than her chest, or simply turning from one side to the other. This is usually enough to cause the baby to move off the cord.

Even in the case of a very serious and extremely rare condition called a cord prolapse, in which the umbilical cord slips down through the cervix before it is fully dilated and the baby's own weight on the cord shuts off the flow of oxygen, the first thing to do is to get the baby to move away from the cord so that the cord is not compressed. The woman should be asked to move onto her elbows and knees, so that her buttocks are higher than her shoulders. This causes the baby to slip back up in the pelvis, freeing the cord. In addition, the birth attendant can put a gloved hand up inside the vagina to keep the cord from slipping down until the baby can be delivered by forceps or cesarean. A cord prolapse can even be handled at home. The woman just needs to remain in this odd position all the way to the hospital. I mention this condition to show how, even in true crisis, there is time for quick thinking and how simple solutions often save the day. Many physicians don't know this simple maneuver.

Let's go back to a situation that occurs more frequently—even in hospitals—and can be a serious problem if it's not resolved. A woman has been in labor for quite a while but, for whatever reason, such as a restrictive hospital policy or the failure of a nurse or family member to remind her to drink something every hour or so, she has not been eating or taking fluids. Her blood sugar will probably drop markedly and she will become seriously dehydrated and hypoglycemic. The common symptoms are that she'll feel very irritable, nauseous, or like she is about to faint. She may start to shake, and her contractions will probably have petered out and be doing nothing except causing her pain, or they may have stopped altogether. She is certainly not progressing at this point, and the baby may start going into distress. Simply giving the woman fluids and a quick source of energy, such as tea with a lot of honey, can change the whole picture. Within minutes she's not shaking or nauseous, irritable, or feeling faint. Her contractions suddenly pick up and become effective.

Physicians and other health workers can panic just as anyone can, but their tendency to rush into major intervention without even trying less-invasive measures is a side effect of high-risk training and habitually being present during crises. Health workers also can be as ignorant as anyone about the benefits of simpler and less-invasive procedures for solving problems. Their ignorance is a product of a particular kind of medical training that is most common in the United States, but that is being exported all around the world. It is training to be aggressive with intervention, an approach that affects nurses and also nurse-midwives. It is based upon an outdated and inaccurate view of childbirth as a disease rather than a natural process.

We should remember that the physician or nurse we count on to know what is best has most likely been trained to believe that *normal* is a word you cannot use until after everything turns out all right. He or she has been trained to think that problems in birth arise out of nowhere, usually without any warning, and that most problems will quickly turn into emergencies unless medical intervention is done immediately. This is simply not true, and a recent ten-year study of birth in the Netherlands is just one of many that has demonstrated the opposite.

The labor of a healthy woman can involve some variations on the norm and still be normal. A skilled physician or midwife can fairly accurately predict which women will have problems and what those problems are likely to be. In those very uncommon situations where an unanticipated problem arises, there is virtually always time to see whether it will correct itself and, if it does not, there is still time to try simple techniques before turning to medical intervention.

Dutch research in a suburb of Amsterdam called Wermerweer shows that among pregnant women who had been prescreened and judged low-risk for problems at birth—80 percent of the general population—approximately 90 percent safely gave birth twenty minutes from a hospital, either at home or at a birth center. The remainder were moved to a hospital in ample time and suffered no added risk by having begun labor outside the hospital. Dutch studies continue to show that skilled midwives are the only attendants needed at 80 percent of all births. Obstetricians can be of value in the other 20 percent, but even at those births midwives can help keep intervention to a bare minimum. The entire maternity care system of the Netherlands is built on the well-proven fact that modern medicine works best when it is used the least. It also costs much less and has far fewer long-term risks to a woman or her baby to avoid medical intervention in birth wherever possible.

SUMMING UP THE RISKS OF CHILDBIRTH

Before women can be expected to insist on a health-care system that supports normal childbirth, we need to know what the real risks of childbearing are and how frequently they occur.

In pregnancy, the main risk to a woman is that of a miscarriage, or spontaneous abortion, which leaves some tissue in the mother and causes her to hemorrhage. Approximately a third of all conceptions spontaneously end in miscarriage. The majority of miscarriages occur either because the fertilized egg has not implanted properly in the womb or because the embryonic cells were not healthy. Heavy blood loss jeopardizes a woman's life. Even if it is stopped, she is prone to infection while recuperating, as it takes time for her body to rebuild its full supply of blood. A rare but very serious threat to the woman is if the embryonic cells do not begin to grow in the uterus but in a fallopian tube. A tubal pregnancy is not normal and usually ends spontaneously. It is usually signaled by sharp pain in the area of the fallopian tubes, which indicates that something is wrong and requires medical help. If the tube ruptures, the woman is in serious danger from hemorrhage or infection.

The main risks to the fetus as it develops within the mother's body are that of deformity or damage caused by something the mother has ingested, or by temporary loss of oxygen to its tissues caused by hypertension, infection, or some other trauma to the mother.

In labor, most of the few serious complications for the mother have always been associated with the placenta. The placenta is the organ connected to the sac that houses the fetus; it is also attached to the wall of the mother's uterus and directly nourishes the fetus. The placenta is expelled from the body after the baby is born. In very rare instances the placenta lies too low in the uterus and covers, or partially covers, the cervix; it will not permit the baby to come down without tearing in the process, causing massive bleeding in the mother and loss of oxygen for the baby, endangering both of their lives. Other potential problems include preeclampsia, a condition in late pregnancy in which the blood pressure rises and the woman suffers edema and severe headache. Women who have this should be carefully monitored and given the correct drugs so they do not have seizures.

In rare cases, the baby lies across the uterus, rather than head or bottom down, at the end of pregnancy and needs to be somehow turned. In this position it cannot come down through the pelvis and no amount of labor will help, unless the baby changes position on its own or is physically shifted by massage from the outside, called *version*. Sometimes, but usually not in a first birth because the uterus is so firm, a baby turns in labor as a woman moves around, walks, or rocks her pelvis. Sometimes it is necessary to turn the baby manually or perform a cesarean.

One interesting fact of nature is that even a very small mother, or a woman with a pelvis that is shaped very flat or very narrow at one end, can usually deliver her baby successfully. This has to do both with the flexibility of the pelvis and the flexibility of the baby's head, which can mold to almost any shape in birth and then resume its normal shape afterward.

After the birth, there is the slight risk that the placenta will not come out or will not be fully expelled, which would result in hemorrhage and possible infection for the mother. If the mother's cervix, vaginal wall, or perineum has for any reason torn badly during the birth she is also likely to hemorrhage. This can happen during the process of childbirth itself, but is much more often a result of forceps delivery, cesarean surgery, or episiotomy. Besides the risk of hemorrhage, the risk of infection to the open womb is the most serious complication for a birthing woman.

For the baby going through birth, the main risk is that its supply of oxygen might be diminished or cut off for a long enough time that it will have brain damage. This can occur if the cord is around its neck too tightly, or if the baby is lying in the uterus in such a way that some part of its own body is compressing the cord. The nature of the umbilical cord, which is thick, tough, sinewy, and very slippery, makes it difficult for it to compress so tightly that the blood supply is shut off. Even when the baby has moved around in the uterus so that it has created a knot in the umbilical cord, it is extremely rare for that knot to be pulled tight enough to cut off the blood flow. Also, the mother's normal movements and her changes in position in the course of labor usually keep the baby from lying against its own cord. These are rare but serious risks, nevertheless.

For the newborn baby, the most serious risk has to do with breathing. For many minutes (perhaps as long as half an hour), or as long as the umbilical cord has not been cut and the placenta has not disengaged from the uterine wall, the newborn baby receives ample oxygen from its mother's blood supply. This is the baby's fail-safe and the reason why it is unwise to cut a still-pulsating umbilical cord until the placenta has fully detached from the uterus or has been delivered. At some point, however, the baby must begin to breathe on its own, or it will die. In addition, there is also the possibility of the baby getting an infection, which can be life-threatening, or of simply not being kept warm and dry enough and thus losing too much body heat. Though serious, these rarely occur.

Bearing a child has always carried elements of risk. Traditionally, women have had various effective ways of stopping bleeding, treating infection, helping a baby to breathe, and keeping a baby from losing too much body heat. Sometimes herbal preparations were drunk or put on the body; sometimes physically compressing the bleeding area with a hand would cause the blood to clot and the site to begin healing. Some attempts were probably made to help the baby begin breathing. All through history, women and men have tried to reduce the risks inherent in childbirth.

Preparing Women and Men for Childbirth

Childbirth education and preparing for birth are more important today than ever. Yet much of what passes for birth classes is not education at all, but a reinforcing of the fear of birth so prevalent in our culture. Much birth education is little more than training in passivity and compliance with the status quo, paying lip service to the concept that birth is a healthy, normal process. Too many birth educators are paid by hospitals or obstetricians and feel obliged to serve *their* needs, not the real needs of the women and men they are there to educate. Too many are afraid to question and challenge women who are looking for the easy way out and say they want the most medically managed births possible.

Authentic preparation for childbirth opens the mind and instills a hopeful attitude and a sense of proportion in a mother-to-be, no matter how difficult her circumstances are. It imparts a proper dignity and a sense of awe toward the birth process, the life a woman is carrying, and the woman herself. It should enlarge a woman's—and a couple's—vision about the significance of what they are undertaking in bringing a baby into the world, give them a sense of what the fetus is likely to experience during birth, and what the baby—and the mother—will need, emotionally and physically, in order to thrive.

Childbirth preparation should include information about the long-term psychic and physical effects of what happens during birth, especially because modern medicine focuses only on the physical and the short term. Much of what people need to know to be in the best position to give birth normally and to provide what a growing baby needs is information not currently discussed or valued in our culture.

Most childbirth classes today are organized primarily around the idea of coping with the pain of labor, and many teachers feel they are not doing their job unless they detail each and every hospital procedure and try to prepare every woman for the possibility of a cesarean.

Some women today read medical textbooks in an attempt to learn everything they can about birth and babies and to know the names for every possible thing that can go wrong. But it's not women's intellect that needs to be addressed— it's their hearts and their sense of courage. It's the primitive, nonverbal part of the brain that is most active during childbirth, and data don't affect that area of the brain, whereas emotions do. The primitive brain is calmed by touch and music and poetry, not numbers or logical thought.

Visual images of birth are especially important in a culture where women rarely see birth before going through it themselves. But there is probably little value in showing images of cesarean surgery or complications. The subconscious mind is simply too suggestive, especially during pregnancy, for a woman to take in these images with any sense of proportion. A woman in pregnancy and labor is affected by her environment, including all the information she gets about childbirth. It is far better to show her normal births—and a variety of them—so she can see the range of variation within "normal." Women today need to be inspired; they need to believe in themselves, their babies, and the birth process. They should be shown images of women rising to the demands of labor, being challenged and pushed to the edge, but finding the strength within themselves to push through what they thought were their limits. They need to find support for what their instinct is telling: labor is valuable and productive work and should not be avoided. How we give birth, how we are born, does matter.

> *Women need to trust their bodies, trust themselves and their support people. They should not blindly trust the medical establishment. There need to be big changes, but in the brief time you have before you give birth it's too hard to make the system change. So you need to figure out ways around it, ahead of time.*
>
> —FAMILY-PRACTICE PHYSICIAN

Giving birth is painful, and it takes a tremendous physical effort for most women, especially a first birth. Women don't benefit from being lied to about the reality of childbirth, but they also don't benefit from education that reinforces abnormality, romanticizes technology in birth, or supports practices that are likely to hurt women and babies and their families. Childbirth education ought to be an antidote to the messages so prevalent in our culture, which women constantly hear from friends and family and doctors, and which they read about. Television and the press and birth stories focus on the drama and risks of birth, and the role of doctors and high-tech equipment in saving mothers and babies. We are seldom given a role model of a woman who is working with the forces of labor and conducting her own delivery.

Childbirth classes should be an oasis to come to after a tiring day at work, or when pregnancy seems to be going on forever and a woman finds her mind filled with fear and her relationship with her partner is under extra stress. Classes ought to be a place where fathers-to-be can find support and reassurance for anxiety and apprehension. While pregnant women become more and more preoccupied with the idea of labor as they get closer to their due date, they need help addressing the psychological changes they are undergoing. They also need to know about the psychological side of pregnancy and birth for the baby.

There are certain times during pregnancy when a woman is especially open to learning about the consciousness of her baby and how to meet its psychological needs. Teachers should take advantage of these windows of opportunity and start classes early enough in pregnancy so that they can do justice to the whole picture of reproduction. Childbirth is a very broad and deep subject if it is looked at holistically. It represents not only a powerful life-changing experience for a woman, but the beginning of her child's sense of itself and the world, and is a major adjustment for the woman, her partner, and the family.

Although I am not a professional childbirth educator, I put together in the late 1970s a course of study called "The Evolution of Childbirth Practices," which I taught for several years to birth educators, would-be midwives, and nurses. In the late 1980s, after being present at more than one hundred births in various settings in the United States and Europe, I decided to offer a series of childbirth preparation classes in partnership with a midwife.

We kept the class size small and made the series twelve evenings, followed by a celebratory picnic reunion, held after everyone in the class had given birth. There was so much we wanted to cover. We tried not only to help the couples prepare for labor, but to give them skills they could use for the rest of their lives. We cooked dinner for the couples to start out the first few evenings, so that they could come straight from their jobs and relax and be taken care of. We taught songs and simple birth chants from other cultures that women have found helpful. In a few of the classes women practiced focused, calm breathing. We talked about ways to keep labor progressing, how to "settle into" contractions despite their distracting intensity, how to keep the spirits up, and how to avoid an episiotomy. Many of the classes included centering practices. At the final class we held a special ceremony to honor each woman for the journey she was embarking on. Each sat in the center of a circle and listened to the good wishes of all the others: "I wish you courage to face whatever comes." "I wish you wildness and the freedom to be completely yourself." "I wish you a sense of humor to keep everything in proportion."

We worked with couples who were going to different hospitals, some of which we knew to be unsupportive of normal birth; couples having home births or going to a nearby birth center; lesbian couples; and single mothers. Several evenings were set aside for women only, and those proved to be particularly meaningful. Previously unspoken fears were voiced, and women talked openly about their doubts and about their relationship with their partners, if they had a partner. We gave each other massages. We tried to explain to the women the concept of timeless time, of seeing labor as just one contraction at a time, of staying in the present and looking neither forward nor backward. Our classes were not the most popular in town, and we exposed many women and men to things they initially thought were strange. But all the women—and some of the men—told us later how much they grew to love those classes, and how much of what they learned there positively affected their births and the way they looked at parenting. And more of them ended up having normal births than even we had hoped for, given some of the choices they had made before they even came to class.

Perhaps the most important thing anyone can do for a woman going into childbirth is to help her shed her misconceptions and diminish the fears about giving birth that she has picked up in the course of her life. We all need to help each other create inner peace in regard to pregnancy and childbirth, for it is vitally important for the baby as well as the mother. Every woman, no matter what her age or circumstances, deserves to know how transformative a process birth and motherhood can be. If she is fortunate enough to have a supportive mate, both of them need to know that each one's experience will be unique, just as the baby's will be. Yet they are connected as they go on this journey.

The best kind of education draws the best from the woman herself and treats every woman's experience as important. It treats every woman's pregnancy, childbirth, and motherhood as a valuable time for learning more about herself and her baby. It does not claim every childbirth is equally safe or equally positive. A cesarean done for "failure to progress" because a woman doesn't make progress in dilating for several hours is not likely to be as positive or as safe as the normal birth that might have happened if the woman had been given more time, more privacy, or more emotional support. A baby being taken to intensive care for tests because he is breathing rapidly and no one is willing first to sit and watch him in his mother's arms to make sure tests are necessary does not have as positive an experience as the baby who is observed and, if need be, given special care while still lying in his mother's arms.

Going to childbirth classes during pregnancy can be the most valuable thing you can do with your time and money. But it pays to check around and find out which childbirth educators are independent—paid by their clients, not by a hospital or doctor—and which have the highest percentage of normal, unmedicated births. Childbirth classes can make the last half of pregnancy much less stressful. The thinking you do as a result of childbirth classes may result in your changing some of the decisions you've made about your baby's birth and what you have planned for the months afterward. You may discover that you have the wrong physician, or decide that you don't want a physician but a midwife and that you don't want a hospital birth unless it is medically necessary.

It's never too late to make a change. One woman I know decided when she was about to deliver that she didn't agree with her doctor. He was about to do an episiotomy and she wanted to push the baby out without being cut. She told her husband, "Get me up and take me out of here!" You can imagine what a stir that produced. In fact, she didn't leave, but she was taken seriously after that and had neither an episiotomy nor a tear.

If you've been led to believe you might need a cesarean, or if you've had one already, or if you are having your first baby after the age of thirty, your choice of childbirth educator is especially important, because you are one of the women who are most likely today to have a medically unnecessary cesarean and have your baby end up in intensive care for no good medical reason. Few doctors are interested enough or supportive enough to help a woman achieve a vaginal birth. Even interested doctors feel pressured to get the baby out as fast as possible.

Your childbirth educator can also give you the names of doulas, women who are skilled in helping other women have the most normal birth possible. A doula can help keep you confident and help protect you and your baby from unnecessary and risky procedures such as artificial hormones to stimulate contractions, anesthesia, forceps, vacuum extraction, episiotomy, and cesarean surgery.

At this time in the United States, women have more choices regarding childbirth than at any other time in history. Unfortunately, they also have a greater chance than ever before of having an unnecessary cesarean, and of their baby undergoing all sorts of painful and medically unnecessary interventions after birth. The difference in the kind of experience a mother and her baby have lies in the decisions she makes before, during, and right after the birth. Women, ultimately, are the ones who have the greatest influence over the kind of childbirth they have and whether the experience is positive or negative for themselves and for their babies.

If you are pregnant or are considering having a child and cannot afford to pay for a good series of childbirth classes, consider asking others for financial assistance. Friends and family may have told you they want to help in any way they can—this is a good way. Several of them can even share the costs, and you and your baby will be the better for it. Real preparation helps a woman enter labor with confidence and at the same time helps her to evaluate the experience afterward.

Many childbirth teachers, especially those who teach in hospitals, believe they are teaching women acceptance when they tell them not to expect a perfect birth. They don't want women to be disappointed when their hopes are not matched by the reality of the experience. It's true that life works better when we have no rigid expectations. But we also need to remain hopeful and to be truthful with ourselves. That way we are much less likely to let ourselves be deceived, we can set about getting the kind of birth experience we desire, and we will be truly ready to accept the outcome, whatever it may be. We must find the balance between having unrealistically high expectations and submissively accepting whatever comes.

The *real* purpose of childbirth education ought to be helping people prepare for the coming of a new soul. We must do whatever we can to open our hearts and adjust our circumstances to fit the needs and pace of this human being for whom every experience will be fresh, and who will be completely dependent on us. Lifelong trust is established by how safe and wanted we feel at the beginning of life. *The path to healthy self-love, self-reliance, and acceptance of our interdependence lies in being allowed to feel dependent during our formative early months.*

Many practices that are considered wholesome in other parts of the world are dismissed in this culture as unnecessary or dangerous. These include such developmentally important practices as responding to babies whenever they cry during the first nine months, carrying babies right next to our bodies as much as possible, and having them in our beds when they are young. We can adapt modern lifestyles to babies, but babies are at risk when *they* are expected to adapt to lifestyles that do not meet their basic needs.

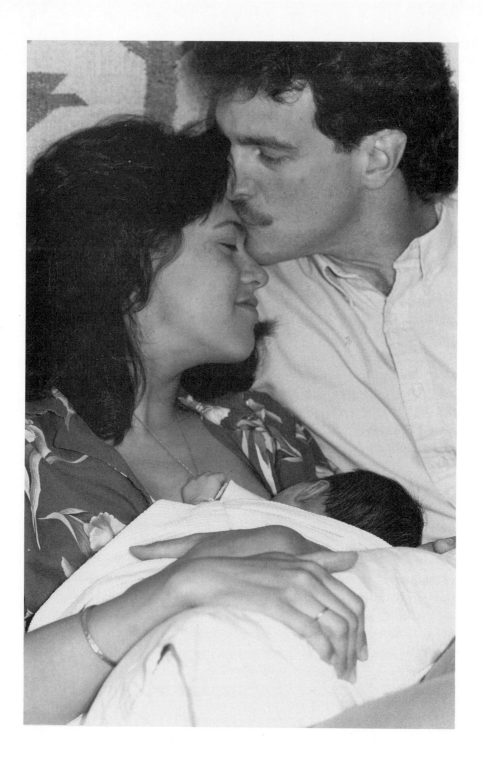

CHAPTER FIVE

Moving Toward Normal Childbirth

Consumer Pressure and Change

THE CONSUMER MOVEMENT in childbirth, also known as the natural childbirth movement and the alternative birth movement, is today a worldwide grassroots movement whose goal is to foster normal childbirth. It supplies women and their partners with information and support for making conscious choices about how, where, and with whom they will give birth. Ironically, the roots of this consumer movement lie in the writings and practices of two renegade male physicians, Dr. Grantly Dick-Read in England and Dr. Fernand Lamaze in France. These men rediscovered what most midwives had known throughout history but in recent years had been unable to practice: childbirth is a normal physiological process that seldom results in problems for a healthy woman.

In the 1930s Grantly Dick-Read gained his insights from watching working-class women in urban England give birth without help from drugs. He also traveled to Africa, where he observed women giving birth on their own in rural villages. He saw the transpersonal and spiritual dimensions of birth and wrote eloquently about women's innate capacity to give birth successfully on their own and without great suffering. His primary point was that modern fear-based expectations of birth led to intensely painful births. Dick-Read promoted the unheard-of concept that fear leads directly to muscular tension (or resisting contractions), which creates the sort of pain that makes a woman feel she cannot cope without drugs. He emphasized the need for modern women to prepare for birth through a series of simple relaxation exercises that they could then use in labor to give a sense of well-being and diminish pain during contractions.

With his associate Pierre Vellay, Fernand Lamaze put together his views on natural childbirth from observations he made in Russia of Ivan Pavlov's experiments with animals. Pavlov, the physiologist and experimental psychologist, developed a technique that made it possible for the brain to override sensations of pain with rapid, shallow breathing. Lamaze referred to Pavlov's technique as a form of self-hypnosis and believed it could be applied to childbirth. If a woman consciously practiced different kinds of breathing for each phase of labor during birth, he thought, her mind could turn off the most painful sensations of contractions and allow her to give birth in reasonable comfort, without drugs.

Both Dick-Read and Lamaze focused on the crucial role breathing plays in pain relief, and promoted its practice during pregnancy to help women in labor. Dick-Read's and Lamaze's approaches were soundly based in physiology, and both worked. They were also strikingly different and took hold on different continents—Dick-Read's in Europe and Lamaze's in North America. The Dick-Read approach was based on a slow, rhythmic form of breathing. The Lamaze approach was based on several different controlled patterns of breathing, including shallow, rapid breathing and panting, which many animals do at the end of labor. Dick-Read's focused on centering by turning one's attention inward, while Lamaze's focused on centering by distraction.

The National Childbirth Trust (NCT), a grassroots organization of women, was founded in England in 1956 to spread Dick-Read's work, which had no name and no formal technique. Also that year, Marjorie Karmel, a mother, wrote one of the first consumer-authored books on birth, *Thank You, Dr. Lamaze*. Karmel, progressive physician Benjamin Segal, and physiotherapist Elizabeth Bing founded the American Society for Psychoprophylaxis in Obstetrics (informally known as ASPO or Lamaze) in 1960 in New York City. Bing created a series of highly structured childbirth preparation classes around Lamaze's ideas.

Both the NCT and the ASPO found success among educated and progressive-minded women who were not satisfied with the idea of routinely taking drugs for childbirth. Both, along with other childbirth education organizations, encountered strong opposition from physicians, waged public campaigns to gain the confidence of pregnant women, and fought difficult political battles for a foothold in hospitals.

The NCT and the ASPO believed that they were championing the rights of women for self-determination in birth and for birth with dignity. However, for many years the ASPO was made up almost exclusively of nurses and physiotherapists and, perhaps because of that, it tended to place value on drugs to control pain in birth. Lamaze-trained teachers tended to focus on breathing techniques as a way to handle labor until drugs were available and for many years made no effort to dissuade women from using them. Over time, the ASPO began to espouse consumer-related causes such as not separating mothers from their babies after birth, family-centered environments, sibling visitation of the newborn, husbands present during cesarean, vaginal birth after cesarean, and siblings present at birth. Today a nursing degree is not required for entrance into Lamaze teacher training, although a college degree is. Most Lamaze teachers continue to teach in hospital settings and are paid by hospitals or groups of physicians. Although the ASPO has been affiliated with hospitals and obstetricians, it has nevertheless played a very important role in making childbirth a more normal process for millions of mothers and babies. APSO's leadership is taking a radical position by supporting home and birth centers, and discouraging drugs, anesthesia, and bottle feeding.

In 1965, obstetrician Robert Bradley wrote what was a radical book about childbirth preparation based upon Dick-Read's ideas called *Husband-Coached Childbirth*. Bradley gave fathers a prominent role in coaching their mate during labor, so that women did not feel the need for drugs. Marjie and Jay Hathaway, a California couple expecting their fourth child, drove all the way to Colorado to have Dr. Bradley help them with natural childbirth. They and a nurse named Rhonda Hartman then helped Bradley found the American Academy of Husband-Coached Childbirth (also called the Bradley Method) and offered the first teacher training in 1970. Two stated goals of the Bradley Method are to have 90 percent of Bradley-prepared women give birth without medication, and to have a very low cesarean rate. From the beginning, the Bradley Method stressed the importance of excellent nutrition in pregnancy, immediate breast-feeding, and continuous contact with the baby after birth.

The more well-known organization that pushed the ASPO to the left of center was the International Childbirth Education Association (ICEA). Founded in 1960 with no ties to the health-care delivery system, ICEA was originally eclectic in its approach to birth, incorporating sociology, anthropology, and midwifery as well as nursing. ICEA was the first organization to incorporate Sheila Kitzinger's recognition that birth is a psycho-sexual experience.

During the 1970s a second generation of childbirth organizations came into being in both Britain and the United States, and the movement spread to many other countries. This second wave focused on alternatives to standard medical and hospital birth practices. Notable among them is the National Association of Parents and Professionals for Safe Alternatives in Childbirth (NAPSAC). The Stewarts, a couple from North Carolina who founded this organization in the mid-1970s, challenged the assumption that a hospital is the best place for birth and created a series of national conferences to support out-of-hospital birth and midwifery. Rahima Baldwin, a Michigan lay midwife, founded Informed Homebirth in 1977. Like many other organizations of that era, its name changed first to Informed Homebirth, then to Informed Birth and Parenting, and most recently to A.L.A.C.E. These more radical organizations recognized the need to reach women who would never consider a home birth or a midwife.

With the skyrocketing cesarean rate in the United States in the 1980s came the Cesarean Prevention Movement, founded by New York State mother Esther Zorn, who, like Rahima Baldwin, understood that birth is political. After CPM came ICAN, aimed at lowering the cesarean rate by educating women *and* empowering cesarean mothers. These teacher-training programs focus on preventing unnecessary cesareans and increasing the number of women having vaginal births after having cesareans. The underlying premise is that women innately know how to give birth successfully; they need to rediscover their bodies' wisdom and learn how to listen to their bodies. The approach is psychological as well as physiological, and the teachings of a number of prominent authors in the childbirth movement have been drawn upon to create a holistic approach.

Doris Haire, a prominent figure in ICEA and a fighter of the overuse of drugs in maternity care, wrote a radical pamphlet in the early 1970s entitled *The Cultural Warping of Childbirth* (still available through ICEA; see Resources) and then created the Maternal and Child Health Foundation (MCHF). The MCHF was a one-woman organization, run from Haire's home. Its unique purpose was to bring news of the risks of modern medical childbirth to nurses and physicians and to expose them to the growing body of research on alternative practices that promote normal childbirth.

During the 1970s attention was focused on the dietary health of pregnant women and the importance of breast-feeding and breast milk. The international movement back to breast-feeding began in 1956 with the founding of La Leche League in the United States. With a series of postpartum support meetings for mothers (where children were always welcome) and the publication of *The Womanly Art of Breastfeeding* in 1963, La Leche took on the medical establishment and the bottle and formula industry, which for years had been promoting bottle and artificial formula feeding.

The number of books on pregnancy, birth, and baby care aimed at the lay public has mushroomed since the mid-1970s. Two in particular stand out for their radical descriptions of birth, and one of them for its frank images of women giving birth naturally in the setting of their own home.

In 1973 California lay midwife Raven Lang (now a licensed acupuncturist who continues to focus on the care of childbearing women) published *The Birth Book.* This unique book included the stories of women and men who dared to birth their babies at home, without any medical or nursing assistance. Their birth attendants were self-trained. Lang also included a brief history of modern childbirth practices and information about lay midwives and a handful of radical physicians who were beginning to teach at classes and conferences in California and other places in the United States. Most dramatic, however, were the photos. For the first time in recent history, pregnant couples could see how women behave in labor when they are unmedicated and in their own homes, and what the birth of a baby looks like. Even today these photographs would be considered challenging by many people—especially the series of a woman giving birth on her hands and knees, her anus distended at the end of pushing and the baby slipping out into the midwife's hands without the woman's perineum intact.

Also revolutionary and even more far-reaching in its readership (it's still in print) was a book of stories from a community in Tennessee called The Farm. Inspired by Stephen Gaskin, a visionary spiritual teacher at San Francisco State University, several dozen school buses full of men and women took off from the West Coast to find land. Along the way a number of babies were born. Gaskin's wife, Ina May, found herself compelled to participate at these births, and from those unself-conscious beginnings she is today one of the most knowledgeable and skillful midwifery teachers in the U.S. Her book *Spiritual Midwifery* and her *Birth Gazette*, as well as Jan Tritten's *Midwifery Today*, are invaluable.

The stories in *Spiritual Midwifery* displayed the creativity embodied in the new midwifery of the 1970s, which was practiced primarily by well-educated, middle-class women who did not stop to consider the powers they were pitted against when they first felt called to assist a friend or neighbor having a home birth. Like Raven Lang, Gaskin yearned for knowledge that only physicians had and displayed an independent spirit and toughness in the face of problems.

In the late 1970s and early 1980s, every English-speaking country and some non-English-speaking countries saw the rise of radical consumer and midwifery organizations that wanted to take back power and autonomy in everything related to childbirth. The purpose of one such organization, the Midwives Association of North America (MANA), was to draw together midwives from all backgrounds into a strong coalition that could work toward maintaining high standards in midwifery, legalizing (or at least decriminalizing) midwifery in all states, defending midwives from harassment, and finding alternate methods for training midwives so that they could be trained in their own communities rather than in nursing schools. MANA earned the respect of the American College of Nurse Midwives who have struggled to gain a foothold in hospitals and improve care for *all* women. The CNEP program of ACNM today offers strong community-based midwife training.

In Britain, the Association for the Improvement of Maternity Care and the Association of Radical Midwives were determined to put British midwifery back on course and out of the back pocket of physicians, and to press for direct-entry training. The Royal College of Midwives eventually had to pay attention. In 1982 the Active Birth Movement was born when five hundred women marched on the London Royal Free Hospital to demand the right to give birth in an upright position instead of lying down. In the late 1980s the First International Congress on Home Birth was held in London, and nearly 2,000 people from 26 countries attended. The grass roots midwifery and home birth movement continues.

The Advent of Birth Centers in the United States

In the late 1970s, a movement toward out-of-hospital birth centers began. The purpose of these centers was to make it possible for women to control the childbirth environment, to have whomever they wanted with them during the birth, not to be subjected to risky hospital intervention, and to have unbroken contact and privacy with their newborn babies. The movement continues today despite every imaginable obstacle, from physicians refusing to provide obstetrical or pediatric backup, to insurance companies refusing to insure the births at the centers, to state regulatory agencies requiring the centers to have insurance if they want to open their doors. Midwives primarily staff these centers.

Maternity homes and small maternity hospitals were common in most English-speaking countries between 1920 and 1940. A transition from home to hospital, these institutions were usually staffed by midwives or nurses. Some provided a homelike, supportive environment. Current birth centers offer women, their partners, and whoever else they wish to include safe and positive birth experiences. Some centers see themselves as family centered, others as woman centered.

Carefully controlled studies of birth centers have repeatedly shown that they can be safer than hospitals for normal births. One study published in the *New England Journal of Medicine* ("Outcomes of Care in Birth Centers," December 28, 1989) included 11,800 births at eighty-four freestanding birth centers in the United States. The women and babies were followed for four weeks after birth. Among the women admitted for labor at birth centers, 15.8 percent were transferred to a hospital for some medical indication, but only 2.4 percent were emergency transfers. The overall rate of cesarean was 4.4 percent, the neonatal mortality rate was a low 1.3 per 1,000 births, and the health of babies was comparable to that of babies born in hospitals.

Research also shows that women who give birth in birth centers, like women who have home births, feel better about their childbirth experiences than do similar populations of women who have hospital childbirths. Other research shows that women who feel good about their childbirths feel better about their babies and think that their babies are more intelligent and more capable because of their birth experience. The rate of intervention in births at birth centers is consistently much lower than the rate of intervention in hospital births among a similar population of healthy women. Partly, of course, this is due to the fact that women are screened for complications during prenatal care and early labor; those who might have unexpected serious problems are sent to a hospital for delivery. Birth centers are not only cost-effective alternatives to hospitals, they support the *concept* of normal birth.

The interest in taking back control of the birth process, which is so intimately female, began in the second half of this century and went a long way toward transforming the face of childbirth. But the alternative birth movement

> *Some people were very surprised I was paying out-of-pocket for a home birth with a midwife, when I was fully insured for a hospital birth with a doctor. I would tell them, "It's worth it!" I knew the difference it would make in the kind of experience I had. I was talking to another nurse at the hospital where I worked, who wanted to know how much my home birth cost. I told her, and she said, "That's all! It would be worth a lot more than that not to have it here."*
>
> —OBSTETRIC NURSE

has yet to achieve its goal of returning childbirth to a healthy, normal process, with birthing women and their partners acting as the authorities and the health-care system there only to support them. Looking back, one cannot deny the many gains that were made on behalf of all women and babies. But in the last decade and a half the alternative birth movement has lost its foothold, in part because of seeming "advances" on the part of hospitals. Many hospitals made an effort to make birth a more positive experience, often installing birthing rooms with wallpaper and other homey touches. Parents were deluded into thinking that they had more control over childbirth, but the truth is that the basic attitudes and policies of the hospitals have stayed unchanged. Control of birth remains in the hands of physicians, and invasive procedures and the unnecessary use of high-tech devices are still common despite more pleasant surroundings.

The Midwife Debate

"I've been placed in handcuffs three times in my life. The first two times were in the 1960s; when I was giving birth I was handcuffed to the de-livery table—like every other woman in labor those days—to keep me from touching my baby. And then in August 1991, I was arrested at my home—my youngest daughter had to watch it happen—and taken to jail for assisting women who give birth at home."

These words were spoken by a forty-eight-year-old woman, an apprentice-trained domiciliary midwife based in Palo Alto, California, named Faye Gibson. Like more than one hundred women since 1973, Gibson was arrested, jailed, and forced to wage a costly defense simply because she had built a practice assisting families who had chosen to give birth in their own home.

Gibson was a nurse for fifteen years in Florida but left the profession after fighting unsuccessfully to change the hospital system. She had been part of too many births in which invasive practices were routine, and she believed these in-terventions were both unnecessary and risky. These practices became so standard that Gibson could no longer continue to be a nurse in good conscience. Most of the midwives arrested for doing home births have not been to nursing school or nurse-midwifery programs, but are skilled through a combination of appren-ticeship, reading medical and midwifery texts, and attending training confer-ences. Even Certified Nurse-Midwives are not safe from prosecution in the U.S. if they attend home births. Like other midwives, the core of Gibson's skill lies

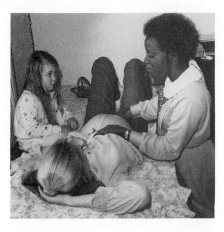

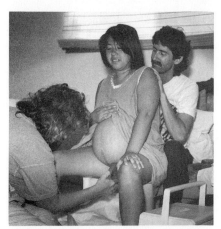

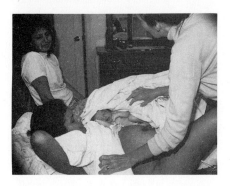

Midwives

Unlike the majority of doctors, midwives *expect* childbirth to be normal and women to be competent. They practice their craft wherever a woman is most comfortable: at home, in a birth center, or in a hospital. Midwives offer prenatal care that is usually more intimate than the care doctors provide. They also spend more time with the birthing mother. In labor they stay with a woman and can anticipate and prevent problems. If problems occur, midwives try to handle them with natural aids instead of resorting immediately to medical intervention.

Midwives pride themselves on caring for a woman's body *and* psyche, and on helping mothers and babies remain together after the birth. They view childbirth as a social, not a medical, event, and the family as a whole unit. Most of the world's babies are delivered by midwives.

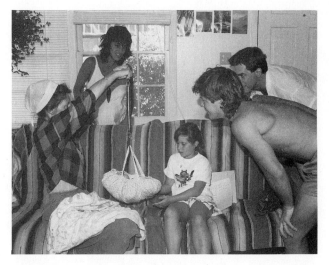

Top: A midwife explains to a four-year-old girl how she is measuring the mother's tummy to see how big the baby inside is. Middle: A midwife kneels and waits to catch the baby. Left: Keeping the baby on the mother's warm skin, a midwife waits for the placenta to come out. Above: An hour after the birth, after the parents have had time in private with their baby, a midwife shows everyone how to weigh the baby in a warm blanket using a fish scale.

in being able to tell the difference between a pregnancy or labor that is progressing normally and one that is not. As is true of a family physician or nurse-practitioner, she is trained to recognize complications immediately, but does not need to know the appropriate treatment for a serious medical condition. She simply needs to refer her client—or if the immediacy of the situation calls for it, bring her client—to a specialist, an obstetrician, or a pediatrician.

The public today believes that subspecialists, such as obstetricians and neo-natologists, are the physicians we need to see when we have a health problem. In fact, the evidence demonstrates that subspecialist physicians, like specialized "high-risk" hospitals, are an ill-fitting match for patients with ordinary medical needs. They tend to administer many expensive, often unnecessary tests, spend their time looking for rare diseases rather than treating the whole person, and far too often prescribe costly and risky drugs and surgery. Subspecialists tend to complicate childbirth rather than make it safer.

In most cases, midwives are prosecuted when they are not licensed nurse-midwives. The catch-22 is that in many states there is no way for someone to legally train or practice as a midwife—there are very few midwifery schools—without a nursing degree. But not even becoming a nurse-midwife will protect you from discrimination. Nurse-midwives are continually refused privileges in hospitals and denied physician backup for their patients. Even family physicians find themselves under attack for attending births if there is an obstetrician in the vicinity. Many rural counties in the United States do not have obstetricians practicing in the area, yet obstetricians have banded together to deny midwives the right to provide care there either.

The arrest of a midwife usually results in the woman either choosing to go through nursing training as the only available means of becoming "legal," or abandoning the craft that she felt was her deepest calling. The loss of a midwife is always deeply felt. It is costly to the individual midwife, to her family—especially her children—and to the community, which is then left with one less person to assist in home births. Fewer and fewer physicians and nurse-midwives dare to do home births in such a hostile political climate.

The case against Faye Gibson, a Mennonite who considers herself a religious practitioner at birth and who only attends women seeking home birth as part of their religious faith, was ultimately dropped. (Midwives are rarely convicted.) But despite the many contributions she received to pay for her defense, Gibson, like every other midwife placed on trial, was left with a heavy personal debt and no well-heeled professional organization to pay it.

Few people who hear about the arrest of a midwife stop to consider what it means. Most assume the midwife must have endangered a mother's or a baby's life. Not true—it usually has to do with licensing. Gibson's case is typical. Having practiced for more than ten years in the same community, she never had a complaint lodged against her by a client and no mother or baby injuries had been associated with her care. She had never been negligent; but she was charged with practicing medicine and nursing and nurse-midwifery without a license. (In the rare cases where injury is involved in a case against a midwife, it is often found that the mother or baby would most likely have suffered the same damage in a hospital, that the injury or death was unavoidable no matter where it occurred.)

The choice of giving birth outside a hospital is being restricted more every day. And everyone's democratic right to quality health care is slowly but surely chipped whenever individuals are restrained from choosing the form of health care they feel is best for them. This is true whether the individual wishes to see an osteopathic, homeopathic, or naturopathic physician, an acupuncturist, or an herbalist to treat a physical ailment, or a midwife to assist in a normal birth.

Physicians tend to frame the argument as a question of whether a parent has the right to jeopardize the well-being of his or her baby by seeking a birth outside a hospital, but that is a completely inaccurate reading of the situation. It is the question of whether, in a society that supposedly protects the rights of minorities, healthy people who believe that a hospital is not the safest or most wholesome place to give birth have the right to make an alternative choice. As it now stands, in most countries where midwives and physicians are susceptible to prosecution, individuals still have the right to a home birth; what they are being denied is access to a skilled attendant. And that endangers their health.

Ever since Yale University Hospital physicians received notice in 1975 that any doctor (or nurse-midwife) present at a home birth will lose the right to practice in that hospital, other institutions have followed suit, telling doctors and nurse-midwives that they cannot attend any birth out of the hospital. Insurance companies, greatly swayed by organized medicine's powerful lobbying efforts,

> *Most of the reasons for hospitalization have to do with physician convenience and have nothing to do with the patient. I always encourage people, "Get out as soon as you can. Take your baby home as soon as you can."*
>
> —PEDIATRICIAN

refuse to cover nurse-midwives or physicians who attend births out of the hospital, even if it is in a licensed birth center. A few doctors and midwives dare to do it anyway and are willing to give up their malpractice coverage. For the most part, they quickly discover that no physician will provide backup or be on-call for them when they go on vacation, need a day off, or get sick.

Several states throughout the U.S. do not prohibit the practice of non-nurse midwives, allowing them to operate birth centers and use physician backup. However, they will never be paid by an insurance company. Any woman who goes to them will have to pay out of pocket. Fortunately, the cost of a midwife is far less than what physicians charge, and midwives' fees include home visits and postpartum care, which physicians' do not.

One of the answers to the midwifery crisis lies in decriminalizing midwives and making it possible for people to train, prove their level of skill, and practice without a license. Licensing health professionals has not kept bad medical practice to a minimum; health-care workers are now fearful of practicing in ways they know are effective and appropriate lest they lose their license for "failure to practice the community standard"—rigid standards set by a few prestigious medical centers that promote a high-tech approach.

Despite protracted and widespread opposition, midwives are forging ahead because they know their services are important. They have created organizations to implement standards of care, offer alternative forms of training, and change the laws. Public health studies have revealed that the United States needs far more midwives than can presently be trained. We must have community-based training.

Today in the United States there are under forty nurse-midwifery programs, but that number is steadily growing. However, these programs take place in high-risk hospitals, and there is little or no training in out-of-hospital settings (home and birth centers), which many students want. Midwives are fighting to get the kind of training they know they need in order to be independent practitioners working alongside, but not under, physicians. They need education that focuses on keeping birth normal, *preventing* problems, and handling those that come up as simply as possible.

In the case of Faye Gibson, the county district attorney, after vigorously pursuing conviction for a year, suddenly dropped all charges and the judge dismissed the case. The public heard much about her arrest but little about why the case was dropped. The district attorney stated publicly that "the interests of justice would not be served in prosecuting (Ms. Gibson). There's no sense in spending taxpayers' money on a trial." And in a complete turnaround, he added, "It's not illegal for anyone to deliver a baby." But, in effect, it is illegal.

Physicians often claim they cannot back a midwife or see her clients because they are fearful of being held liable in case of malpractice. Creating a system in which midwives are autonomous—that is, do not have to work under the "supervision" of a doctor—as in the Netherlands, will aid and protect physicians. Creating a clear distinction between the practices of medicine and nursing, and the practice of midwifery, would allow midwives to be responsible for conforming to the standards of good midwifery care rather than medical care. The difference is vast.

As the debate on how to ensure universal high-quality health care currently rages in the United States it should be obvious that the traditional practice of midwifery—supporting normal childbirth—could be a large part of the solution.

Mothering the Mother: A Case for the Doula

If midwife is the first word pregnant women should be well acquainted with, doula is the second. Doula (pronounced "*doo*la") is a woman who provides continuous support during labor and who may also help out in the first days home after the childbirth. A doula helps a nurse by giving the pregnant woman or new mother the attention she so desperately needs.

Today, nurses find themselves unable to provide that attention because so much of their time is taken up charting, handling equipment, and participating in cesarean surgery, and because there is often inadequate staffing.

A doula stays with the woman at all times throughout the childbirthing process. As an outsider, she can be more objective than a family member, and as a nonmedical professional, she is not forced to enforce hospital policy, as nurses often must do. Most of all, a doula's primary function is to ease the childbirth experience, enabling the woman in labor to give herself entirely to the process of childbirth. Afterward the doula provides the mother—and also the father and any other family members present—with an umbrella of protection, guarding them against hospital procedures and regulations that so often block intimacy. The first few hours after birth are a precious time, a state of heightened consciousness and vulnerability for both mother and baby. This bubble can be broken so easily by any number of intrusions. Unfortunately, hospitals are often infamous for intrusive and sometimes unnecessary procedures done for their own records. The new family needs privacy to focus their attention on being with their new baby, not to be dealing with external details. And the presence of a doula extends this much-needed support.

In the early 1990s a series of papers was published on the outcome of several doula studies conducted in Texas, Guatemala, and South Africa. The results illustrated the dramatic impact that a woman in a nonmedical, non-nursing role—present throughout labor—can have. Pediatrician/researchers John Kennell and Marshall Klaus and psychotherapist/teacher Phyllis Klaus conducted this research by comparing a control group of women who did not have a doula with a group of women who did. The doula was not a person familiar to the laboring woman.

The results of these studies reveal that simply introducing doulas into the current hospital system could transform childbirth. Women in labor reap the benefits of having a doula; here are just some of the reasons why:

1. On average, the length of labor was significantly shorter with a doula (by 25 percent for first-time mothers).

2. There was a dramatic reduction in the use of artificial hormones to speed up labor. This is significant—not only because oxytocic drugs make labor harder to handle and result in women taking more drugs for pain relief—but because the use of artificial stimulants during labor is associated with medical complications in newborns. (These complications include increased incidence of jaundice, the treatment of which usually separates a baby from its mother.)

3. There was a marked reduction in the use of epidural anesthesia and the number of mothers asking for it. Not only are fewer women exposed to the known hazards of spinal anesthesia, but fewer babies land in the intensive care nursery as a result of possible systemic infection.

4. In seven trials, the cesarean rate was reduced by 60 percent!

5. Fewer babies had to stay in the hospital after the mother was discharged.

6. Twice as many women breast-fed their babies and continued to breast-feed longer than those in the control group.

In the South African study, researchers observed the new mothers for six weeks after childbirth and conducted thorough psychological studies on them. The women who gave birth with the aid of doulas were significantly less anxious about their baby, both the day after birth and six weeks later. The number of women who experienced depression six weeks after birth was cut in half. The sense of being supported and valued during labor—a feeling that a doula helps to bring about—has positive and lasting effects on a woman's self-esteem and her confidence as a mother.

A mother's feelings of self-worth have a great deal to do with how she views and treats her baby. When the doula-supported mothers were compared with the control group, they ranked their own baby as much more capable than other babies of the same age. And so did the fathers!

For years many observers of the childbirth scene have strongly recommended to women giving birth in hospitals—especially first-time mothers—that, in addition to a partner, or family members and friends, they bring a woman who will be with them throughout labor to advocate on their behalf. Many demur, naively believing the hospital staff will grant them privacy, and whatever support and care they need. "Oh, my husband and I are very private," women often say. "We don't want to have anyone else there." But the doula studies illustrate what an advantage it is to have a woman companion during labor.

A doula is not a replacement for the baby's father. Instead, she frees him from feeling totally responsible for his partner's well-being. Childbirth classes in the past have focused on the father as a coach. This may fit with the old cultural view of a man as a protector, but it doesn't serve the real needs of most fathers. A man needs the same emotional freedom during labor as the mother does; he is becoming a father. If we want men to participate fully in the nurturing of their children, we must make room for their experiences.

Women who are fortunate to have a midwife while giving birth—especially those who have already established a relationship with the midwife during pregnancy—probably do not need a doula. But with the continuing campaign in the United States to restrict or eliminate midwifery, most women will give birth in a hospital with a physician who only appears at the end. For these women, the single most important decision they can make during their pregnancy may be to find a doula. For more information about doulas, read *Mothering the Mother* (see Bibliography).

What We Share with Other Animals:
The Need for Privacy

A Dutch physician and researcher named Cornelius Naaktgeboren was through the 1970s and until the early 1980s professor of animal physiology in the department of obstetrics in the Netherlands' largest and most prestigious medical school. There he studied and documented the impact of lack of privacy or interruption on the birth process of animals and compared human and animal birth. This may be the only known case of an animal researcher being placed as a tenured professor in an obstetric teaching department. He was there because the chair of the department was Dr. G. J. Kloosterman, a man renowned for his consistent support of birth as a normal process and the central role that midwifery plays in keeping birth normal, as well as his resistance to the takeover of Dutch maternity units by technology and intervention. Professor Kloosterman believed that there are many similarities between human birth and animal birth and that the study of animals could teach doctors a great deal about how to support normalcy and prevent problems in childbirth.

Naaktgeboren (whose surname aptly translates as "born naked") produced a series of short films on animals in birth. In one enlightening film of a wild red deer in the process of giving birth, we see just how an animal's fear of imminent danger creates tension in her body and completely stops her uterine contractions. Her body's need to prepare for immediate flight halts all progress, even though labor was active and birth imminent. Her body cannot do two contradictory things at once: be on guard and let go. She quickly abandons her place in the trees to search for a safer place. The hidden camera quietly tracks her. Once she finds a place of privacy where she feels safe, her body relaxes and is drained of tension, and her contractions renew without interference.

There are two key points to this film. It shows how privacy is essential to a sense of security for a birthing animal. And it shows how the uterine muscles and all of the hormones that are engaged in the process of birth act in a coordinated fashion and will actually stop labor, even when it is far advanced, in order to permit the animal to focus her entire being on preparation for flight.

From other researchers of large mammals we hear stories of how elephants create a ring of protection around a female in labor. One of the elephants may even push her over onto the ground, a position in which she is helpless to protect herself from harm. The other elephants then turn their back to her from the periphery of the circle, and in that ring of security and privacy the female elephant delivers her baby.

Naaktgeboren found that he himself was, on more than one occasion, the cause of fear-initiated obstruction of the birth process in the laboratory.

> I observed that one young rabbit was already expelled, and I tried to catch the rest of the births on film. Although I waited for over two hours nothing happened, whereas normally the expulsion phase for an entire litter of rabbits does not take more than about ten minutes. I decided to leave the room for a short time. Upon my return twenty minutes later, I found thirteen newborn rabbits.

Rabbits, unlike large animals or humans, have babies that are much smaller than the size of the mother's pelvic outlet. Thus ordinarily there is hardly any labor at all; the babies are more or less squirted out. On the other hand, in humans and other large mammals labor normally takes some amount of time, because the size of the baby is very close to the size of the pelvic outlet and the baby must be slowly squeezed and pushed through a rather tight-fitting pelvis and down a rather narrow birth canal, the muscles of which must stretch and open to allow the baby out. Anyone who has grown up on a farm has probably had an experience similar to Naaktgeboren's, where a person's presence caused a delay in an animal's labor. A mare will often deliver her foal only when the nervous breeder or farmer, or a well-intentioned veterinarian, momentarily disappears from sight and the mother can no longer smell the foreign presence. Because the process of human birth is physiologically longer than for most mammals, owing to the relatively tight fit of the baby's head through the mother's pelvis, there is even more opportunity for it to be disturbed.

AN IMPORTANT LESSON TO LEARN:
DO NOT DISTURB

Modern women may not like to be compared with other mammals when it comes to natural physiological functioning in childbirth. But we are more like other mammals than we are dissimilar, and there is much we can learn from animals about how to have uncomplicated births. Naaktgeboren's classic studies of sheep illustrate how unnatural disturbances during labor can cause such severe delays in uterine contractions that the animals need veterinary assistance to deliver. At that point, without some assistance or intervention, a ewe might deliver a dead lamb or die herself from protracted labor. In his studies of cattle, dogs, and rats, Naaktgeboren also found that disturbances of the maternal environment created by mere observers or helpers not only prolonged labor but resulted in a much higher death rate among newborns.

As women, we need to give each other information, especially about the possible consequences of different choices. When a woman is under lots of pressure, in a situation she may feel she has little control over such as giving birth, she needs information more than anything.

—FEMALE PHYSICIAN

Convinced by his research of the importance of a woman having privacy during labor and of the important role a midwife rather than an obstetrician could play in protecting the normal process, Naaktgeboren in his final film on birth showed a woman giving birth at home. She uses relaxation techniques based in yoga practice to put herself in a mental state conducive to a natural, normal birth. In the film you see a woman who is secure in her own natural environment—her home—freely moving around and spontaneously choosing positions that facilitate the birth process. Much of the time she is on her feet or squatting. There is no need for intervention of any kind. She simply needs reassurance that all is well from her midwife or her husband at those times when she loses confidence. She gives birth on her own and you can see, hear, and palpably feel the ecstatic response she has right afterward as she cradles her newborn child in her arms, knowing that she has accomplished this amazing feat all by herself.

Physician-researcher Naaktgeboren finished his long career in obstetrics feeling certain that most of the pathology we hear so much about in modern childbirth is created by hospital environments and physician intervention. He wrote, "In textbooks it is written that contractions, when irregular, frighten women. Women then become anxious. This is not true. It is the other way around. Even if the woman herself is convinced of the importance of being in a hospital, the changing surroundings may influence her inner biological rhythms."

The Ecology of Birth

Ecology, the study of the interrelationships of organisms and their environment, is based on the principle that we are connected with and dependent on each other and the world around us for our survival.

Our bodies also have a natural ecology. For many years we have been systematically destroying that ecology in the same way that we have been destroying the earth. Nowhere is this more clearly demonstrated than in childbearing and the mother-baby care. Women whose bodies seem to be going into early labor spend months on a regimen of bed rest and drugs. The drugs they take produce a constant flow of adrenaline-like substances that produce a continual state of anxiety. These same drugs flood their babies' bodies. Today most women go through labor numb from the waist down. One out of four women is anesthetized and prepped for major surgery, cut open, and has her baby pulled out. Even when life-saving, it's traumatic to the human body.

Mothers and their babies are separated for every conceivable excuse after birth and spend much of their hours or days apart. After they return home with their baby, mothers and fathers find themselves isolated, unprepared, and unsupported for the major adjustments they must make to parenthood.

Many babies come through birth with drugs in their bodies that were never intended for them, or with drugs that were intended to force their intrauterine development. Many not only find themselves separated from their mother's body, but are given artificial nourishment; it is nothing like breast milk, and they must take it from plastic and glass containers and through silicone rubber or plastic nipples that are nothing like a fragrant, soft-skinned mother's breast. Sucking from a bottle does not satisfy either their physiological or their psychological needs. If they are baby boys, and they live in the United States, they most likely will have a vital part of their penis surgically removed without anesthetic. Babies of both sexes have routine tests and procedures done to them that are painful and have negative side effects, and they often spend time in brightly lighted and noisy hospital nurseries where the physical environment is upsetting to the natural rhythm of their bodies or can cause outright trauma.

When babies leave the hospital they find that many of their basic needs for nourishment, comfort, and affection continue not to be met according to their natural rhythm but are subject to the clock or an adult's convenience. As adults,

"Feminizing" Maternity Care

"Feminizing" maternity care means bringing qualities traditionally associated with women into the way we care for birthing mothers, babies, and families. The ability to listen and be receptive and nurturing are the primary qualities birth attendants need.

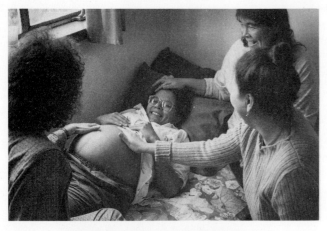

A childbearing woman cannot expect a more "feminine" approach simply because she chooses a female care provider. Some men are supportive and protective of the natural process; some women won't stand for a patient disagreeing with them and intervene aggressively when a problem arises.

It is imperative that the midwife, doctor, or nurse does not take advantage of a woman's vulnerability in childbearing and her need to trust those around her. The power needs to remain firmly with the woman, her body, her baby. Whether or not she knows it, the mother is the expert.

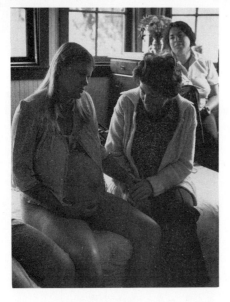

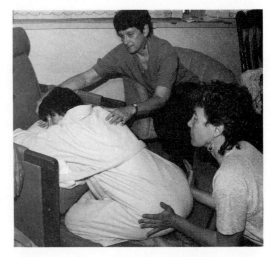

Top: Women need help making room for a baby emotionally; this requires some time and a lot of listening. Left: Sometimes a woman's own mother is the best support—here, a midwife sits quietly in the background, her mere presence reassuring. Right: Acupressure can help relieve the pain and tension of labor.

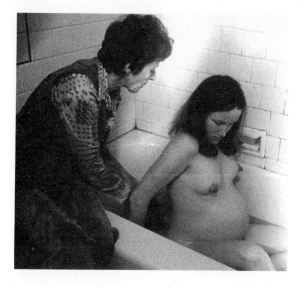

Feminizing birth means that those who assist take the lead from the woman (which may mean helping her discover what she instinctively knows) and stay in the background, allowing mother and baby to conduct the experience. When problems require birth attendants to be advisers and/or skilled technicians, they must ask themselves: Am I acting out of a need to be in control or am I acting in the true service of the mother?

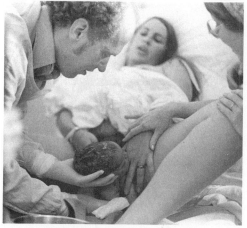

A woman needs the support and care of others before, during, and after childbirth. Her body should be lovingly attended to. After the birth, home visits by a midwife, nurse, or home health attendant who also checks in with other members of the family can be especially supportive and beneficial.

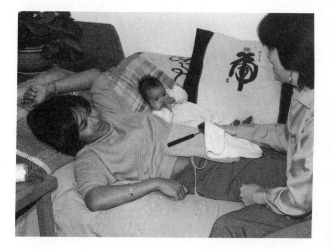

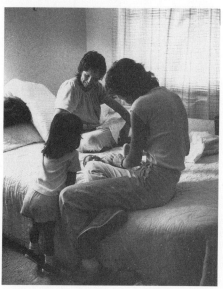

we often come to our babies so disconnected from ourselves and from them, and with so many other priorities, that we find it difficult to interpret their pleas. We are encouraged at every turn to place physical and psychological distance between ourselves and our babies, in the mistaken belief that this will make our babies more independent.

Simply stated, we are numb to how much we have deformed the processes of childbirth and child care and ignorant of the harm that we inflict on ourselves and our babies. The saddest victims are the babies themselves. So much of what parents and health workers unwittingly do causes them to feel afraid, isolated, and abandoned. The nurses, midwives, and mothers who are aware of the situation find themselves deeply frustrated by a culture and a health care system that are guided by one overriding principle: maximizing production and profit with the least amount of human involvement. The medical care system responds to changes in technology and procedures much faster than it does to the need for humane and ecological health care.

> *A mother's breast milk changes to meet the needs of her baby. Its content is different during various times of the day, over the months as the baby grows, and with each individual mother for each individual child. No formula can duplicate this perfect primary food.*

Drugs, technology, and surgery should be used in the service of the whole person and the whole relationship of mother, child, and the entire family. Not to do so creates human beings who are disconnected from their bodies and from the earth. Today childbirth and parenting may be the worst ecological disaster areas of all. With all the medical technology at our disposal, we've lost sight of what a human needs to remain healthy and vital. Physically, we have an increasing incidence of immune-system breakdown and chronic degenerative diseases. Emotionally, we see increasing numbers of detachment disorders, child abuse, and neglect. By living, giving birth, and parenting without regard to human needs, we become disconnected from our bodies and the earth. Then we behave in ways that do damage to both. It is by being intimately connected to one another that we can learn what it is to be connected to life as a whole. We must pay attention to what is natural and normal and follow that course, or the long-term price we pay will be dear.

Modern medicine cannot duplicate the authentic experience of childbirth or child care. No system, no hospital, no professional can ever give us the joy that comes with having completed the journey of birth ourselves. Our task is to re-learn respect for the entire process of birth, beginning with conception and ending when the baby begins to toddle away from the mother and explore the world on its own. At the heart of the ecological crisis in birth is the splitting apart of the mother-baby diad. Such splitting began with the industrial revolution, when a person's worth was gauged by how much they produced and how many goods they consumed. In such a world babies have no real value, and neither do mothers. The human body is simply a complex piece of machinery and a mother, and father too, is replaceable by almost any other adult.

Ecologically, mothers and babies (and fathers) benefit in every way from close physical contact, rhythmic movement, eye contact, and the continuous presence of each other during the first year of life. Breast-feeding is a fundamental part of this bond, increasing intimacy, but the mother must be nurtured and supported by the adults around so she can give easily to her baby. Not only is this the best, easiest, and least costly way to meet the baby's needs, it is also the best, easiest, and least costly way for a mother's body and psyche to recuperate from the huge physiogical changes and demands placed upon it by pregnancy and childbirth. From this ecology comes whole people, capable of living joyfully, even in the midst of great hardship.

By moving birth away from the home, work away from the neighborhood, and men and women into the workplace without their babies and children, we damaged human ecology. Society's way of caring for mothers and babies in two separate domains creates a uniquely modern crisis—human beings as an orphaned species, separated too early from their mothers, fathers, and community, disabled by a wound to the soul. This wound creates a sense of loneliness and isolation, where we are cut off from our source, and what begins as an ecological crisis becomes a spiritual one. If we are fortunate, we make our way in the world and, with great effort, find ways to fill the longing for connection that began at birth. If not, we turn to anything that dulls the pain.

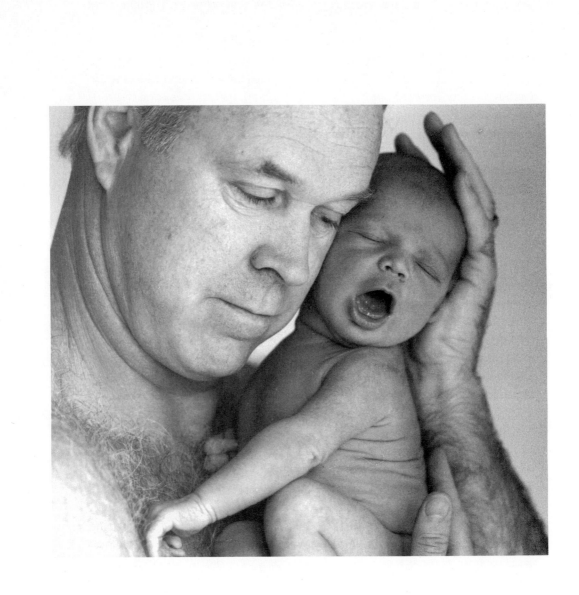

CHAPTER SIX

The Care of Babies:
Before, During, and After Birth

The Paradox of Babies: Separate Yet Dependent

EVERY BABY IN THE WOMB is an astronaut of inner space. The umbilical cord connects it to the mother ship and its life-support system. Although the baby depends on its mother's body for survival, the baby's body is not simply passive. As a simple organism of just a few cells, it began to grow its own placenta, the blood-filled organ connected to the water-filled sac in which the fetus lives while in the womb. The placenta attaches itself to the inside of the womb and transmits oxygen-filled blood from the mother to the baby until after the baby is born. Only then does it shear off and leave the mother's body, after which the open blood vessels at the raw site of the womb close down, stop the flow of blood, and are reabsorbed into the mother's body.

It is an elegant, symbiotic process, and it is now understood that a baby is not immediately separate from its mother even after its birth. It continues to need the bacteria from her skin and the colostrum and breast milk she provides to be protected and to thrive. A baby's hormones and patterns of dreaming during its first few months outside its mother's body are synchronized with the mother's. The baby may even need the vibration of her body's energy and the sound of her heartbeat to keep its heart beating regularly when it is asleep. The mother is calmed by the hormones produced in her body when she knows her baby is nearby and safe. Each time she breast-feeds, if feeding is going well, she is internally bathed with hormones that produce a feeling of well-being. And breast-feeding does the same for her baby, providing the baby with much more than nourishing liquid.

We can truly say that a baby and its mother continue to be a symbiotic unit, each benefiting from and being deeply affected by the presence of the other for many months after birth. Unlike the offspring of most large mammals, human babies cannot stand, follow their mothers, or forage for food until many months have passed and much development has taken place in the nervous system and brain, and in the musculoskeletal system. During those months we are truly dependent on others for our survival. More than that, infants require a close relationship with at least one adult in order to develop a sense of trust.

The Baby's First Task Beyond Survival

The development of trust, it has been shown, is the human being's first psychological and spiritual task in life. It cannot do this unless it is cared for in an intimate way. Merely seeing that an infant is fed adequately and kept warm and dry does not automatically meet any of its emotional needs, as research in orphanages has clearly demonstrated. Not only that, human babies need to hear language spoken in order to develop language. The capacity to speak lies within every baby, but if the child is deprived of warm human contact—the stimulation and comfort of tender touch and spoken language—it may never be able to trust another person and it may not develop speech. Babies develop trust most easily when they are lovingly cared for by one or two individuals over the first year of life. It is during the first two years of life that babies learn the most and learn most rapidly. But the time just after birth is now believed to be the greatest potential learning time of all.

People often ask why this should be so. Why is what happens at the time of birth so important, and why does it make such lasting impact on us, since we have no language at that time and have no memory of what happened to us then? First of all, it is now understood that babies are learning language and are communicating constantly from the time of birth. Second, being unable to say words does not keep a baby from forming lasting impressions or patterns of behavior right from birth. Third, it is being documented more and more that we *do* have strong impressions and even memories of the things that happen to us during the time of birth, but for most of us those memories are not conscious. Parents are shocked when their two-year-old, who has just begun to talk in full sentences, will say something about an incident that they know happened long before the child was able to talk. How could this be? The answer lies in the way our bodies receive and store sensory input, and the fact that we are able to communicate with our body long before we are able to use language.

Brain physiologists now understand some of the mechanisms by which early experiences leave their traces in our brain and other parts of our body. These primal experiences affect the way our system organizes itself. Later experiences of a similar nature continue to affect us in later life, whether or not we are conscious of the roots of our reactions. Early experiences of a similar nature create lifelong patterns, tendencies to respond to similar situations in the same way we responded when we first experienced them. Why should this be so? The simplest answer is that first impressions tend to last. Think about the first impression you had of some place or some person; it is indelibly imprinted on your mind, even though later experiences might alter that impression.

Babies Are Just Like Us

Early in this century, before the pediatrician Dr. Spock conceived his first book on baby care, a physician named Robert Aldrich wrote the book *Babies Are Human,* in which he entreated people to stop and look at the inhuman way we were treating infants. Today, in an age where there is a much more widespread understanding of the nature and prevalence of child abuse and neglect, and a strong interest in parent-child bonding, we continue to treat babies as if they weren't fully human.

Today we know a great deal about the phenomenon known as PTSD—post-traumatic stress disorder—and we allocate resources to treat soldiers traumatized in war, rape victims, or schoolchildren suffering from the shock of a classmate being murdered in the school yard. Yet the culture does nothing to treat infants traumatized during fetal life or at the time of birth. Most people, including health workers, do not even consider the possibility that a baby might need to have psychological healing. Yet the perinatal experiences of many babies are traumatic.

Not all unpleasant experiences, even when physically painful, are traumatic, and pain alone does not necessarily produce long-lasting harm or trauma. Trauma consists of physical or mental pain combined with an element of shock, along with the inability to get away from whatever is causing the pain. How emotionally sensitive a person is at the time an event occurs also makes a difference. Just as an adult's threshold for tolerating pain changes along with his or

Babies in the Womb

Although there has long been speculation that babies in the womb are much more conscious than we have given them credit for, it was not until the late twentieth century that scientific research revealed their capabilities.

Modern technology provides us with the ability to document fetal responsiveness. Through ultrasound one can see into the womb, and by inserting instruments into the amniotic sac one can observe, from early on in gestation, a baby clearly responding to its environment. Numerous studies have documented expressions on fetuses' faces and their attempts to get out of the way of unpleasant stimuli, such as the poke of a needle. When it comes too close to them, babies have even been observed to bat at a needle taking amniotic fluid from the sac.

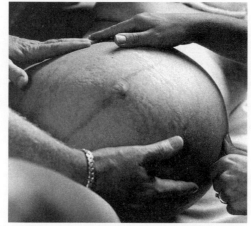

The fetus, who can taste by fourteen weeks, will swallow amniotic fluid more often when it has been injected with something to make it extra sweet. By the time the mother feels her baby moving inside her, usually sometime between the fourth and fifth months, the fetus is already reaching for and grasping its umbilical cord, scratching, opening its mouth, and rubbing its hands and feet.

Vision, too, develops before birth. Though the eyelids are shut until the twenty-sixth week, the fetus responds by movement to light flashed onto the mother's abdomen. As for hearing, research has proved that babies can hear while in the womb; they can distinguish—and do prefer—their mother's voice to all others. The sense of smell develops last, but, within days after its birth, a baby can distinguish between its mother's scent and that of any other woman.

Research also shows that babies become socially oriented in the womb. They like stimulation, but they can be overstimulated as well as neglected. Just as ancient people believed, a crucial relationship develops between baby and mother long before birth.

With thought and planning, much can be done to improve the quality of a baby's experiences within the womb, during the birthing process, and in the first days of life. Pregnant women must insist on receiving the services and support they need to have comfortable pregnancies and diminish the stress of birth. After the birth, parents and their babies should have uninterrupted private time to get to know each other. Procedures should be kept to a minimum. If a procedure on a newborn is necessary, it should be done in a parent's presence whenever possible, and the baby should be comforted afterward.

Preventing and healing trauma in the pre- and perinatal periods may well lead to a happier and healthier child and a closer parent-child relationship. For more information on how pregnancy and birth can affect babies, read David Chamberlain's book *Babies Remember Birth* (see Bibliography). □

her mental state, a baby may or may not find a painful situation tolerable or a particular experience traumatic. How the baby reacts depends on a number of things, including how sudden and unexpected the event is and how vulnerable the baby is at the moment when it happens.

As we discussed earlier, all human babies are born in a very immature state in which their organs, and especially their central nervous system, are not able to function at full capacity for many weeks or months. A newborn baby is innately vulnerable. Physically, it is particularly susceptible to lowered body temperature and infection, but it is physically vulnerable largely because it is so totally dependent on someone outside itself to provide it with food and keep it warm and dry. For example, if a newborn's head remains wet for very long, the baby will lose enough heat from the head alone to go into dangerous hypothermia. Yet a baby cannot protect its own head and must rely on another person to keep it warm and dry.

Fortunately, the mother's body naturally provides just what her baby physically needs. Snuggled up skin-to-skin against its mother, a baby remains warm, and in her presence it is less likely to pick up a bacterial infection, because her skin, the first fluid from her breast called colostrum, and her breast milk all give the baby protection from bacteria.

Every newborn is also vulnerable psychologically. A baby emerges from the womb prepared for the sight of a human face and the sound of the human voice, but not just any face or voice. What it searches for is the face

At the special-care nursery of the hospital where I gave birth, they weren't going to let me breast-feed my daughter for at least a week. They said she could have pumped breast milk but that breast-feeding would burn up too many calories. I'm a doctor. I called the director of the hospital nursery at home at eleven o'clock that night and told him, "You have to get me out of here." I went to another hospital where they were far more progressive. They let me nurse and even allowed grandparents and siblings into the special-care nursery.

—PEDIATRICIAN AND MOTHER

and the voice of its own mother. Each newborn is biologically organized to need physical and emotional contact with its mother. And it has amazing abilities right after birth to interest its mother in taking care of it.

We are only beginning to look at evidence—including our own gut feelings—that human beings are particularly sensitive at and around the time of their birth. A newborn baby is definitely not a blank slate, as it was thought to be just a century ago in our culture. A baby comes into the world with its own temperament and tendencies toward responding to its environment in certain ways. Beyond that, it is continually affected and shaped by everything that goes on around it. A newborn infant is a highly impressionable creature. Labor does not dull its sensitivity; it heightens it.

Human babies are born in a heightened state of awareness, unless they are born unconscious or numbed due to drugs given to their mothers. If a baby has been allowed to go through the entire labor under its own power, being squeezed and pushed down the birth canal has stimulated and stressed it in a particular way that produces its heightened state. A baby is meant to emerge from its mother's body aware of everything that goes on and geared for survival.

Studies over the last several decades have shown just how capable newborn babies are, especially in getting the attention of the adults around them and getting their needs met. A newborn baby who has not had the disadvantage of having drugs in its body is very discriminating. It can distinguish between the scent of its own mother's breast milk and the breast milk of any other mother after just a few times at her breast. It also prefers the sound of its mother's voice to any other voice.

In a remarkable study done in Sweden in the early 1990s, newborns were immediately placed naked on their reclining mother's abdomens. The mothers were instructed not to respond to or touch their baby in any way, in order that a camera could document on film what the babies did entirely on their own. First they seemed to take the time to get a sense of where they were. Then, after a few minutes, they would begin to smack their lips, in the same way that some adults do when about to eat something very pleasurable. A few minutes later a high proportion of the babies began to move. They astonished everyone, including their mothers, when they literally crept up their mother's body until they were level with her breasts. Once at the breast, the babies began to turn their heads from side to side until they finally opened their mouths wide and latched onto the breast nearest their face. Babies who are not drugged and are therefore in full capacity of all their senses are determined little beings who know what they need to do to survive.

A newborn baby, it has been proved time and time again, is also highly resilient. Babies emerge from the womb with an innate ability to adjust to new stimuli and then to correct any imbalance within their own body. They usually need little help and can recuperate physically in an astonishing way. Resilience is part of human nature. Think about the true stories you've heard of babies born very prematurely and weighing only a couple of pounds in the days before hospital intensive care nurseries. Many of them survived by being placed on a piece of cloth in a shoe box that was put on the door of a warm oven.

Yet some babies can be stressed beyond their tolerance. For the majority, simply being held close in the mother's arms, against her warm body, is the perfect environment right after birth. Any special care given to a baby should be done while the baby is resting on its mother's body, even the procedures done to resuscitate a baby, that is, to get it to breathe. Once in a while, however, a baby will need treatment that can best be done in an ICU setting. The question is which baby and which specific procedures should be used. Modern newborn medicine assumes that every baby who seems to have any kind of problem can benefit from all of the advancements of high-tech medicine. This simply is not true. If these advancements did not carry risks along with potential benefits, it might be true. But all tests and procedures, whether or not they are painful, impede the normal flow of events: the baby's relationship to its own body and the delicate dance between mother and child, father and child, and family and child. Any alteration in this natural process can adversely affect a newborn. We must learn when to intervene and when to simply observe and trust.

A great deal of research has been done in recent years on the nature of stress and its impact on individuals. Even happy occasions like weddings and births are stressful, but stress is not necessarily a negative thing. For example, normal childbirth is a naturally stressful event for both the mother and the baby. It is the stress of labor that creates a heightened state of consciousness for the baby, and this stress creates a hormonal environment in the mother that readies her to bond with her baby to protect and nourish it. To understand the valuable role of stress in birth we need to understand the critical role hormones play.

It was not so long ago that researchers pinpointed a category of naturally occurring hormones called endorphins, which produce an extraordinary state of emotional well-being or bliss. Certain kinds of experiences are known to release endorphins to flood the body. At the same time they bring a sense of calm to the body, they also inhibit or diminish feelings of pain. It is now known that people who engage in physical activities that push them beyond a certain point of stress find themselves in a state of joy or peace. It's a high many people become hooked on and the reason why someone who is used to jogging and is unable to because of an injury goes into depression. Although it is seldom talked about, mothers and babies going through birth and during breast-feeding are able to have similar endorphin-produced experiences, especially if their senses are not dulled with drugs or numbed by too much anxiety.

Recently researchers discovered another category of hormones called stress hormones, or catecolamines. Physicians took it as an alarming sign when they found high catecolamine levels in laboring women. The high rate of catecolamines was immediately discussed at obstetric conferences and used as one more argument for recommending medication or anesthesia in labor. It was thought that the stress hormones of the mother would harm the baby. The history of modern obstretrics is full of instances in which physicians have wrongly blamed birthing women for problems encountered by their babies.

Fortunately, with regard to the catecolamine story, sanity was regained when it was discovered that stress hormones have a positive role to play in birth, as long as they are in balance with other factors. Obviously, too much stress over too long a period of time isn't good. It's a matter of balance. And, once again, medical science made the serious error of not looking at the whole system, but instead looking at one tiny piece and blowing it all out of proportion.

Neonatal physicians are now doing their best to assess fetuses in labor to determine whether a sign such as increased or decreased fetal heart rate shows simple stress or true distress. The distinction between a baby being stressed and a baby being in distress can be subtle. What is an acceptable—and even useful— stress to one baby may be too much for another. There is always a point along the spectrum at which stress turns to distress for a baby, just as there is a point during contractions when serious discomfort for the mother suddenly becomes pain that is very hard to cope with.

Once again, both physical exhaustion and mental attitude play an important part in determining the difference between stress and distress. That is one reason the practice of midwifery has always focused on making sure the mother gets enough rest and nourishment in labor and maintains a positive, hopeful attitude. This is another reason why using machines to monitor a pregnancy or a laboring woman creates problems. Machines, and the limited data they produce, can never show the whole picture and, at the same time, they tend to undermine trust in the natural process and confidence in the woman's ability.

I was recently at a prenatal clinic for low-income women and followed several pregnant women through the process of being weighed and measured and having blood drawn and then seeing the nurse practitioner. Each woman was seen by a minimum of five people, including the person who set up her next appointment and the representative from the federally funded Women, Infants, and Children program (WIC) that gives food supplements to pregnant women and mothers. At every turn the focus was entirely on getting some pieces of data and charting it. I observed virtually no eye contact between the health workers and the women they were supposed to be caring for. All the time was taken up in finding bits of information that could be put on a graph or noted in the records. None of the women had any opportunity to sit and talk about their feelings. The question "Are you having any problems?" was tossed off as if each woman were expected to produce some instantaneous list. There was no meaningful interaction at all between the health workers and the women. And this does not go on just at clinics for low-income families.

I have seen the same behavior time and again in private physicians' offices in North America, and in hospital obstetric and maternity units, and in hospital nurseries on several continents. We are obsessed with recording data that can be put down as numbers, and we have no time for the whole person, no interest in the whole picture. Today there are machines that can give hundreds of pieces of information about a particular body. Many people are excited at the prospect that one machine reading information from a pregnant woman's body will be able to tell what her labor is going to be like and what medical procedures should be done on her and her baby. Women are slowly being prepared for this substitute for true care early in pregnancy as machines replace human interaction. And the larger the volume of women or babies seen at one place the worse it tends to be. Much of the problem with childbirth today directly relates to scale. Bigger facilities do not mean better care. This is why traditional midwifery and home visits and home births have proved time and again to be high-quality, safe care when balanced against a high-tech hospital and specialist physicians. It is also why there is so much unnecessary stress and anxiety connected with childbirth today in the modern world. We must remember: Anything that overly stresses the mother will negatively affect her baby.

Research done by American and European psychologists, in which adults are "taken back" to their births, shows that when a mother was in a constant state of fear during labor or dulled with drugs, the message the baby received was one of fear. A baby is continually receiving messages from its nervous system, and its body is constantly trying to gauge the situation and respond appropriately. What prenatal and perinatal research shows is that these impressions, whether they are positive or negative, become a part of our stored memory and can affect the ways in which we view ourselves, our mothers, and the rest of our world.

In the 1920s and 1930s psychiatrists Wilhelm Reich and Otto Rank called the time of birth the "primal stage" of life. Their pioneering work lay largely unnoticed for nearly half a century. Then, in the 1970s, psychiatrist Arthur Janov pioneered primal therapy, termed "primal screaming" by the media after Janov's book *The Primal Scream* and reports of people screaming uncontrollably when they reenacted the trauma that occurred at their birth. The premise was that what happened to us before we could speak affects all the rest of our lives. Most people dismissed the notion that what happened to us in the womb, in birth, or in infancy could have any lasting impact.

Now there is a growing body of evidence that the fetus in the womb and in labor is aware of, and affected by, its mother's physical and emotional state. This is one more reason why giving women drugs is no better than abandoning them totally to labor alone. It is also a reason why machines are not a substitute for a thinking, observant, sensitive human caretaker. If a fetus in labor can be so affected, just think about how impressionable a newborn is, since it is viewing the world from outside the safety of the mother's body for the first time and having to cope with all sorts of new stimuli and function in new ways, beginning with having to breathe air and to get the attention of adults to satisfy its most basic needs.

The Paradox of Being Human: Resilient Yet Vulnerable

One of the basic paradoxes of human existence is that we are both resilient and vulnerable. This fact remains true throughout our lives, though at any given time we are either more resilient or more vulnerable. Nowhere do we see this more clearly than when looking at the newborn baby.

Resiliency is a special kind of strength that comes from flexibility. If all is going well in our life, if our body is in good shape, and if we are getting enough rest and sleep, then we are more likely to be resilient. Our capacity to rebound from an accident or shock of any kind is probably strong. We are like a willow tree, which can bend any direction in a strong wind but is unbreakable. On the other hand, if we have been under a lot of stress, if issues of survival are in the forefront, if we are feeling alone and unloved, then any kind of stress is likely to put us over the edge. We are then more like a dead tree, brittle and easily broken. If we understood this basic fact we would not continue to treat women and babies the way we do. We would certainly begin to question our dependency on machines and tests, and the data they give when it comes to matters of well-being, especially in pregnancy, childbirth, and recovery.

In 1972, U.S. pediatrician-researchers John Kennell and Marshall Klaus published the results of a series of studies on newborns and their mothers at Stanford University that brought the concept of bonding to the general public. Although there has since been some controversy over their findings, they did a lot toward liberalizing hospital policies with regard to newborns.

Kennell and Klaus observed the behavior of mothers who were given unstructured private time with their newborns in the first days after birth, and followed these mothers and babies in order to determine the quality of their later relationships. As they reported in the *New England Journal of Medicine,* they found that the first hours and days following birth are the optimal time for a mother and her baby to bond. Mothers who, for any reason, miss out on the first days of intimate contact with their babies *can* go on to create a healthy attachment with them. However, it may require extra effort on the mother's part.

The Kennell and Klaus research was conducted at a time when all mothers and newborns were being routinely separated in hospitals across North America. In their study one group of mothers had unbroken contact with their babies for one hour during the first three hours after birth and for five hours during each of the next three days. The other group of mothers had standard contact, holding their babies for the first time six to twelve hours after birth. Not only did the researchers find that separating a mother and a baby during the first days can make their relationship more difficult for a while, but that the effects could sometimes be seen a year or two later.

Kennell and Klaus also studied prematurely born babies in intensive care nurseries whose mothers were allowed to visit and touch their babies. Even minimal contact between mothers and babies made a great difference in their relationship. The standard practice at the time was not to permit mothers to see or touch their premature babies until the day they were to leave the hospital, which was often weeks after the birth.

The developing field of prenatal and perinatal psychology has drawn together researchers, physicians, nurses, psychotherapists, teachers, and parents for the first time in history in an international effort to focus attention on the processes of gestation, birth, and the first months of life. Their research shows that the entire time around birth, perhaps even beginning with conception and going right through the first eighteen months after birth, is a sensitive period for a human being and meant to be a time of heightened awareness and learning. This is a crucial time of great change and possible transformation for a woman becoming a mother, a man becoming a father, and the beginning of life for a child and for a family together. If any of the relationships within the family are damaged, the dynamics of the entire family system are affected.

It is important to know that if damage does occur at this crucial early time in an individual or family's life, it can be healed. Sometimes healing occurs spontaneously. Because human beings are so naturally resilient, often the mere process of living and having positive experiences heals psychological wounds. The human body is organized for health and recuperation from injury. A baby or mother who has had a very difficult time in pregnancy, during the birth, or shortly afterward can get a lot of healing simply from the process of breast-feeding. But because healing does not always occur spontaneously, we need to become much more aware of the possibility of psychic as well as physical trauma for both mother and child. There are therapies specifically effective for healing perinatal trauma. For children and adults, these include psychotherapy, hypnosis, regression work, and art and other expressive therapies. There are also physical therapies, notably various kinds of massage or touch. Infant massage is currently being taught to nurses and parents in many communities.

The Sensitivity and Awareness of Babies

A newborn baby takes in the world primarily through what it sees and what it touches, since the largest sensory organ is the skin. Being human is all about the basic need for contact and relationship. A baby first grasps the world through its eyes and ears. But its mouth is its most sensitive part, and as soon as a baby is able to, it attempts to put anything with which it comes into contact into its mouth. That is how we first explore our world.

A newborn baby that senses some threat in its environment will begin by crying loudly to alert someone to come and help. If no help comes and the baby still feels threatened, it may attempt to block out the unwanted stimulus by withdrawing. Since it cannot physically escape, it will withdraw within itself. In the early 1960s researcher-physicians began noticing that some babies in hospital newborn nurseries who looked as if they were asleep or at rest were actually in a state of great anxiety, with a rapid pulse and other bodily signs of distress that could be documented. It was discovered that when babies cannot escape an overly stressful environment or situation, such as brightly lit, constantly noisy nurseries, being stuck with needles for tests, or being harmed in their own homes, they will try to protect themselves any way they can. If crying doesn't produce the right response in the adults around it, the baby may then block awareness by shutting down, physically withdrawing, even though it cannot run and hide.

There is now a large body of evidence showing that hospital nurseries, especially intensive care nurseries, are particularly stressful environments even for a healthy baby. Babies do have the ability to cope with noxious environments, but it taxes them to do it. A newborn, or a baby of any age, subjected to continual stress from which there is no relief, may over time develop a pattern of responding to new situations in a fearful way, either by fighting or withdrawing. These are the roots of aggression and despair.

Today we have advanced to the point where there is little disagreement, in theory, that newborn babies experience discomfort, pain, and shock in the same way adults do. There is still disagreement as to whether babies are also capable of giving meaning to physical sensations such as being taken away from the mother. But researchers and physicians now admit that babies have the same range of emotions as adults. This ought to affect the way we treat newborns.

Because babies receive everything through their mothers while in the womb and in labor, we should begin transforming the way we care for pregnant women and women in labor, since so much of what we do heightens anxiety. And every hospital intensive care nursery and every pediatric unit ought to be designed so that there is a parent's or a surrogate parent's bed right next to the baby's. It is not only humane for the baby, but keeping sick babies with a parent and providing care that the parent can observe and participate in will help parents feel more secure about their ability to care for their baby when it leaves the hospital.

Reputable studies done on babies within a few weeks after birth show that babies can be made angry and even depressed by what happens to them. If babies are known to be able to feel sadness, fear, or confusion, just as we can, then we must acknowledge that much of current maternity and newborn care is likely to cause trauma to many babies, and that hospital maternal-newborn care should be reorganized to serve the whole family system.

There is not yet agreement in the culture, or in the medical world, that trauma experienced in the prenatal or perinatal period can have lasting effects on people. Yet it is known that early experiences leave their traces on the neural pathways of our brain. You could rightly say that we have been imprinted with our perinatal experiences—negative or positive—whether we ever remember them or not. Furthermore, you can see how these very early experiences can become the basis of many of our behavioral patterns as adults.

We live in denial about what babies do experience for two reasons. If we were to look at babies and allow ourselves to feel what they are feeling when they appear to be in distress from things we do to them, then we would not be able to continue doing what we do. Second, if we stopped denying a baby's capacity to suffer, we would then have to face the feelings we carry deep within ourselves of the trauma we experienced during our own birth and infancy. Because of the routine obstetric practices of the past century, few individuals alive today are free of psychic wounds dating from the prenatal and perinatal periods.

BABIES FEEL AND BABIES REMEMBER

The period just before, during, and soon after birth may prove to be as influential in the course of our lives as genetics or later environmental factors. Because most parents and health workers often are not yet aware of this, or of what they can do to prevent or heal trauma early in babies' lives, we need to reexamine everything done to and for women in maternity care, and to remember that the treatment of mothers always directly affects the treatment of babies.

In the early 1970s, pediatrician-researcher T. Berry Brazelton conducted several important studies of newborns to learn whether babies could feel depressed or hopeless. In one study he filmed a series of babies and their mothers. Each baby was placed in an infant seat so that the only thing it could see was its mother's face directly in front of it. The mother was instructed to maintain a completely blank expression on her face and, no matter what her baby did, not show any emotion or response.

In a heartrending series of videotaped sessions, each baby can be seen trying to elicit a response from its mother and, failing to do so, working even harder. After a number of minutes of making all kinds of faces and trying to make eye contact, each baby finally reaches its level of tolerance and begins to look away from the mother, finding it too difficult to continue making an effort with no response. The baby eventually turns it face away from its mother's face. Then it turns toward the mother again and tries to rouse a response. Each time it turns

Is Circumcision Necessary?

Today the world's pediatric associations unanimously agree that there is no medical reason to circumcise and many insurance companies now refuse to pay for the procedure, yet circumcision is still performed on 60 percent of newborn males in the United States each year. Some babies are circumcised for religious reasons, some for the cultural belief that it makes the body more attractive sexually, and many others are put through this unnecessary surgery because it is erroneously claimed to promote hygiene and prevent infection.

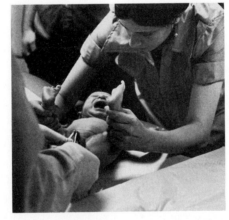

In circumcision, the delicate covering of the head of the penis is pulled away, crushed, and cut off. For many years people believed that babies—especially newborns—did not feel or remember pain. Because of the known risks of giving babies anesthesia, all kinds of surgery used to be performed on conscious babies. Today, it is understood that a newborn baby *does* feel pain and is traumatized by undergoing surgery without anesthesia; circumcision is the only surgery that continues to be done without it.

I recall the first circumcision I saw. The parents had gone to great lengths to birth their baby without drugs or other interventions so that he might have a peaceful beginning. He had spent his first week at home, breast-fed and cuddled, before arriving at the pediatrician's to be circumcised. The couple had argued over whether it should be done at all, but the boy's father prevailed. He felt his son's penis should look like his.

Both parents were present, and the mother held the baby down. The moment the doctor put the clamp on the foreskin, the boy began to scream. His father went pale, turned away, and left the room. Holding her son's legs apart, the mother bent over him and tried to calm him as the doctor cut quickly. The baby, awake and helpless, continued to scream. It took less than a minute, yet during that time, the baby had arched his back, grabbed his mother's collar in both hands, and tried in vain to pull himself away from the source of pain. Afterward, his mother picked him up and put him to her breast. He suckled frantically, crying and gulping air between swallows of warm milk. Turning to me, the mother said, "I'd never have allowed it if I'd known it would hurt him."

"We were told it was a simple procedure, that few babies find it painful, and that if they do, they get over it," the father later said.

I've since witnessed a number of circumcisions. In each case, the baby obviously feels pain and makes a strong effort to escape. Parents trying to decide whether to have their infant son circumcised need to know that the foreskin is a normal, healthy, protective tissue, and that the circumcision procedure carries the serious threat of hemorrhage and unintentional mutilation. Even if the procedure is successful, the wound is raw for ten to fifteen days. Circumcision is painful and potentially traumatic, and the imprint of that trauma can be lasting. For more information, contact NOCIRC (see Resources). □

away for longer and longer periods. Finally, each baby slumps down, drops its head, and shows all the signs of hopelessness. This and other studies clearly show that babies have very strong reactions to not having their expectations or needs met.

Any approach toward improving childbirth would have to eliminate the routine use of numerous painful and frightening just-in-case tests, procedures, and treatments that are currently used on newborns. We would have to find gentler alternative approaches to treating babies who actually require intervention, and we would have to be willing to follow up babies who we think may have been traumatized, whether spontaneously or as a result of medical intervention.

Swiss psychiatrist Alice Miller, whose provocative books *The Drama of the Gifted Child* and *Thou Shalt Not Be Aware* are the result of decades of clinical research with patients, has attempted to awaken therapists, physicians, educators, and the general public to the widespread injury and abuse of children done in the name of helping them. Miller is a pioneer in the understanding of how certain cultural values promote abuse and blind people to the fact that many common behaviors toward children are in fact abusive. She does not extend her observations to the newborn. It is time we do that.

Fear-Based Just-in-Case Obstetrics and Newborn Care

From the late 1970s on, physicians were trained that all women should get sugar water IVs in labor. This was done just in case the woman became dehydrated. For a decade, this resulted in standard hospital policies in the United States of not permitting women in labor any food or liquid by mouth. Doctors did not want any women to simply eat and drink what they wanted during labor, just in case one of them might be one of the rare women who suddenly develops a complication that might require general anesthesia. Anesthesiologists don't want to give anesthesia to a woman with anything in her stomach, just in case she might vomit. After all, she might then breathe the vomit into her lungs, get sick, and die.

Depriving a woman of all food and drink once she enters the hospital for the duration of labor causes dehydration. Dehydration makes a laboring woman anxious and agitated, and makes her labor longer, more difficult, and more painful, or stops its progress altogether.

Physicians and nurses were not ignorant of the effects of dehydration. But rather than feeding and hydrating women to prevent it, they came up with the novel solution of giving all women intravenous drips of glucose. This IV drip was intended to provide every laboring woman with sufficient calories to give her all the energy she needed in labor. But the IV caused several problems: first of all, it was not sufficient for many women; second, it subjected women to the risks of having an IV in their arm; third, it resulted in women having lots of acid in their stomachs due to the absence of liquids or foods. This meant that if a woman did vomit, she vomited up acid, which was even more harmful to the lungs than undigested food or drink. So anesthesiologists came up with the solution that all women should not only have IVs but be forced to take an antacid like Pepto-Bismol in labor, to neutralize the stomach acid. This bizarre scenario was common in the early eighties in prestigious hospitals in Boston, New York, and other major cities. After five or ten years (depending on the hospital) of this insanity, hospitals loosened their restrictions on what a woman in labor could have by mouth. First it was ice chips only. Now most hospitals permit juices as well, or even light snacks.

What we see in this example is one intervention leading to another. When it was found that babies of the mothers given IVs and antacids were born with their pH out of balance, they had their stomachs washed out with saltwater in the first minutes after birth. During the same year, physicans in training all across the United States suddenly began to routinely intubate and aspirate all babies who were born with any sign of meconium. In this procedure, metal blades are inserted into the throats of newborns to spread their vocal cords apart. Meconium is the tarry blackish-green substance that plugs the rectum of the fetus in utero and thereby keeps the intestines empty and sterile. Babies sometimes discharge this during labor, especially when stressed, or being born in the breech position. A baby lying in amniotic fluid with meconium in it can suck it into its lungs in labor, and a tiny fraction of babies who get meconium in their lungs die each year from what is called "meconium aspiration syndrome," a dangerous form of pneumonia.

So in an effort to protect all babies from the possibility of meconium aspiration, pediatricians were suddenly being trained to treat all babies with any meconium in their waters, no matter how fresh or how light it was, in the same aggressive manner, first suctioning out their delicate lungs and then putting water down them and "washing" them out. Unfortunately, a risky side effect of this procedure, called lavage, is a pneumonia-like condition called wet-lung disease. The possibility of this side effect resulted in many newborns being separated from their mothers and put in high-risk nurseries. While there they were

How Doctors Can Instill Fear in Parents

Upon finishing his residency at a renowned hospital, a pediatrician I know was so steeped in aggressive newborn care that he could recite the names, symptoms, and treatments of every disease listed in pediatric literature.

Shortly after entering practice, he saw a baby whose mother had brought her in because she had signs of an ear infection. He listed each and every disease that could possibly have the same symptoms—a red, painful ear and a sore throat—rather than examining the baby and discussing the mother's concerns. Highest on his list was encephalitis, or brain fever, one of the rarest and deadliest of all illnesses.

Shaken to her core, the mother complied with his recommendation that her daughter of one month be hospitalized for all applicable tests. What else could she do? She was afraid for her child. Nearly a week later, after the baby was subjected to a myriad of painful procedures, all done "just in case," her baby was allowed to come home. This mother brought home a distressed baby whom she had difficulty breast-feeding and comforting, and she found herself no longer trusting her instincts and judgment.

In the next year, whenever her baby showed any sign of illness, she wasted no time before seeking medical attention. If her daughter's pediatrician was not on call, she panicked and went to the hospital emergency room. She was continually afraid the baby might be suffering from some rare, acute disease.

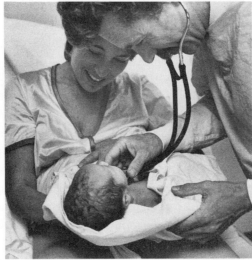

This conscientious doctor was doing what he'd been taught to do as a specialist, to search for a needle in a haystack. It was the legacy of his training. While it had the positive aspect that he would no doubt recognize a rare disease if he came across one, this approach unfortunately had the negative side of scaring parents, causing babies a lot of needless pain, and separating parents from their infants.

Several years later, this physician spent some months traveling through Africa, paying particular attention to the rural health-care system there. The trip opened his eyes, and he began to trust the human body's natural capacity to thwart disease. He developed a more relaxed approach in his practice and did not jump to "what if?" conclusions. Now, many years past his high-risk intensive training, he always weighs the possible benefits of aggressive hospital-based newborn care against all of its accompanying risks—which include undermining a parent's sense of competence and subjecting infants to traumatic procedures. He continues to be a thorough, meticulous observer but is now more aware that problems often work themselves out without the need for high-tech pediatric medicine, and he is a much better doctor as a result. □

deprived of breast-feeding and the mothers' physical contact and usually sub-jected to at least one painful spinal tap. Many other babies ended up with bruised and painfully sore mouths and tracheas from aggressive suctions with tubes beings pushed down their throat. A baby's mouth has such sensitive tissue that even suctioning with a light syringe, regardless of the amount of meconium or their condition, can be enough to cause injury or pain and sore throat and impede breast-feeding. Putting a tube down a baby's throat also causes a reflex that slows the baby's heart.

Women and babies suffer greatly from the fads that blow through medical training hospitals. These procedures or policies become ingrained in the culture and are difficult to get rid of. Physicians who are trained in the "do everything just-in-case" approach spread those practices all across the country and continue the practices long after research is published that clearly shows that the benefits are outweighed by the hazards. The story of modern obstetrics can be seen in the long list of practices that became routine, only to be found unwarranted and eventually dropped or altered: shaving women for birth, doing rectal exams dur-ing labor, rupturing membranes, using IVs, speeding up labor artificially, using silver nitrate on babies' eyes, giving epidurals in early labor, and now using ce-sareans to treat any unusual occurrence in labor.

These procedures on an adult normally would require anesthesia, but no anesthesia was—or is today—used on infants who have these procedures done to them. Usually a baby must be held down or it will fight, gagging and flailing its arms and legs. There was always the risk of the metal blades or the tubes puncturing the side of the windpipe, which sometimes happened, causing a pneumothorax in the baby that was as life-threatening as the meconium-aspiration pneumonia that the procedures were intended to prevent.

IN DISTRESS? OR SIMPLY STRESSED?

We often misinterpret the needs of newborns, believing that babies who are simply tired and stressed require medical care. Like their mothers, babies are often exhausted from the birth; often all they need are to be closely observed in a quiet, calm environment, to be given the chance to rest and recuperate. In order for this to take place, ideally a baby should remain with its mother or an-other family member after birth.

This physical closeness isn't difficult to achieve. Almost any procedure that is truly indicated can be done with the baby lying next to its mother or in a parent's arms. Too often we further traumatize an already stressed baby by separating it from its parents and subjecting it to myriad painful procedures. We tend to forget the risks involved as we focus on the possible benefits of each procedure.

Look at our high-tech approach from the baby's perspective: bright lights, loud noises, rapid movements from one place to another, sharp needles, tight bands around our body, many different people touching us. When a baby has been physically or emotionally traumatized, constant touching, remaining close by, massaging, and special healing techniques are crucial. But first we must observe the infant, paying close attention to the signals it sends. If a baby has been truly traumatized by the birth, there will be signs: persistent feeding or sleeping problems, an inability to calm itself or be comforted.

BABY IMMUNIZATIONS AND TREATMENT

Another trend that began a few years ago in the United States is to routinely put babies back in the hospital for jaundice just days or weeks after birth. Jaundice is a normal physiological condition in many babies. It's the result of the baby's system quickly throwing off the extra red blood cells they needed while in utero. One little-known fact is that when the artificial hormone stimulant oxytocin is used during labor, the baby is at increased risk for developing a form of jaundice after birth. Jaundice only rarely results in a serious health hazard for a baby, when what is termed the baby's bilirubin rate becomes very high. Pediatricians began to disregard the level at which jaundice is serious and to treat more and more babies aggressively, who had less than critically high bilirubin. The trend—until the risks of hepatitis and AIDS became too great—was to do blood exchange transfusions for lower and lower rates of bilirubin, out of fear that if physicians did not act aggressively they might be sued or lose a baby.

Today, a few women, physicians, and midwives are challenging the prevailing belief that all babies should be immunized against diphtheria, pertussis (whooping cough), and tetanus (DPT), polio, and measles. This is a complex issue, because in the days before such immunizations existed, many children became infected and perhaps 20 percent of these sick children died. There is growing evidence, however, that the immunizations, which do carry a small but serious risk, weaken the immune system, particularly when done before the age of six months, and that is a serious problem that must be weighed against the obvious value of eradicating or controlling serious infectious diseases.

Our immune systems can usually handle what is present in our own home and family, but when babies are put in day care and begin interacting regularly with nonfamily members, they are exposed to many sources of infection. What we now see as public-health policy is the routine practice of giving babies their "shots" beginning when they are only six weeks to three months old. Immunizations used to be given around six months of age, by which time a baby's own immune system has pretty well developed, especially if it has been continuously breast-fed. Current pediatric thinking is that immunizations must be begun just weeks after birth because older babies may not be seen by a health worker. Two to three months old is well below the age at which a baby's immune system begins to function at full capacity, raising the issue of whether the benefits do outweigh the risks.

Few parents are told that it is possible, and perhaps much wiser, to divide immunizations into smaller doses given over a longer period of time, and to start them when the baby is six months or older, in order to allow the baby to develop to the point where it can handle the immunizations better. And few parents realize that they can choose to have some immunizations done and not others.

Caring for Newborns: Developing Trust

For several decades, it has been known that the primary task of a baby in its first months is to develop trust. Anything that impedes that process or teaches a baby that it cannot trust is dangerous and has long-lasting implications. Current studies clearly prove that the one crucial factor in determining a child's resiliency in the face of difficulty is whether that child has a primary caretaker who is a constant figure and whom that child can count on and feel safe with. The age for receiving this quality and quantity of care is from birth through the first several years of life. This does not mean that a person needs to spend eight or ten hours a day giving rapt attention to a baby or toddler. Research has shown what tribal cultures have long practiced: that children of all ages, even babies, actually benefit from a fair amount of benign neglect, times when they are left to their own devices, without any outside distraction. Allowed this time, children naturally daydream and drop into meditative states and learn to meet their own spiritual needs. But benign neglect is something altogether different from failing to meet an infant's or young child's real needs for human contact and stimulation.

In most tribal cultures babies spend many hours a day bound to an adult's or older child's body and, during this time, the baby is likely to have no special attention focused upon it whatsoever. The babies' needs for food and touch, warmth, and a feeling of comfort and safety are naturally met while their mothers or other caretakers go about their daily business. The baby is constantly bathed in the sounds of its mother talking or singing, and in periods of silence it listens to the rhythmic sounds of her heartbeat. It feels the swaying of her body as she walks to the stream to fetch water or stoop in the garden or the calm stillness as she rests against a rock or a tree. Meanwhile, it is free to wander through its own thoughts or feelings. It is not on show or expected to perform to please others. For many months, it seldom tries to express unmet needs, for its needs are met so quickly.

Western visitors to tribal cultures and to countries where babies and children are almost constantly in close physical contact to an adult as he or she goes about daily life remark on how rarely they see young children cry. And adults in these cultures do not find caring for their young to be difficult and stressful. These cultures support people in maintaining close ties with their young and offer ample social support to parents.

Today, many parents who want to do the very best for their babies and children make a conscious effort to be close and loving and provide stimulation whenever they are able. But most of their day they are separated from their young children and consumed with work, so that they are exhausted during the time they can be with their children. Their attention is tainted with tension. It is difficult to be a good parent to an infant or young child in a culture that requires us to spend so much energy apart from our children, trying to earn the money required to live. Taking leave from work in the first few months of a baby's life nurtures not only one's baby but one's self as well. This is one of the best ways to begin a process of healing, whether it be for a baby who had a traumatic birth or time in a hospital or a parent who long ago was traumatized as a baby.

INNOVATIONS IN NEWBORN CARE

Some innovative hospital pediatric units around the world are now practicing "kangarooing": mothers and sometimes nurses carry babies in a pouch against their chest for periods of time each day to provide the warmth, comfort, and stimulation these babies would normally get from being still in the womb. Some nurseries are placing newborns on natural lambskins or lambs-wool mats, because this practice—common in Australia and New Zealand—has been shown to result in babies gaining strength and weight more quickly.

A newborn intensive care unit (called by the British a "special care baby unit") in High Wyckam, England, has rooms for mothers right off the nursery, to allow babies to spend large amounts of time in intimate contact with their mothers while in intensive care. Because of the pioneering efforts of pediatrician Donald Garrow, many of these babies spend the major part of their time with their mothers, in a simple, small clip-on clear plastic cot attached to the mother's bed. The mothers can have all the privacy they need with their babies by closing the blinds on the door that separates them from the nursery.

In Pittsburgh, Pennsylvania, there is an out-of-hospital intensive care nursery on one floor of the Children's Home Society. Some pediatricians elect to move a baby to this unit as soon as it is stable. The unit uses miniaturized portable equipment. Parents of these babies are taught to use the equipment, which is then loaned to them so that they can care for their babies at home. The purpose is to normalize the intensive care experience for parents as well as babies.

These are hopeful models, but standard newborn medical care has a long way to go before it admits its excesses and risks. Nothing is likely to change significantly in the way babies are treated in hospitals until parents raise their voices and begin to demand humane treatment and to protect their babies from being separated from them while in the hospital.

The Personal Politics of Feeding a Baby

Feeding forms much of the foundation of an infant's reality. How we are fed and what and when we are fed teach us how it feels to be satisfied or frustrated, to feel pleasure or discomfort. How we feed a baby is both a personal and a political statement, reflecting our beliefs and values as well as our preferences.

Breast milk is precisely designed to meet the needs of the developing brain and body of a baby. In fact, it is so precisely fitted to a baby's needs that the composition of the mother's milk actually changes in direct response to the needs of her baby. No one yet knows how exactly this happens. A prematurely born baby receives breast milk of a very different composition—in terms of the protein and fat content and trace nutrients—than a full-term baby, and the milk a mother produces when her baby is two weeks old is different from the milk she creates when it is six months old.

As the name *mammal* suggests, breast-feeding is an integral part of our nature. We are meant to thrive by breast-feeding. Research shows that breast-fed babies receive the benefit of special hormones released by suckling, which help stimulate the baby's growth and calm the baby. This should be particularly important to a woman who recognizes that her baby has suffered trauma in the course of its birth, whether from forceps, cesarean surgery, or drugs received from the mother during labor.

How we hold a baby's body and the way we feel as we feed it are transmitted to the baby as much as the food it takes in. How and when we feed a baby forms an underlying pattern of satisfaction or dissatisfaction with food and nourishment of all kinds for the rest of a child's life. How we feed a baby also has economic and social implications, because what we do with regard to food affects not only our family and friends, but people half a world away, and the world's natural environment as well.

If a woman chooses to bottle-feed her baby with anything other than her own milk, it will certainly cost her money. That money goes to profit a large industry that is not run to make people's lives easier or to improve people's health but to make money.

Consider the marketing practices of formula manufacturers. For years they attempted to convince new mothers that their product was superior to and more convenient than the mothers' own breast milk. In advertising today they do their best to sell women on the idea that formula-feeding, while maybe not *better* than breast-feeding, is really just as good. For decades they convinced hospitals to buy starter kits of formula and bottles so that every new mother left the hospital with one. When they discovered new markets in the developing world, they thought nothing of trying to undermine breast-feeding in those countries, even though doing so brought tremendous financial strain to families who barely

---

> *Breast-fed babies are often given bottles of sugar-water in the hospital, even though this practice has no benefit and can make breast-feeding difficult. For their records, nurses must know the baby has taken in a certain amount of fluid.*
>
> *I am working hard to change this practice. In the meantime I tell mothers, "Take the bottle of sugar water, pour an ounce down the sink, put the nipple back on, and put it in the bassinet and say nothing." Nurses will see the bottle has been partly emptied, write the amount down, and they'll have done their part. The mother doesn't have to do what she and I both feel is not good for her baby, and there will be no battle. It should not have to be this way, but that's the way it is.*
>
> —PEDIATRICIAN

earned enough for necessities, much less expensive bottles and formula. At the same time, this practice caused the deaths of millions of babies. Families who could not afford to buy enough formula diluted it with water, not realizing they were diluting vital nutrients, and in many cases they mixed formula powder with contaminated local water.

If a woman chooses not to breast-feed her baby, that decision sends a message to doctors, nurses, midwives, and health educators that breast-feeding is something modern women do not want to be bothered with. If a poor woman on government assistance elects not to breast-feed, the message she unconsciously sends to her government and social service agencies is that money that could be spent on crucial needs such as housing, education, and job training should be spent instead on buying vast quantities of artificial milk. That money lines the pockets of those companies that manufacture formula, bottles, and plastic nipples. It does not help poor women.

By choosing not to breast-feed, a woman sends a message that her physical presence is not required by her child. This allows the government and employers to assume that it is not necessary to provide women with either paid maternity leave or day care at the job site.

One of the most negative side effects of the Industrial Revolution was that it removed fathers from their children during the working day. Now the same thing is happening to mothers, and it is happening sooner and sooner after birth. Your government and your employer see no reason why women should be allowed—much less encouraged—to bring their infants to work with them, even in jobs where the presence of a very young baby would not be a problem for other workers and might even be a pleasure. Women whose jobs do not permit a baby to be with them should have day care that permits them to spend some time during the working day with their baby.

Middle-class or upper-middle-class women have the ability to pay for someone else to provide day care for a baby. That person will not be paid wages anywhere near what their employers are paid. That, too, is not only a personal but also a political statement, for it sends a clear message to everyone in the culture that it is all right. When a mother is not breast-feeding her infant as nature designed—which is continuously during the day—she can be separated easily from her baby, with negative results for each of them. So the separation of mothers and babies goes hand-in-hand with artificial feeding practices, including breast-feeding according to the clock.

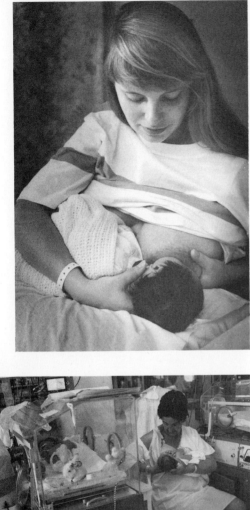

Breast-feeding

Breast-feeding not only affords an infant the best nutrition possible and provides essential immune factors that no formula can match, but also gives mother and infant time together to bond. Breast milk is something only a mother can provide and it is free.

At the start, breast-feeding takes patience and practice. It is not instinctual. It is a dance both you and your baby must learn. Breast-feeding shouldn't hurt. Once it's going well, you can even sleep while feeding your baby.

For more information on successful breast-feeding, read *Bestfeeding: Getting Breastfeeding Right for You* (see Bibliography) and contact La Leche League (see Resources).

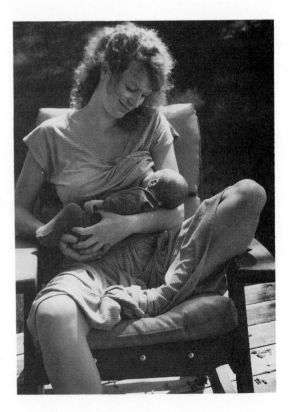

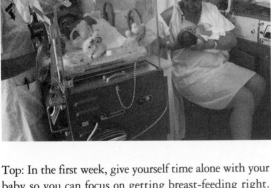

Top: In the first week, give yourself time alone with your baby so you can focus on getting breast-feeding right. Above: You can still breast-feed if your baby is in intensive care, although you may need to express your milk if your baby is being tube-fed. Right: One of the good things about breast-feeding is that it's easily portable.

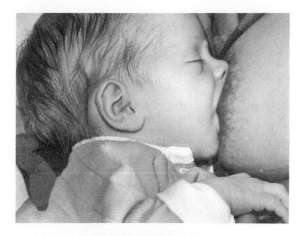

The baby on the left is on the breast well. The baby just below has let go of the breast, full and contented. The photo to the right of that shows a baby nipple suckling, which leads to sore nipples, breast infections, and insufficient milk.

Lying on your side, you can feed your baby while resting. You can also learn to express or pump your milk, so someone else can feed your baby when you are away.

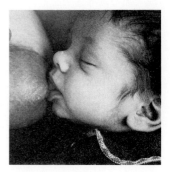

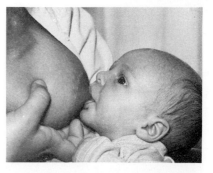

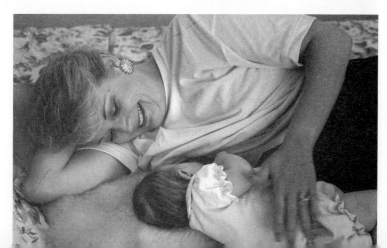

Breast-feeding is on the decline in North America again. Having dropped to a low of 10 or 15 percent in the 1950s it slowly increased, especially among middle-class and well-to-do families, almost totally as a result of the efforts of a mother-to-mother support group called La Leche League (see Resources). Breast-feeding was helped by the back-to-the-earth movement of the late 1960s but continued to decline among women of color, especially poor and very young women. Breast-feeding steadily declined during the 1980s. Although on the rise, only 20 percent of babies in the U.S. are fully breast-fed at six months. Yet *all* babies need it at least that long and would benefit from being breast-fed for two years.

BREAST-FEEDING MATTERS

It is not just babies from developing countries who suffer when they are not breast-fed. Babies born to middle-class and wealthy parents in developed countries suffer too.

When we talk about breast-feeding, we really need to recognize the two components: what is in the milk itself and what happens in the course of the baby suckling at its mother's breast. The two can and sometimes have to be separated. A mother can express or pump her milk, let someone else give it to her baby, and then let her baby suckle for comfort as well as for milk when they are together. It is quite possible to feed your baby only on your milk while never being able to put the baby to your breast. It is also possible to feed your baby someone else's milk or an artificial substitute—even out of a cup or spoon or bottle—and to still give your baby the many benefits of being held with its body tucked in close against its mother's body.

In the United States, virtually all of the three million babies born every year spend at least a few hours in a brightly lit hospital nursery, away from the protection of its mother's body and milk, and exposed to strangers' germs, some of which, like hospital staph infections, can be life-threatening. Babies are born without any bacteria of any kind—good or bad—in their stomachs. It is essential that good bacteria set up home in a newborn's stomach; otherwise harmful bacteria will take over and the baby will sicken or die if left untreated with drugs. Where does a newborn baby get the kinds of bacteria it needs most? From its mother's milk and from her skin, which are also the sources of the substances that create a strong, healthy immune system that the baby needs for the rest of its life. We need good immune systems, especially now, in a world filled with pollution and stress.

A baby is actively involved in the breast-feeding process: the amount of its suckling determines the amount of milk that is produced in the mother's breast for the next feeding. This is not true in bottle-feeding, which is a much more passive activity. The baby's jaw and mouth muscles are fully involved and active in suckling, but not when taking milk from an artificial nipple. Research is now being done to determine the way breast-feeding helps a baby learn to calm itself, which allows the baby to have a sense of well-being and trust in its own body.

Mothers also benefit physically and emotionally from breast-feeding. Having your baby suckle at your breast contracts your womb, helps it and your entire body return to its prebirth state, and even assists you in losing that extra weight without effort. In addition, it has now been shown that breast-feeding causes a woman's body to produce special hormones that calm her.

Although successful breast-feeding also allows a sense of well-being for the mother as well as reinforcing the bond between mother and baby, breast-feeding does not always mean ease and comfort to the modern woman. In fact, breast-feeding failure is the biggest reason why women today choose not to breast-feed at all. Too many women have experienced pain and frustration, have felt helpless and inadequate in the face of a crying and hungry baby, or have heard myriad similar stories from other women.

There are no accurate figures on how many women in the Western world actually intend to feed their babies their own milk. Health professionals estimate that figure to be between 50 and 65 percent of all women giving birth. We do know that many women put their babies to breast only once or twice to please an enthusiastic hospital nurse or a member of their family, or to be able to say they "tried," but never attempt to breast-feed once they are in their own home.

The percentage of women having home childbirth and childbirth in birth centers (both in and out of the hospital) who not only choose to breast-feed but succeed at it is much, much higher than the average, close to 100 percent. But these women and their babies represent a tiny fraction of all mothers and babies in North America, no more than 7 to 10 percent.

LEARNING TO BREAST-FEED

Breast-feeding is not primarily instinctual but learned. Each generation of babies learns how to breast-feed by suckling at their mother's breasts, by following what she shows them to do. How do mothers learn to do it correctly? By having been breast-fed, by having seen it all around them as part of their culture, and by having the baby itself as her body's teacher. The main reason why so many women today are not breast-feeding is that we are preceded by three generations during which bottle-feeding was the norm. People have come to believe that artificial milk substitutes are good for their babies, and that sucking on an artificial nipple is just as good as suckling your mother's breast. Some people actually believe artificial formula is superior to mother's milk.

Why has breast-feeding become so fraught with problems for many women? Because after observing bottle-feeding all around us, we try to use the breast as if it were a bottle. We even speak of emptying the breast, as if it were a bottle, when a breast that is producing milk is never really empty. Women who have seen only bottle-feeding commonly place a hand on the breast, squeezing it between thumb and forefinger, or scissoring it between the forefinger and middle finger. They are unconsciously trying to relate to the breast as if it were a bottle with a firm nipple, attempting to push the breast into the baby's mouth or hunching up and leaning over the baby try to drop the breast into the baby's mouth. All of this is an unconscious mimicking of bottle-feeding. You never see it in countries where breast-feeding is the norm.

In addition, women in our culture routinely press a finger against the breast near the nipple alongside the baby's nose when it feeds. Women in breast-feeding cultures don't do this. It is not necessary, because all babies' nostrils flare to the side, which is nature's way of ensuring that they will not have trouble breathing while breast-feeding. Pressing on the breast makes it harder for the baby to take in enough breast tissue to feed well.

* * *

Having women and babies spend their first hours and days after birth separated from each other or without getting the privacy and support they need to establish breast-feeding, plus running breast-feeding by the clock, have probably done more to damage breast-feeding than any other factors. These often significant factors include the drugs that many babies have in their systems from medication and anesthesia given to their mothers in labor, which make them sleepy or inhibit their sensory motor skills, greatly affecting their ability to suckle.

Modern hospital childbirth practices have ruined breast-feeding for many women and babies. Not only are women in many modern and developing countries seldom given the instruction many of them need to get breast-feeding established, but they are leaving the hospital before their milk is fully in, and going home to no postpartum care.

Despite the skillful help given by volunteer breast-feeding counselors through La Leche League and other breast-feeding support groups, and despite the growing number of professional lactation consultants, most women do not get the help they need when they need it. If they did, they would not be quitting in frustration.

Health workers around the world do not see breast-feeding problems among traditional cultures where bottle-feeding has not become established. That is proof that the problems we encounter are not a result of something wrong with women or with babies but with our culture.

Why do women who go to midwives for childbirth so rarely encounter serious problems with breast-feeding? It is not because midwives are more skilled in helping women get breast-feeding right. The difference is in the fact that midwives respect the natural process of birth and consider breast-feeding an intrinsic part of that process and of a woman's sexuality. They also understand the need for a mother and her newborn baby to have privacy after birth, time alone where the mother is not distracted and has no responsibilities. We have underestimated the need for privacy both in labor and its role in establishing good breast-feeding.

Michel Odent, French physician-surgeon and author of a modern classic, *Birth Reborn,* observes, "It has been my experience, in thirty years of obstetrics, that when a mother and her baby are allowed to be alone together in the first two hours after birth the mother will learn how to put the baby to her breast correctly, without anyone's help." This is difficult to achieve when hospitals are organized around schedules by the clock, when doctors are rushing to stitch up an episiotomy immediately after the placenta is delivered, when nurses feel compelled to tag and footprint the baby and get its vital statistics down on the chart in the first minutes of life. It is even more difficult to achieve when women (between a quarter and a third of birthing women in the United States) are undergoing cesarean surgery for birth, and when as many as 20 percent of all newborns spend their first hours or days in an intensive care nursery, and virtually all of the rest spend at least some time in the first days separated from their mothers.

If we are going to turn the tide in favor of breast-feeding we will have to begin to structure hospitals around the real needs of mothers and babies, not staff convenience or doing things simply to keep elaborate written records in case of lawsuits. This will require some consumers and health workers taking a strong and vocal stand.

It is understandable why so many women are not breast-feeding their babies.

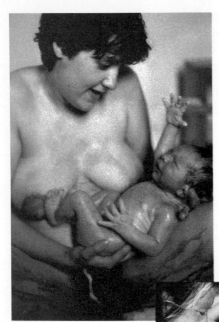

Bonding

Bonding—or attachment—is the crucial exchange of love and trust that develops between a baby and its primary caregivers. Strengthening this connection, which begins in the womb, takes time and effort.

To develop into a resilient and healthy child, an infant must be able to trust someone else to provide what it cannot yet obtain for itself. Bonding helps in this development. These photographs show the joyful bonding of babies, parents, and siblings right after birth.

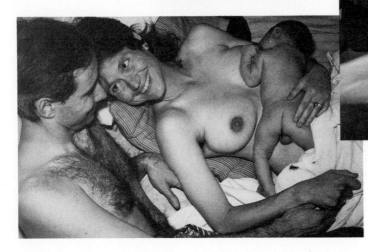

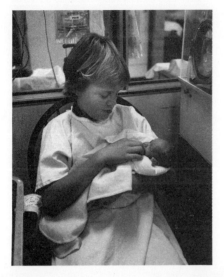

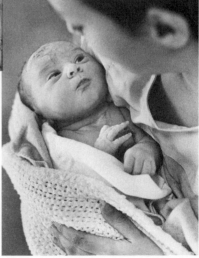

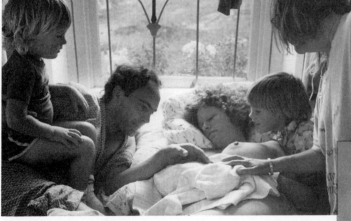

The keys to bonding with a baby are spending uninterrupted time together and having close physical contact. A welcoming face, a warm voice, and a gentle reassuring touch show a baby that we seek, accept, and return its love.

Now we must unlearn what the culture has erroneously taught us and make it possible for all women to breast-feed their babies successfully. When we support women and babies by making it easy for them to breast-feed we will right an imbalance that has existed for three generations.

Attachment and Attachment Disorders in Modern Society

The pattern of insecure attachment between parents and their young children has become a serious concern in highly developed societies, especially in urban cultures. Children who feel insecure about their parents' or other primary care-taker's attachment to them and who have no person in their lives committed to their emotional and physical well-being often grow up to be alienated and de-pressed or violent. The failure of women to breast-feed is just one more contri-bution to the general pattern of separation of parents and their babies and young children. This should be of great concern to all of us who care about the health and welfare of children.

The World Health Organization and health workers in developing countries are well aware of the worldwide trend for women to copy Western women and to bottle-feed rather than breast-feed. This is part of a worldwide pattern: wher-ever tribal members begin to move out of the village and away from agriculture, they abandon traditional family and tribal values, including their connection to the earth, their bodies, and their babies. Soon after, they begin to lose close con-nection with other people. They replace these relationships with becoming con-sumers of goods and services. The move from home birth to hospital birth, from breast-feeding to bottle-feeding, and from parental or home care to institutional day care is all part of the same syndrome.

Other factors that contribute to the decline of parenting and the neglect of children are that women are not paid for their work as homemakers and mothers, and that when they do enter the paid labor force they earn only a little more than half of what men earn for comparable work.

Modern culture encourages the separation of babies from their mothers and fathers and isolates parents from community support. Working parents try to make up for the lack of time they have to spend with their babies and children by doting on them. They buy them every conceivable toy and comfort object. Some parents are desperate for the contact they themselves are missing, while others are so disconnected that they have no desire to be with their children. Our culture promotes parents who do not feel torn between work and family life but who choose work over all else.

Short periods of so-called quality time, when adults find the time to focus intently on their children and attempt to restore the balance, do not make up for long periods of absence each day, especially in infancy. As if this were not hard enough on parents and children, most parents come home so stressed that the attention they do give is not from a full cup but a drained and empty one. Children, even babies, know the difference between attention that is given easily, out of joy, and attention that comes with the price tag of stress and exhaustion. We are teaching children from infancy that they should not expect much from other people. Instead, they learn to take pleasure in toys, TV, and video games, and grow into adults who turn to adult toys and high-priced recreational activities, or to work, rather than focus on personal relationships.

What are termed "attachment disorders," so common now in the United States, are at last being recognized as important factors in child abuse, especially incest. Adults are much more likely to neglect or harm a baby or child that they have never felt strongly attached to. Children who are unable to bond with their parents, or who feel insecure in their connection to their primary caregiver, can be overly needy or can resist affection entirely and be unable to form close relationships in later life.

There has never been any public outcry against the routine practice of separating newborn babies from their mothers, despite the fact that it has never been shown to be either safe or healthy for either mothers or babies. Quite the contrary, many studies have shown that babies—and mothers—are healthier when they are together. This is only logical, because they are still functioning as if they were physically connected long after the umbilical cord is cut.

Many Southern European countries such as Spain, Italy, and Greece, and those in Eastern Europe now proudly show visitors from the United States their large hospital newborn nurseries in which all newborns spend most of their day lying alone in their beds. Row upon row of babies. Each is suffering from the lack of being held and cuddled and cooed over, deprived of the sound and smell of their mothers, as well as their innately preferred food, mother's milk.

In Northern European countries such as Holland, Sweden, and Denmark, healthy mothers and babies continue to room together routinely from birth until they leave the hospital, just as they have always done in hospital maternity units. A visiting North American would be surprised to discover that in those countries what is called a "nursery" is a small, unpretentious room containing only extra baby beds and other basic supplies, or an occasional baby who will be sent back to its mother in an hour or two. Unlike nurses in American "well-baby" nurseries, nurses in these countries do not carry out stressful and painful procedures on babies in these rooms, "just in case" a baby might develop a problem that requires treatment. Instead, babies are quietly observed or held. When a baby there cries it is brought to its mother or picked up. When a baby is in such a nursery during the night, the room is darkened so the baby will not have its sleep-wake cycle disturbed. This is something much appreciated by a new mother who will have enough difficulty adjusting to the nearly constant needs of a newborn without being kept awake all night because her baby's sleeping pattern was disrupted.

This modern trend toward separation and isolation is threatening all of us. Changing the way we approach childbirth and infancy will not solve the problem entirely. The solution must be political, social, and economic, as well as personal. It begins with opening our eyes and hearts and becoming aware of how one thing is connected to another, how one thing often leads to another. We can tackle the problem anywhere, but it is easiest to tackle it at the beginning of life.

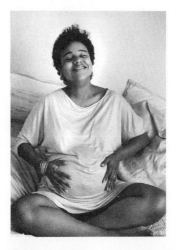

Pregnancy

Pregnancy is a time of preparation. As your baby grows and develops, you have many months to get yourself mentally, physically, and emotionally ready for childbirth and the task of caring for a newborn. Read as much as possible and talk to mothers and birth professionals about birth and childcare—especially if you're a first-time mother. Even if you've already had children, you can always learn more to make your experience the best it can be. Take this time to nurture yourself: become as physically healthy as you can, try to rid your life of undue stresses, and enjoy the love and support of those around you as you wait for your new baby.

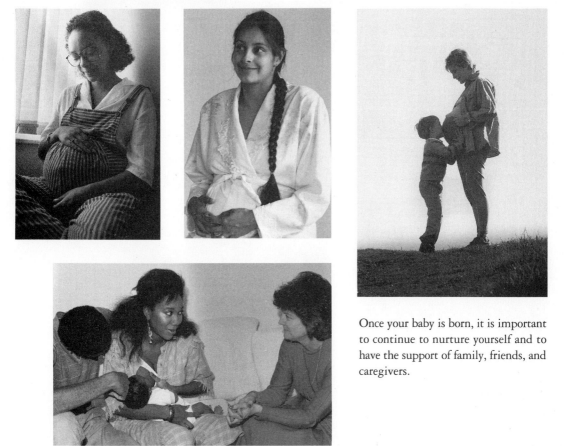

Once your baby is born, it is important to continue to nurture yourself and to have the support of family, friends, and caregivers.

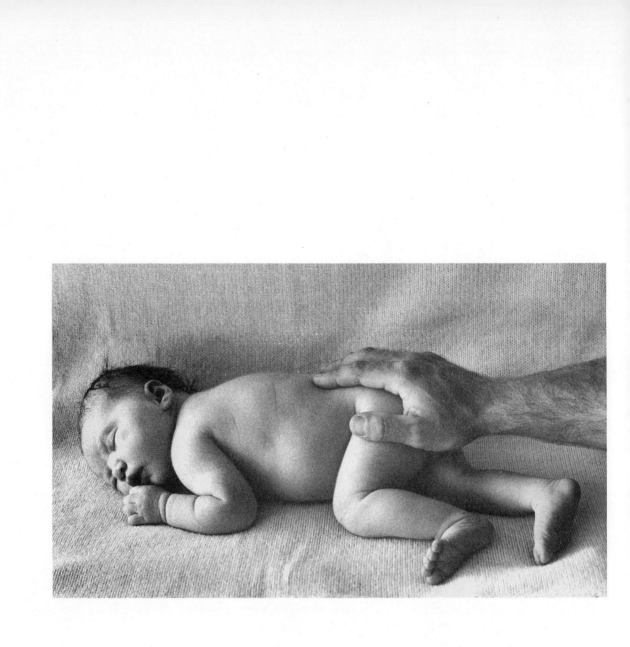

Where Do We Go from Here?

What Has Changed in the Last Thirty Years?

ALTHOUGH A LOT OF THINGS IN childbirth have changed since 1963, when the fictional Marion first gave birth, very few of those changes have supported or protected normal childbirth. During that time, general practitioners lost their role in assisting in childbirth. Good, small hospitals that could have provided individualized care for all but seriously ill mothers and babies were forced to close as more and more births took place in huge facilities set up for high-risk patients. Some drugs and routine procedures were eliminated, but others took their place. Mothers are still being routinely offered pain medication or anesthesia in lieu of real labor support, and therefore their babies are starting life with drugs in their bodies. Labor and delivery rooms are becoming combined into one room and attractively decorated, but all the modern medical technology packed into them will never give a birthing woman the kind of emotional and physical support she needs to have a normal birth.

The United States now trails far behind other countries who have neither our technological resources nor our numbers of subspecialist physicians in perinatal and neonatal care. While the mortality rate among premature and low-weight babies is declining, it is not due to the amount of money we are pouring into high-risk medical care. We still have one of the highest rates of small and premature babies among technically advanced countries. Despite all the resources we have thrown at intensive care, we have slipped continuously in the past decade in the number of healthy babies born in this country. We've gone from ninth to twenty-first place. We have one of the highest rates of infant mortality in the developed world, and we continue to slide toward the bottom. This is despite the fact that we boast the most sophisticated medical care in the world. People who don't need high-tech medical care are given it anyway, while many of those who are medically at risk receive little or no care because they have neither money nor health insurance.

High-tech medicine has proved to be valuable for between 5 and 10 percent of all mothers and babies. This includes complications of all kinds, the vast majority of which are not life-threatening. That means that 90 percent of all mothers and babies are today subjected to emotional neglect and physical over-treatment and to the risks of high-tech childbirth and newborn care. The only reason we have been able to get away with this much intervention is that child-bearing women and their babies in this country are in reasonably good health to begin with and are able to tolerate a certain amount of unwarranted intervention. But that does not make it right or beneficial.

To most people today, "normal childbirth" means that the woman has had an intravenous drip of glucose and water and an electronic monitor throughout labor, some form of drug or anesthesia to cope with the pain, and an incision to enlarge the vaginal outlet at birth, after which her baby spent some time in the hospital nursery for observation. To some, a normal birth is anything short of a cesarean. To others, it even includes a cesarean, as long as the mother and baby go home from the hospital together. Many women today see nothing wrong with scheduling a cesarean birth to fit a busy work schedule—theirs or their physician's—or just to avoid having to deal with the pain of labor. Childbirth practices, while they have evolved to benefit the rare woman or baby who truly needs intervention, have actually gone backward for the majority of mothers and babies. For them, modern childbirth practices complicate and obstruct an otherwise normal process and make it all but impossible to experience it fully. The majority of mothers and babies have been unnecessarily harmed by the modern medical assumption that childbirth is a catastrophe waiting to happen, and most people aren't even aware of what is going on.

As we have seen, electronic fetal monitors, IVs, artificial hormones to stimulate labor, drugs, and epidural anesthesia are used routinely in hospital childbirths despite the fact that they alter labor and risk harming the mother or baby. They are used because they are there, because they permit hospitals to staff the unit with fewer nurses or midwives. They are used because birthing women and their families, as well as juries in malpractice lawsuits, believe such things equal quality care. They are used because they make money. Private physicians buy expensive equipment like ultrasound machines and then tell their patients they need to do scans on the baby every few visits to make sure that the baby is growing well or that the placenta is not too near the cervix, when the real reason is to be able to charge extra fees. Obstetricians rush to do cesareans but fail to be present during long labors when mothers need their encouragement, because they earn much more money in much less time doing cesareans than in helping a woman have a vaginal birth.

Many otherwise-liberal-minded obstetricians who say they believe in normal birth and women's rights to make decisions about their births are afraid to stand up to nurses in the hospital on behalf of their patients and go against routine hospital policies such as electronic monitoring, IVs, or nursery visits for babies, for fear that incident reports might be written up on them and that they might have their hospital privileges taken away. They won't stand up to anesthesiologists or the neonatology staff when it comes to supporting a mother in her insistence on keeping her baby with her. Most doctors won't stand up to their medical associations and insurance companies and show their support for normal birth by attending births at out-of-hospital birth centers or by providing medical backup for midwives or women having home births. And many don't try to interest their clients in alternatives when the women insist on drugs or epidurals or cesareans for which there is no medical indication, or when they say they are going to formula-feed the baby. Nurses allow themselves to act as police for hospital policies that have been set up by administrators and lawyers for the purpose of avoiding malpractice lawsuits. They carry out doctors' orders that don't make sense to them out of fear of making waves and possibly losing their jobs.

Hospitals give lip service to birth being a normal process and even state that mothers and babies need to be together. But they do everything in their power to bring the process under control and to manage it according to their ideas of what works. If the latter part of the 1800s saw a leap forward in scientific advancements and those advancements quickly applied to childbirth, the latter part of the 1900s has seen a leap in the medical community's ability to design and refine technology and apply those advancements to childbirth, the care of women, and the care of babies.

Today conception can be manipulated in many ways; pregnancy can be maintained in women whose bodies are attempting to miscarry; labor can be stopped, started, or accelerated artificially, or circumvented altogether by scheduling cesarean surgery to occur before the onset of contractions; fetuses in the womb can have their lung development forced and can even have surgery performed on them; and the lives of babies born at twenty-four weeks' gestation or earlier and weighing just a few ounces are being saved by elaborate technical care. It is amazing how fast the medical community has moved in the direction of manipulating life at birth. Unfortunately, it has not been equally aggressive in investigating the nature of health and the human spirit, and the body's own innate capacity to thrive and to rebound.

Childbirth today is more artificial and disconnected from the rest of our lives than at any time in history. This disconnectedness and artificiality sets a pattern that continues when we bring our babies home and through the first two years of life, which is known to be the crucial time in which a child's sense of self is formed, a mother's sense of self is enhanced or diminished, a father's sense of worth within the family is fostered or weakened, and the family is strengthened or weakened. As we stand on the threshold of the twenty-first century, with childbirth more unnatural than ever, it is vital that we think about what we are doing to this natural process and where it is leading us.

*   *   *

We have ignored the unconscionable treatment of women and babies for too long. It is time to make fundamental changes in our attitudes about and practices of the perinatal period and maternity care. How a woman gives birth is of vital significance to her physical and emotional health, and to her relationship with her child. The experiences we have as babies in the womb, during birth, and in the first days and months following birth are crucially important. These earliest times affect our relationships with family, friends, strangers, and especially our own children. They ultimately shape our very culture. The way the perinatal period provides the lifelong foundation for relationships has yet to be *fully* comprehended. However, if we gave full respect to this period in a family's life, we would certainly approach childbearing in a very different way. We would care for every childbearing woman—and every baby who is born—with appreciation, tenderness, and respect.

First impressions do not dim with time. Think about how vividly you can still recall your first day at school or in a new home, or your first love. Early life experiences actually lay down pathways in our brain that determine how we think and feel, and how we act within the world. Just because we cannot recall our conception, our life in the womb, our birth, and the care we received in those first hours and months does not mean that these events do not matter. If we were to examine the habitual and unconscious ways in which we react from moment to moment, we might be surprised to learn just how much of the way we think, feel, and behave today is rooted in the past, when we were just starting out in life.

Perinatal experiences are as important as genetic factors and environment in determining the kind of person a child is likely to become. There is always choice, which we call "free will." However, once our basic character and way of dealing with the world is formed, it takes courage and a lot of effort and help to make significant changes. Our tendencies toward trust and openness, or mistrust and being closed, are created early on. We greet each new experience that comes our way with either curiosity or fear. All of us know where we fall on this spectrum.

*   *   *

For the most part, people have believed, *as they were taught to believe,* that they were doing the very best for childbearing women and babies. That this treatment was based on ignorance and fear, not cruel intent, is no justification for denying that people have done much harm by failing to fully acknowledge the human soul and other subtle dimensions of life during this formative experience. What people have been taught about childbearing women and babies has become institutionalized in modern maternity care. Since society has fundamental difficulty in questioning its own institutions, the inhumane treatment of childbearing women and babies remains one of the great, unacknowledged crimes of modern times. The resulting wounds—and their long-term effects— find expression in the alienation, victimization, troubled relationships, and violence that characterize modern life.

The nature of society makes it especially hard for us to confront these ills. Few of us today would dispute that we benefit greatly from living in a society whose patterns of thought, codes of ethics, and standards for behavior are passed from one generation to the next. Few of us would wish to return to the time when we lived in caves and had only the most rudimentary tools with which to make our lives more comfortable. We are grateful for the improvements of civilization, among them the technology and medicine that we believe keep us safe and healthy, adding years and quality to our lives. For the first time in history, birthing women in many parts of the world can be assured good medical backup if something goes wrong and they, or their babies, require emergency care. (Paradoxically, in the United States today, one of the richest countries in the world, many are denied care and attention because they do not have the money to purchase it.) In terms of bearing and caring for children, however, it is time to admit that all our technological and medical sophistication is harming as well as helping. We have not learned how to use judiciously, and in the service of life, the technology we have developed. In effect, we are prisoners of the fancy tools we've created and feel compelled to use.

We have paid dearly for every "advancement" because each step has altered our worldview. What have we lost? Respect and reverence for nature and all natural processes, including birth. The sense of belonging to the whole and of each part of life being inextricably connected to every other part. We have many riches, but we have lost our way in the spiritual sense. Most women today want to have a baby without having to go through pain, and hope their babies will fit into their already busy lives with as little interruption as possible. Whatever a woman gains or loses in terms of competence in the course of giving birth and caring for a new baby goes with her for the rest of her life. Birth is a challenge. It is time to see it fully and treat it with the respect and reverence it deserves. We need to respect the natural rhythms of life before intervening in birth in the name of improving it. From that place—bringing the sacredness back into the start of life—we will find ourselves walking the path that will lead us to a better future.

The way to ensure the future is to serve the needs of children today, and the needs of the women and men having children. The decisions parents make about the births of their children are much too important to be handed over to others in the mistaken belief that "experts" know best. True authority lies deep within ourselves, for we each know what is best for us and what we can live with. Reclaiming our own authority does not mean being left alone and unsupported when it comes to bearing and caring for our children, but the decisions must be our own. Just as every pregnant woman needs to be discriminating about the care of her body and spirit so that she can create a nourishing environment for her unborn child, every childbearing woman has the right to choose where, how, and with whom she will give birth. Women need information and support to be able to make the best decisions.

A woman deciding who will be her birth attendant should consider carefully. Even if she is receiving care in a system that tells her she has no choice, she *does* have a choice. She may have to be assertive or demanding and ask a lot from the people around her. But she and her baby deserve the best; she needs to be cherished for committing herself to another life. Three equally important questions for a woman to ask when choosing a birth attendant are: Is this person experienced in keeping birth normal? Is this person able to handle serious problems if they arise, or get someone who can? Does this person have reverence for the process as well as for me and my baby? Look at the person's hands and ask: Can these hands be gentle yet sure? Look in the person's eyes and ask: Can you care for me, my body, my baby? We need birth attendants and caretakers for ourselves and our babies who know that they are in service to the birth, not in control of it.

Nurturing qualities have been identified by many cultures as exclusively female. They are not female; they are human qualities we all need to develop. The important role of the father in a child's life, in supporting the childbearing woman, is being understood and valued in new ways. Men going through the process of becoming fathers must also have the information and support they need. There are times when a baby's father plays a more central role than its mother. Fathers must be allowed to take on the primary care of babies and young children and be granted as much respect as mothers.

Throughout history, childbearing has presented enormous challenges both to individuals and to the entire social group. The responsibility for raising a healthy child is a collective one. Patriarchal cultures the world over have devalued the worth of females and allotted them less of the society's resources and rights. For many years, it was accepted that in a difficult birth it was more important for the baby to survive than the mother. Today, health workers make equal efforts to save mother and child. In this country we give lip service to the idea that all people are important, yet we allow financial, racial, and social status to bias the kind and quality of care received.

Childbearing and early childhood is such a brief and crucial time in each person's life. Surely we can, individually and together, do a great deal to make this time optimal for every childbearing woman, baby, and father.

A Blueprint for the Future of Maternity and Infant Care

I envision a different world in which the needs of mothers, babies, fathers, and families are treated with respect. The following are my recommendations for what we as a society must do to make the process of childbearing a normal and healthy one and to improve the care of infants:

1. Birth educators need to work independently of practitioners (especially obstetricians) and hospitals. This is so that they are able to advocate optimal care and tell the truth without being inhibited by people or institutions who have their own expectations, such as getting compliant patients.

2. Birthing women need to understand that midwives are essential to the protection of normal, natural childbirth. We all need to support our local midwives, get involved when midwives are harassed or wrongly prosecuted, and lobby to bring midwives into communities and hospitals where there are none.

3. Communities need to establish out-of-hospital, independent birth centers that specialize in natural childbirth and women-centered births. Policies at these birth centers, whether profit or nonprofit, should be determined by boards whose membership includes a balance of women, consumers, physicians, and midwives. States and communities must make it possible for birth centers to operate.

4. Our government needs to establish a national policy that instates midwives as primary health workers in childbirth. Midwifery must be designated and protected as a profession that is separate and distinct from both nursing and medicine. Midwives should not have to work under the supervision of physicians and other health workers but should be able to collaborate with them to provide a full range of services to clients.

5. Obstetrics, perinatology, and neonatology must be understood as specialties that treat serious birth-related problems. All women and babies, regardless of their ability to pay, must have access to specialists and hospital care if they need it. The number of obstetricians trained must be limited to the number actually needed to handle cases requiring a surgeon's care.

6. The number of family physicians must be increased, and family physicians must be allowed to take extra training to attend births and act as consultants or backups to midwives. Physician assistants and nurse practitioners should also be offered additional training to provide care for pregnant, birthing, and postpartum women. This will expand the number of skilled people available in locations where there are not enough midwives or physicians providing care to childbearing families. It will enable more women to safely give birth where they live, and it will reduce the cost of delivering care.

7. A variety of training options must be available to those who wish to become midwives. These options include direct entry into the field as well as through the field of nursing. All training should include apprenticeship, fieldwork consisting of home visits and home birth, and course work at community colleges. Not only will a variety of training options make it possible for more people to become midwives, but they will better ensure that there are midwives in all parts of the country, since health workers tend to take up practice where they train.

8. Health insurance needs to cover equally all health workers skilled in attending births and all sites, including homes and out-of-hospital birth centers.

9. All forms of birth and care for babies should be paid for at the same rate. There must be no financial incentive for health workers to do unnecessary tests, procedures, or cesarean surgery. It must be understood—and the public must be educated—that there are risks, as well as possible benefits, for every test, procedure, drug, or surgery and that in childbearing the risks are compounded by the fact that what is done to the mother directly affects the baby and vice versa.

10. Quality, humanistic maternity and infant care must be provided in all hospitals. The size of hospital maternity units needs to be scaled down, and so does the number of intensive-care baby beds. It has been well documented in maternity and infant care that bigger does not mean better and that the more facilities and beds designated for high-risk or intensive care, the greater the likelihood that healthy individuals will be treated as high-risk. Especially in maternity care, which is more of an emotional and family event than a medical one, bigger means more impersonal and usually more

unnecessary, costly, and risky tests and procedures. The number of acute-care facilities needs to be spread out across the country so that they can be used appropriately. Hospitals must be monitored to determine whether they have the personnel, rather than simply the medical technology, to adequately care for patients.

11. We need to encourage the reestablishment of small hospital maternity units—with emergency transport available to take people to high-risk centers—and to discourage the use of intensive care for babies who do not require it. All nonsurgical hospital births should take place in LDR rooms (one room in which the mother labors, gives birth, and stays with her baby until she leaves the hospital). Every baby needs to remain with its mother after birth, even in intensive care settings, which require the mother's bed to be alongside the baby's cot.

12. Well-baby clinics need to be set up in every community—augmented by mobile units that go to sparsely populated areas. These clinics need to focus on providing a place for mothers and fathers to gather and offer help to each other, and on providing education and support rather than tests and medical procedures. The health records of a baby need to remain in the parents' keeping.

13. A system of health educator and child-family advocates needs to be set up to work with nurses at well-baby clinics and follow all babies through childhood. It would be their responsibility to see that children are not being neglected or abused and that children and their families are receiving the information and the health and social services they need.

14. Bonding and breast-feeding must be solidly endorsed and supported. A financial incentive must be given to all mothers who breast-feed for at least six months and to at least one parent who is with the baby most of the time during the first year. It must be understood that fostering healthy bonding between parents and babies is the surest way to prevent child abuse, neglect, and antisocial behavior in older children.

15. A system must be established to provide universal postpartum care for women, babies, and their families through the first year and longer if necessary. The primary care can be provided safely and affordably by

community health workers, midwives, nurse practitioners, and physician assistants.

16. There must be a national policy supporting maternity and paternity leave for the first six months after birth—for both natural and adoptive parents. Because there is a national crisis in family bonding today, parents and employers must be given incentives for job sharing and flexible hours. There needs to be day care at the workplace or time-off during the workday for parents whose babies cannot be near them, so babies aren't separated from a parent for more than three to five hours at a time.

17. Education in infant care and infant and child development—psychological and physical—needs to be offered free of charge in every community to anyone and required of all child-care workers.

18. A compassionate rather than adversarial system needs to be established to handle all situations of injury or death around childbearing. A primary focus will be to limit malpractice claims by taking most complaints out of the hands of lawyers and courts and placing them in the hands of local consumer/health worker boards. These local boards will listen to all parties and decide whether the injury or death should be treated as "an act of God" for which no one is blamed, or as something for which an institution or health worker must make amends. For example, a health worker might be required to improve skills, work under supervision for a time, or have a license suspended or revoked. Criminal cases would be turned over to judges, courts, and attorneys.

19. Overall, mothers and babies through the first year must once again be respected as the symbiotic unit they are and cared for as a pair. Birth must be treated as the primary family event that it is. All medical decisions need to be made with the parents fully informed of their rights, choices, and responsibilities and actively involved in the process. When there is a dispute between parents and health workers, the parents' rights to privacy and choice need to be respected, except in cases of child abuse. When there seems to be good cause for intervening against the wishes of a parent, there needs to be a process similar to that which is beginning to occur in situations related to dying, in which the decision is made with the help of local individuals who are able to weigh the ethics and all other aspects.

20. Since healthy pregnant women require little or nothing in the way of medical or nursing care throughout pregnancy, prenatal care should be given instead to those who need it most. For all women, attention must focus on education, counseling, and support rather than on medicine and technology. Doing the most good with the least intervention must be the standard. The money saved from dropping unnecessary tests, procedures, and doctor visits can be put into providing full postpartum care for all women and babies.

Let us follow this blueprint in order to foster healthy individuals, families, and communities. The true sense of community lies in understanding our interconnectedness and acting from a sense of relatedness. It is a challenge. Let's begin at the beginning. That is where we can start to reweave the sacred web of life, which has been torn, so that it once again becomes whole. In the process, we will discover our part in the balance of nature and find greater peace and joy in our humanity.

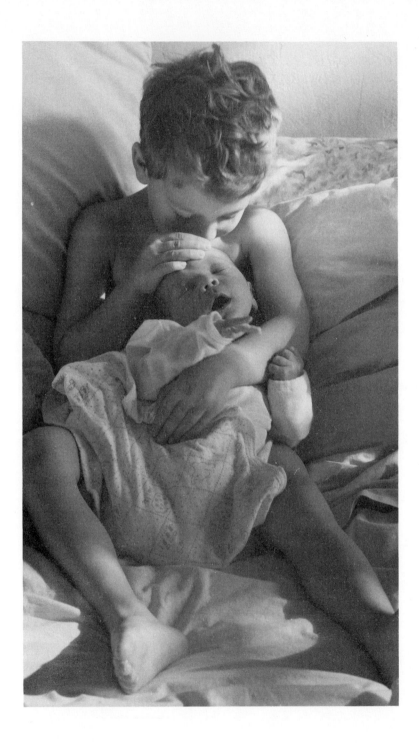

Stories and Interviews

THE FOLLOWING INTERVIEWS and personal stories reflect a wide variety of voices and experiences with childbirth, from first-time mothers to noted doctors to young siblings to respected midwives. While most are from the United States, there are several representatives from other countries as well.

As you read through these accounts, you will see quite dramatically that a birth can be either a positive or a negative event, and that what happens depends largely on the attitudes and perceptions of those involved—the mother and her birth attendants, whoever they might be.

I have included these personal accounts and interviews because I feel that no matter how many facts and opinions one may read, one gets the *real* story by hearing about people's experiences in their own words. A story may strike a chord with you if it is similar to your own, or it may bring one of the points of the book to life for you. It is my hope that this section, together with the rest of the book, will help you make informed decisions about your own childbirths.

KRISTINA

Kristina, eight, has a four-month-old baby sister named Natalie. Natalie has been sleeping in their mother and father's bedroom, but tonight she is going to move into Kristina's room. Kristina is very excited. She is very close to her little sister and was there when she was born.

Q: What was it like when your mom was pregnant?

Kristina: It was sort of hard to be in the shower with her. She took up all the space.

Q: Your mom told me you were there when Natalie was born. Can you tell me what that day was like?

Kristina: It was the day before Thanksgiving. We had a party at school. My dad came to get me early.

Q: What was your mom doing when you got home?

Kristina: She was putting a plastic sheet on her bed, getting ready for it. The midwives were there.

Q: What did you do while your mom was in labor?

Kristina: Most of the time I just watched TV in the other room. It took about four hours. My friend Erica and I—she's six and she came because her mom was going to be there, and her mom used to baby-sit me—sometimes me and Erica, we'd go into my mom's room.

Q: What was your mom like in labor?

Kristina: She made lots of noise.

Q: What kind?

Kristina: Ooohhh. Ooohhh.

Q: How did you feel when she made all that noise?

Kristina: Well, it was a bit noisy. But we were watching a movie on TV about animals and they were making lots of noise, and sometimes I couldn't tell if it was her or the animals.

Q: Did you feel scared at all?

Kristina: No.

Q: Why?

Kristina: I knew it was gonna be sort of noisy. Me and my mom watched tapes of ten different ladies having babies, and three of them made lots of noise.

One time she was in the bathroom. Me and Erica went to see, and she was going "ooohhh," and me and Erica were about to start laughing, so we just ran out of the room.

When she started having the baby and she was having really, really strong contractions I was sort of crying.

Q: What did you do then?

Kristina: I came back and started watching the movie. Then I went back and watched my mom. The head was showing *that* much [her hands make a circle about four inches across]. I was sort of mad that no one told me it was starting to come out. I wanted to see when it started to come out. Then I felt happy. I was waiting for it, and it was taking sort of a long time.

Q: Where were you when you were in the birth room?

Kristina: Mostly I was on the midwife's lap. At the end I just sat next to Sheila—that's my mom's friend—because the midwife had to help my mom.

Q: What was your mom doing?

Kristina: My mom kept on praying, for some reason, that it would be over very soon. The midwife stood next to her, and my dad helped her deliver it. He was the one who picked her up when she was born and passed her under my mom so she could hold her. My mom was on the bed, like this [she gets on her knees and elbows].

Q: What did Natalie look like when she came out?

Kristina: Her head was sort of blue at first and her body whitish. The cord was around the neck, and they had to take it off. Then she was very pink. I cut the cord.

Q: What happened then?

Kristina: My mom holded her—held her—some more. Then my dad held her. Then I got to hold her.

Q: What was she like?

Kristina: She was warm and she smelled good. She squinted and then she opened her eyes. When she first came out she didn't cry, but then she started to go "aaah." We have a picture of me holding her and afterward a picture of Natalie and me both asleep and our heads are turned the same way, and her and my face look really shiny.

Q: Did you tell other kids you saw your sister being born?

Kristina: I called my best friend Jennifer three times. When my mom started to be in labor and when the baby was already out—but then they called me and asked if I wanted to cut the cord—and then I called her back again and I told her my sister was a girl.

Q: Where did you sleep that night?

Kristina: I slept with my mom in her bed. The baby and my mom slept in the middle and me and my dad were on the sides.

Q: What happened when you went back to school?

Kristina: On Monday night we have to each write something about a current event. I wrote about my baby sister and I talked about it on Tuesday. My teacher was glad.

Q: Were the other kids interested?

Kristina: Some of them. Mostly the girls.

Q: Would you like to go to another birth?

Kristina: Yeah! I was hoping my mom's friend Veronica would let me come. She's due tomorrow. She didn't ask me, but I wish she had.

Q: Why would you like to?

Kristina: I want to see what it would be like when it's not my mom.

Q: Did seeing Natalie get born make you think about what it would be like if you have a baby?

Kristina: Not really. It was interesting. I want to have a boy and a girl.

Q: If you have a baby, how will you do it?

Kristina: At home, if I was brave enough. Lots of times I climb up walls and sometimes I fall or get cut. I can do it if someone dares me. But Jennifer is more daring than I am.

Q: What would you say to other kids if their mom was going to have a baby?

Kristina: I'd tell them it was fun. That they'd probably have fun watching their brother or sister get born, if their mom said they could watch.

Q: What else would you tell them?

Kristina: Don't worry about the noise.

MIKE

Mike, father of four, is a forty-six-year-old physician, certified in both family practice medicine and pediatrics. His practice has been devoted to bringing quality health care to the underserved. He founded an inner-city pediatric clinic. In the early 1970s he assessed babies born at home with lay midwives for a public health study in a county whose medical society was trying to get physicians to deny prenatal, backup, and postpartum care to women planning home births. For two years he was in practice with a nurse-midwife and a lay midwife. To get additional experience, he worked in the busy emergency room of a large HMO hospital. For fifteen years he has been in a busy cooperative of physicians, physician assistants, and nurse-practitioners.

When I did my medical training in Wisconsin in the 1960s, it was easy to get a lot of experience in births because the Catholic hospital where I worked did five hundred births a month. All of the babies were born to moms under twilight sleep. Women didn't know who was pushing on their bellies and pulling their babies out. They never even saw any of us; they were unconscious throughout.

I have vivid memories of a three-hundred-pound male anesthetist named Rudy. He would pass the gas mask to each woman as she began to push and the gas would put her completely out. Then he'd raise up his three-hundred-pound bulk, lean over the top of the delivery table, put his hands on the unconscious woman's abdomen, and lean his entire weight on her uterus while one of us pulled the baby out.

Every baby at that hospital was resuscitated with a bag and mask because they were all narcotized! That was the way birth was done at hospitals across the country for decades. Babies were usually born pale and blue, and all the babies I saw were floppy when they came out, which meant they were in bad shape. As if this were not enough trauma for

the babies, if it was a boy he was circumcised within thirty minutes. This was so the babies "wouldn't have to feel the discomfort" and so the mother "wouldn't have to deal with it." Fathers were nowhere to be seen.

All the babies went to the nursery. Rooming-in hadn't even been heard of. Mom saw the baby—it was brought to her, well wrapped, for viewing—when she woke up from anesthesia. Then it went right back to the nursery. All babies were given nothing to drink for at least twelve hours, usually twenty-four. Few mothers breast-fed. That's how it was right up until the early 1970s.

The medical approach to the care of newborn babies has not really changed much in this country over the past twenty-five years. The technology is more efficient and may be more physiologically sound. But physicians' mindsets about newborns—such as how babies who might need resuscitation should be cared for—have not changed at all!

The standard resuscitation approach to babies in hospital that I was taught—and that I've seen ever since—is not "above all do no harm" but "take no chances." We called it the "maxi-min" theory. Do the maximum amount of intervention needed to prevent the minimally likely, but most dangerous, complication. It's just-in-case pediatrics.

Let me give you some examples of this, of what we're still doing in hospitals across the United States. We routinely do blood sugar, or hematocrit, tests on every baby born in the hospital. These tests are done with a stick in the heel or a puncture of a vein and are uncomfortable for babies. They should not be done routinely.

Why not? First, because the chances of a healthy-looking newborn needing treatment of any kind are very small and the chance of getting a false positive rate always exists—meaning the test will show there's something wrong with the baby when there's not. A false positive always leads to other unnecessary tests! Generally speaking it's more blood tests, but it can also involve therapies that are more painful and isolating, such as giving intravenous antibiotics, performing a full septic workup, doing a spinal tap.

Another thing parents should know about before birth is phototherapy—putting babies under bili lights whenever they have a bilirubin level over a certain amount. In the 1970s it was even worse. Babies were put under lights if they had a count of ten, and it wasn't uncommon for babies to get blood transfusions with a count over twelve, when the danger point is over thirty. Almost everywhere, babies are subjected to phototherapy when they don't need it.

This is a potentially harmful treatment, in addition to which it makes the baby uncomfortable and takes it away from the mother. The harm is in the chance of dehydration and the possible interference with the baby's normal chemical mechanisms, including changes in the blood chemistry, which can have long-term effects.

Two of the problems of doing tests and treatments on babies who don't need them is that (1) parents lose confidence in their own ability, and (2) they label their baby as fragile. The message the baby then continues to get is, "There's something wrong with you." Even if the parents feel confident about themselves, parenting a child with "problems" creates a self-fulfilling prophecy.

Modern newborn medicine simply doesn't take into account some important facts. Most important, every newborn baby is basically reorganizing itself after birth. A baby's nervous system has a systematic approach to adjusting to its new environment: to breathing air, to coping with the force of gravity on its body, and so on. If a baby is stressed neurologically—if it suffers from any lack of oxygen—its ability to respond and adjust to its environment is diminished to some degree for some time.

Being able to help or resuscitate a baby goes beyond the cookbook approach of what decisions to make. A newborn, if given the chance, is innately able to correct by itself a large percentage of the problems that asphyxia can create. There's so much fear and panic today in our culture about babies supposedly needing resuscitation to help get started breathing. The public, especially birthing parents, should know what is really needed, so they don't fall victim to "physician panic."

A person who has been at the birth has the advantage of knowing before the baby is born how much chance there is that this baby might not be able to start breathing on its own. There's a big difference between a panicked approach and a reasoned approach. In a reasoned approach you prepare for the worst but, when the baby is born, you look at the baby as an individual, not a page in a resuscitation book. You do only what the baby needs.

The point I am trying to make is this: there is time. Time to think and observe. Time to act slowly and carefully. Panic is unnecessary unless a baby looks horrible and continues to look horrible, which occurs very rarely. Except in extreme circumstances—which are *very* rare—a skilled person has fifteen to forty-five seconds after the baby is out to evaluate the baby and give it normal positive support.

The main dangers in the medical care of newborns are panic and reacting in an aggressive way. Doctors and nurses are trained only in the mechanical aspects of resuscitation, not in the importance of remaining calm and being patient. Panic can cause more harm than the resulting resuscitation efforts will help.

A lot of what I've learned is from my experience attending home births and helping people who've had home births, not from my training in pediatrics and emergency medicine. The most important things I have learned are what I've learned from women. Women *know* what is going on with their babies.

Having a baby should be fun! It should not be full of fear. When women are supported in pregnancy and birth, so that their motherhood can flourish, they fall in love with their babies much more easily, and the first three months after birth is usually much more fun for them.

I've also learned a lot from babies. Babies grow better—both physically and developmentally—and thrive when they are given loving care that trusts their innate ability to survive. From being a father I've learned that the love you expect to have for a baby is nothing compared to what you come to feel when the baby is there. The feeling defies explanation, it runs so deep. But all parents need support.

From practicing in a rural area I've learned that people who do not go to physicians seem to get sick less often than people who regularly go to physicians. And when they do, they get better faster, with less intervention and medicine.

I have learned a lot from working with midwives. Their role is central to the childbearing experience, and I believe midwifery will survive as a profession much longer than obstetrics. Midwives treat birth as a normal event, which is what it is.

There is one piece of advice I would offer pregnant women. Honor your pregnancy. Honor your birth. Honor your postpartum. Make these your priorities, despite your busy and distracting life. It is too precious to let this time go by without allowing it to take you over.

To mothers and fathers of infants, I say: Don't miss your baby's infancy! Revel in it. Even the hard parts. The work you put into those early months with your baby will result in a secure and healthy little person who'll be independent and able to cope with life.

Marji

Marji is a physician instructor at a family practice residency program in New York. When she made the decision to breast-feed, as a full-time working mother, it was partly because both she and her husband had been bottle-fed babies and both of them had a history of allergies. Breast-feeding her baby made her life much more complicated since she had to find a way to do it while continuing her teaching schedule. She has breast-fed all four of her children throughout their infancy.

My husband used to call it demand feeding. Mommy demands that baby eat according to mommy's schedule. Luckily some kids will tolerate being put on someone else's routine. I arranged for a baby-sitter who lived near the hospital, and she would either bring my baby to me for feeding or I'd go to her house, depending on whether I had a lunch meeting or not. I would feed the baby in the morning before I left for the hospital. She'd give him a bottle of breast milk in the middle of the day, then I would feed him again around six and again later in the evening.

Residents saw me teaching and nursing a baby at the same time. Sometimes I also had to give additional seminars around the six o'clock feeding. It became accepted around here that nursing babies could be part of the program.

My last kid was only four pounds at birth and could not adapt to my schedule. She really needed to nurse every one and a half to two hours. So I brought her to work with me. I always asked patients' permission, when I was in clinic, to have her there. Almost no one objected. My daughter was in a bassinet in my office for several months, until she was able to tolerate an extended period of time between feedings.

I would not recommend this ordinarily, but in order to work—which I needed to do—and feed my child the way she needed, I had no choice. It would have been very difficult to do this in a hospital that didn't support me.

I had many patients, teenage girls especially, who commented that seeing me talk to them while I breast-fed made them see how important breast-feeding is and that it didn't need to tie you down. At that point I wasn't even thinking of the positive impact it might have on patients. I was just surviving.

Most of my colleagues were just glad to have me back seeing patients, even if it was in a slightly preposterous capacity. I think it made a big difference here. Within the department, people now often bring their older kids to work, especially for lunchtime or evening meetings. They bring young children and they breast-feed their babies. It's accepted. But I didn't do it to make people change. I had a life to lead and kids to feed, and I wasn't willing to make compromises about the well-being of my kids.

ADAM

Adam is a Dutch obstetrician currently teaching at a large hospital in Amsterdam that is one of the three training schools for midwives.

I worked for five years in West Africa. That's where I learned how doctors actually *cause* public health problems. I was mainly doing radical gastric surgery—taking out large parts of people's intestinal tracts. We were only interested in our heroics, not in the cause of the ill-health of the people we were treating or how the surgery impacted their lives back in the villages. It was nice work. I was dismayed to find out when I visited patients in their villages several years later that they could no longer eat the village diet. Now I can relate what I learned there to what's going on in modern obstetrics.

The obstetrics I saw in Africa was pretechnological. When I came back I began obstetric training in a clinic that was technologically oriented. It was very fascinating, but the main interest was clearly not in the woman, but in her body and blood chemistry. A labor was judged a success and the child considered normal if there was a nice pH and all the test results were "correct." We weren't taught to listen; we just measured. Even if our measurements weren't correct, many women were reassured simply because we told them everything was all right. That's not the same thing as knowing for herself that everything is all right. Everyone has a magical belief in laboratory tests and technology. We're all victims of the same misbelief.

When I came to work in this hospital the midwives considered me the enemy because I'd trained in a place where midwives are being turned into assistants to the doctors. I brought in ultrasonic equipment and I'm not sorry about that, because it's important. I persuaded people here that it was necessary to have all the modern things on hand, but I tried to remember the message of Dr. G. J. Kloosterman, director of Obstetrics and Gynecology at the University of Amsterdam Medical School: "Labor is a normal physiological event and we should, as much as possible, keep technology away from it. Once in a while you need technology; but then, apply it correctly."

Doctors in the Netherlands have not been able to resist modern trends in obstetrics; we are not an island. Our cesarean rate is rising. When I arrived a decade ago, the rate in this hospital was 2 to 3 percent. Now it is 9 or 10 percent. Perhaps we are dealing with more pathological cases now than a decade ago, because of other changes in the population. But we're also doing a lot more diagnostic tests. When you do more tests on pregnant women you always discover more so-called pathology, or things that can be interpreted that way.

Today we have a home birth rate in the Netherlands of more than 30 percent, but in the 1970s it was 60 percent! I think we doctors are to blame for the lower home birth rate, the rising cesarean rate, and a lot of other problems in childbearing. It's our attitude. We're trained for pathology, and it's more satisfying to perform an operation than to stand aside. My hands itch when I have nothing to do but watch. I'm glad that much of my work is gynecology now. I don't have the self-discipline to keep my hands in my pockets at births.

The real issue is still what Kloosterman always said: We doctors always have the inclination to turn labor into some kind of operation. We love to do something heroic. It is too bad that, in general, the women are very grateful. We stop the pain of labor and deliver a live child, but when a woman receives her child from the hands of a doctor, it is less her child than when she has delivered it herself. In the long run that's negative. When you consider that we've changed a physiological process into a pathological one, we've made a mess. The pain of labor is not a negative process. It's a positive contribution.

The main theme in prenatal care needs to be preparation for birth and parenting—not medical management. Women need to talk with midwives and other pregnant women about their common experiences. The medical side is of minor importance. It has not been established that prenatal care prevents pathology. We believe it, but it may not be true. Prenatal care should be at a place where women can meet each other, talk with each other, exchange experiences. As much as possible the father should be included in the care, to foster his bond, not only with the mother but with his child. Birth is primarily a social event, not a medical one.

Vigilant observation is always called for in obstetric care. Here we too follow a system of different levels of care for different levels of risk. It is important that we not become reactionary and refuse all medical tests simply because they are medical, but obstetricians should only care for truly risky cases. Even in certain cases of increased risk we still leave the care to midwives. Some people say primary care shouldn't be left to midwives, that only doctors can spot problems. That's nonsense! Every day I see examples of how midwives spot complications in time. We obstetricians overestimate our specialness.

Medicine is not all that complicated. It's usually more a question of common sense than sophisticated knowledge or fancy technology.

Physicians forget that it is possible to do a good job in medicine without all the technology. The most important instruments we have are still our own nose, our eyes, and our hands! It's so easy to take refuge in technology, so reassuring. A woman and child who have been through a normal pregnancy and start of labor will almost certainly be all right. You have to watch, and trust.

In the Netherlands there's no financial incentive for the obstetrician. Our salaries are the same whether we work hard or are lazy. Financial reward for doctors ruins obstetrics, although most of my colleagues wouldn't agree with this. Because I keep my hands in my pockets when I am not needed, some of my peers would say, "You are lazy. You should be doing more surgery. That is what you were appointed for."

Postpartum care is very important and should be left to midwives. Once you start treating newborns as patients, as is now being done in the United States, then you create two victims. In the Netherlands, every postpartum woman is offered a "home help" for a few dollars a day. They are trained well, do daily checkups, and keep records for the midwife to see when she does her home visits. A woman can choose to have someone two hours a day, four hours a day, or more. The person also helps with cleaning, shopping, and caring for older children. In my experience, every woman needs help, and it should extend for at least seven days.

I believe that all maternity care should be free to those who are poor. Everyone should have access to the full range of care—home birth, as well as physician care and hospitalization if needed. Immediate postnatal care must be well organized, with routine home visits. Birth with a midwife should be emphasized.

I also believe that the central authorities in obstetrics should be the midwives. Every pregnant woman should first see a midwife, who will refer her to an obstetrician if necessary. Ideally, even if an obstetrician were required at the birth, the midwife would also be there.

Physicians in training need to come in contact with midwives. We can learn a lot from them. Also, physicians in training should see a lot of normal births. In our hospital, physicians in training go to home births and learn to do the work a midwife does. It's very important that a country not train too many obstetricians. If you train too many they will be in competition with midwives.

I am happy that in this country, people are be-coming more and more critical of high-tech births. The mood has shifted. Women do prefer less technological care. The number of births is up at hospitals like this one, where midwives do more of the births, and there's less technology used by physicians.

I would like to see home birth for at least one in every three births. I'd like to see even more, but that would be difficult here because it's easier for the health system to work if women deliver in the hospital. This is unfortunate, because in a hospital, birth will always—in the end—be considered a medical procedure.

Modern obstetricians may say: "Birth is a normal physiological event." But their actions belie their words. Their actions tell women that birth is not normal. Women must remember that it is.

ANGIE

Angie is a single twenty-nine-year-old college graduate in training to become a doula, a skilled labor support and advocate for birthing women.

I once lived next door to a nurse-midwife. That was the first time I'd ever heard of one. Then, a couple of years ago, I heard from a girlfriend about a center called The Birth Place and something called a "doula." It sounded really interesting, so I applied and got accepted for the course. There are a dozen women, all very different, eighteen to forty-six, some with kids, some without. I'm the only black woman.

First we learned mostly about the physiology of birth and how an out-of-hospital birth center runs. Now we're learning how to support women in labor, how to help keep birth normal. We are advocates for the mother and her family, to help make each birth the best it can be, to help the woman achieve what she wants, not what we think is best. Different speakers come to our classes. We talk a lot about the politics involved in birth, how hard it is for midwives practicing independently to get physician backup, about the influence of malpractice insurance companies on birth, and how doctors and midwives who do home births or work in birth centers can't get insurance.

My girlfriend took me to a lecture by Suzanne Arms at the Stanford medical school. It was about bringing normalcy back to birth and about the different experiences that women and babies have. She showed lots of slides. For the first time I could see that, right from birth, babies are aware human beings and that how people are born and treated around the time of birth can have lasting effects.

You know how it is in high school when you have all these dreams about what you are going to accomplish in life? And then you get out in the real world and get lost in everyday things? Well, for the first time since high school, I was inspired. I realized I might actually have a calling, and that it might be midwifery. But for now, it's being a doula.

I am surrounded by a lot of powerful women. There are so many things I want to know, so many things I need to ask! I don't think I ever recognized my inner strength before. Until now my associations with other women—except those in my family—haven't been trusting or compassionate. I learned growing up that you can't trust other women—not with your men, not with your deepest secrets. In these classes we open up. There's a bonding I've never felt before. We listen to each other and are learning how to support each other. It feels like a family, like being sisters.

I think it's important that women become much more responsible about the choices they make in birth and for their children. We are the first teachers of our children. What we are teaching them? About the land? About themselves? About creating a community? About social consciousness?

Women need to get back to their own art forms—like quilting, cooking, canning, knitting, sewing, gardening, singing, dancing. And they need to get back to normal birth. I see women who want to have babies and don't want to work for their births, don't want to feel any pain. Too much fear about the birth process has been instilled in us. We've been taught not to trust our own bodies.

A month ago I went to a birth where the woman gave in totally to her body; she gave *in*, she didn't give *up*. She had what is called "back labor," the baby lying posterior with its face toward the pubic bone. Back labors are longer and more painful, but her husband was there for her and I was there for both of them. As the baby came, there was no screaming, just animal groans, and I saw that I'd been lied to. All I had ever heard was how every woman needs drugs or anesthesia and an episiotomy and a doctor to deliver the baby. It's not true. This woman allowed herself to give birth, and the baby really delivered itself.

OLIVIA

Olivia is a physician in her late thirties, senior administrator in a state department of public health, and mother of a seven-month-old daughter. She participated in many births as part of her medical training and thought she knew what to expect at the birth. She was surprised by the intensity of her feelings after her birth.

My husband and I went to classes together so we could share the birth experience. I was looking forward to a natural birth. I chose my doctor carefully. He is warm and compassionate and seemed to understand the feelings of an older mother. I told him what was important to me: natural childbirth if at all possible, having both my mother and my husband there, and keeping the baby with me as much as possible afterward.

I worked until the day I went into labor. After timing irregular contractions for a whole day, I called my doctor. They were still eight or nine minutes apart, but I was getting very tired. He suggested that I take a sleeping pill. I chose not to, but I couldn't sleep either. The next morning I went to his office. My cervix was 90 percent effaced (thinned) and about four centimeters dilated. I don't know why, but he wanted a "biological profile" on the baby, a sophisticated version of a sonogram. It had to be done in the hospital.

They found some decelerations in the baby's heartbeat after contractions. My doctor came and looked at the monitor and said, "I think we should go ahead and do the C-section right away." He didn't ask anyone else to look at the strip. The pressure was on. I was really worn out and upset that things weren't working. Everything happened so quickly. I told my husband, "There's not much of a choice. We'll just do what we have to do and deal with our emotions afterward."

I had the cesarean about twenty minutes later, under spinal anesthesia. My husband didn't want to be there, but I needed him to hold my hand. They held my daughter up as they passed by with her on the way to the nursery to "observe" her. She had an Apgar score of 9, which meant she was fine, but for unexplained reasons I couldn't have her.

That was what was especially difficult about my birth—waiting almost twelve hours before I could hold my baby. I still feel upset. I should have insisted more! I *knew* what was going on in the nursery. Everything is so traumatic there. I just wanted to hold her and tell her, "Don't worry. You will be back with me soon."

I can't believe I am still so upset about not having her with me—and having the C-section. There is a good rationalization for everything that happened. My mind accepts it, but not the rest of me. I try just putting it aside, but it doesn't work. I go to conferences and hear people talking about these issues and it brings up all the feelings that are still there.

I have fought for other people as patients, for their rights. I have always been involved in maternal health issues and have been a strong advocate for women. I fought the system. But when it came to something very personal to me, I let myself down, and I let my baby down. I didn't push the system.

Another negative thing that happened to me was the spinal. Technically, the anesthesiologist was one of the best in the hospital. But there I was, on the table, doubled over with intense contractions, and while he was putting the spinal into my back he was telling me I had to lose weight. It was one of those situations where I'd like to have punched the son-of-a-bitch. But he had that needle. How do you bring sensitivity into the system when it's not designed that way?

My husband and I are still talking about it, in bits and pieces. It's not something we can just easily lay our hearts open about. It was traumatic, maybe more so for him. The way he deals with problems is to slow everything down and think about each part of it. With my medical background I understand what an emergency is. In labor I wasn't able to make the decision whether the C-section was really a medical emergency. That's why you have a professional, to be able to make decisions if they need to be made quickly. That's when trust comes into play, why it's so important to feel right about who you've selected.

It is hard for me to judge whether the cesarean was necessary without looking at my chart and the monitor strip. I want to look for myself. I have to, but I'm not ready yet. When I do I'll try to separate my emotional self from my physician self. Then I'll have to resolve both parts—what happened, and how I feel about it. I have to find a way to bring them together and heal myself.

Part of it means talking to my doctor, telling him my experience and my feelings about it. He's a good person. Maybe what I can share with him will help him be better with other women. And that will help me. I'm afraid, though, that if I go in and I'm emotional, then he'll label me "an emotional woman."

My husband has to be part of this process. He too has to express his feelings in order to heal. My mother says, "Let's be thankful that the baby is okay and that the doctor was smart enough to know he had to do the C-section." It's true, what is most important is that she is here, and she is healthy. I have the wherewithal to cope with whatever trauma I have, but I wish I'd had more support than I did, right from early pregnancy. I needed someone to spend more than three or four minutes each visit, someone who would talk with me. It's one thing to say, "I am here. Call if you need me." It's another to say, "Let's talk. How are you going to manage after the baby comes. What do you think you'll need?"

As a physician, I should have known what I needed and how to ask for it. But I wasn't being a physician. Just a woman. I have the same emotions as anyone. It is one thing to talk about it. It's another to experience it.

I want to see women get a support system and advocacy within the system. People need to know ahead of time their rights and what they may need emotionally, as well as financially and physically, and where to find it. This should be accessible to all women, regardless of profession, age, education, or economic status. One should not be victimized by the system. It's so easy for that to happen! It is not that the individuals in the system are necessarily bad, it's the way the system is set up.

Giving birth is probably the biggest thing I have ever done, and is the most wonderful thing that's ever happened to me, even though it was not how I wanted it. I am rather anxious to go through it once more, so I can do it right. Now it seems incomplete. I wonder how many other women are out there who have trauma from giving birth and don't even realize it. If something triggers it and all their feelings come up, they may wonder, "Am I just nuts?" "Am I just PMS?"

A negative experience giving birth affects your relationships with other people and with your child, as well as your feelings about yourself. If you have to go back into the medical system, even for just the routine exams you need as a woman, you're reluctant. You do not want to be traumatized again.

VICKI

Vicki is a mother of three, licensed psychotherapist, well-known lecturer, and teacher of Native American shamanic practices.

My husband and I talked of moving to Arizona. I woke up one night, hearing the rain, and felt this sense of urgency. I woke Jonathan. "We've got to go." The day the moving truck arrived I was nauseous. I was thirty-seven and knew I was pregnant with my third child.

We found a beautiful little house in the desert near a creek, and right away I began experiencing contact with the earth that I'd never had before. One day we stood on the cliff looking down at the creek beneath and at our house in the distance, and a great blue heron flew just a few feet over our heads. In many cultures, cranes, herons, and storks are believed to be related to birthing. I took it as a wonderful omen.

I had Robin, my first, in 1966, when I was nineteen. They called it "natural childbirth," and it was considered a radical experiment at the University of Iowa Medical Center. When I arrived in labor, my pubic hair was shaved and I got an enema. Labor was induced with a drug, I had a long needle inserted next to my spine. They taped a catheter to my skin, and anesthesia went into my body. It was termed "natural" because I did controlled breathing and was awake. In the process of putting the needle in and taping the catheter down, they must have pinched the tube because I never did get the anesthesia. It was so odd. I was experiencing all the pain of labor, while everyone assured me I wasn't feeling anything. Luckily all my babies came easily and fast.

One day I was nursing Robin and a resident came in and told me she'd been spitting up in the nursery and there was blood in my milk so I would have to stop nursing. I didn't know then that some babies spit up a little blood because of a broken capillary. Nobody approved of my nursing, anyway, in my family. I stopped nursing her, but it broke my heart. For a long time I thought there was something wrong with my breasts and feared one day I'd get cancer.

My second birth, two years later in a Navy hospital in New Hampshire, was worse! I didn't have any power, even though my entire labor was only two hours. They did an enema and a shave and kept me flat on my back in bed when I wanted to be up moving around. I wasn't allowed a drink of water. They said I might throw up and swallow it if I had anesthesia and die. I could only suck on a small amount of ice chips. Because I was upset that they wouldn't give me water, they gave me a drug called Demerol. I hardly remember the birth, just being on the table, getting stitched up, and having the doctor say to me, "Don't fall asleep, Mrs. Siegler. We're almost done." Although I was unconscious, I remember being so mad!

I didn't even see the baby, but she must have suffered from the drugs I got because she was completely noninteractive. I didn't try to nurse her because I could not bear the disappointment of having something go wrong again and having to quit. I spent the first five years of Brook's life trying to bond with her. I'd asked the universe for a baby who was quieter than Robin, who was very active, but this baby was too quiet. For ten years I had to intrude through her barriers and force contact or she would just zone out. I believe Brook's passivity and lack of bonding were definitely related to all the drugs she got through me at birth, and to our not seeing each other for the first twelve hours after she was born. Maybe not all babies would react this way, but she did.

After each of my births I went numb. I was just glad I had had a baby, glad it was over. One of the reasons I wanted a third baby was a sense that I had to complete something that was unfinished.

When I was five months pregnant with my third child, I woke up one night with a feeling of fire in my belly. There was an electrical storm, no rain, just tremendous thunder and lightning that moved across the sky. I took a walk in the darkness out to the cliff. The lightning was coming in big fingers across the sky. I stood on that shelf of earth, looking out over the creek, and felt exhilarated. Something made me want to pledge myself and my baby to the Mother Earth. I raised my arms and said to the sky and earth, "We belong to you. We are totally in your hands." I found myself thinking, "I am just like every woman who has walked across this desert pregnant. I have been here before and I will be here again."

I'd taken us to live in this remote place because I needed to protect my baby and myself. I told everybody, "I will squat under the willow tree if I have to, but I will do it on my own!" It was not a vow I'd made in my head. It was in my womb.

I did have doubts. I was afraid that I wouldn't be able to do it, that something bad would happen and I would die. I expressed all my fears. Jonathan was a little worried, but I'd bring out a book I was reading called *Birthing Normally* and say, "Jonathan, I'm not creating negative images. I am doing the work of worrying. I'm just releasing fear." It is a very fine line, but I knew the difference. Because of the vow I had made to the earth, I had someplace to give my fear. I kept reminding myself that whatever happened would be all right. My biggest fear wasn't death but having to go to a hospital at some point.

My son came three weeks early. I ended up delivering him standing up. The most interesting thing about his birth is that, at one point during pushing, the urge totally went away. An hour passed. My midwife said I needed to push, even without the urge, for the sake of the baby. But I had no urge at all. She sat for a minute, then said, "This must be where they used forceps before." And it was true! Unconsciously I had no inkling I could do it myself. I wanted somebody to do it for me, just like they had before. I pushed and hollered and pushed, and he came. The whole labor was only six hours. I felt so good, so integrated.

Aaron was quiet and a little blue and looked like

an elf. He began to breathe and turn pink, but could not nurse. The midwife said, "Don't worry. When your milk comes in he will." They had seen what it was right away. They weren't positive, because he didn't have the Simian lines on his hands and feet or have all the facial features. They told us later, after we found out what this meant, that they didn't want to be the ones to tell us. They wanted Jonathan and me to discover it, after we had already connected with him as a healthy baby. It took a week until we were ready to see. No one could have prevented Aaron's being a Down's syndrome baby. It's a genetic condition. I am glad we didn't know ahead of time. Instead, he was just Aaron, the baby we loved, not a label.

My milk came in, but he still could not nurse. He'd latch on but not suck. We bought a breast pump and an eye dropper, and I began feeding him my milk with an eye dropper. As he swallowed he began to suck a little. Getting him on my breast was so difficult, so frustrating. I would cry. But in the night, when I held him and tried to feed him, I would think to myself, "There are mothers all over the world feeding their babies right now. And I am going to draw on their energy." I put it out like a prayer, "Please help us! We can do this." And it helped.

Aaron was born on March 14. A week later, at the equinox, I was rocking him at five in the morning, and a voice came through me that said, "Be patient with this one!" I'd been up all night, trying to teach him to nurse, and I was patient. We went to the doctor that day because of Aaron's lack of interest in sucking. He was the one I'd gone to for blood work in pregnancy. He hated people like us who gave birth at home. He brusquely did a checkup on Aaron, turned to me, and said, "He's Down's syndrome."

I started crying, but it was from the experience with that doctor more than anything. For six months I had to work with my dual feelings, loving Aaron for the elf that he is, and fearing how others would look at him.

We moved back to Berkeley. It was the right time, because there are special places here for Aaron. He is two now and goes to a preschool where there are twenty-five children, five of whom are handicapped. Aaron's only been there a month and they've already taught him sign language. He is so pleased with himself. A special education therapist works with him. She has a Down's syndrome child herself and is in love with Aaron.

My pregnancy with Aaron, giving birth to him, and nursing him were so strengthening. On a cellular level, my womanhood is restored. If I had given birth like that when I was nineteen, I would be a different woman today.

GABRIELLE

Gabrielle is twenty-one years old. She was interviewed four days after the birth of her first child, who came one and a half weeks after his due date and after eleven hours of normal labor. Gabrielle's reaction to giving birth is quite unusual in our culture.

I loved giving birth. I miss it. I've been thinking about it all the time, wishing I could do it again. It was like a dream state. The pain actually felt good. I went to my deepest parts, which I'd shut off long ago. My husband and I have been in bliss ever since.

Contractions started in the evening during a summer storm, right after we made love. They were sporadic, and felt like intense waves passing over my body and gripping me. I called the midwife the next morning, and she said just to ignore them until they became regular or much closer together. I'd have contractions every ten minutes for a few hours, and then there would be none for a while. They didn't get strong for two more days.

On Wednesday, I went for a swim in the ocean, the first time I'd done that during my pregnancy. It was warm, and the waves were very mild. I felt nervous, but good too. We went home, and I fixed dinner. I had to sit down constantly. I was having contractions, and was out of breath. I also resented that I was cooking; I could have asked my husband to, but I didn't. I didn't even eat anything. After dinner, I felt something coming, and the contractions began to get harder and closer.

At first, my husband wasn't there for me the way I wanted him to be. I knew it bothered me, but he was tired and wanted to go to bed. Finally, he began to pay attention to me, rubbing my back with each contraction. I'd fall asleep after each one and be shocked awake with the next.

At three in the morning I called my mom. She had already sensed something was going on. She suggested that I call my midwife, but I was hesitant. It was the middle of the night. I decided to call, and she said she'd come. I had two contractions while talking on the phone.

When the midwife arrived and checked me, she said I had already dilated to six centimeters. "Wow," I thought, "I've made it this far, and it hasn't been bad yet."

My husband was great by then. I didn't know he had it in him! He was so loving. He anticipated everything, and he stayed awake.

I don't know what made me do it, but during each contraction, I started pretending that I was making love. You can do that with your mind. I was making those noises, and it really helped ease the pain. It made it enjoyable, *good* pain. Normally, I'm not someone who is totally in my body when I make love. I tend to be in my head. But when my husband rubbed, soothed, and kissed me, it felt so good. I remember our faces pressed together, like a nice blur.

Sometimes, the midwives sang to me. That helped so much. It felt like a dream—the dark night, candlelight, and the contractions—it felt exciting. There was the pain, but I kept saying to myself, "This is *good* pain." That's what worked.

Pushing was *serious* pain! When the baby's head appeared, I said, "I can't do this." I didn't think that part was going to be so hard, although I think it had to do with becoming a mother. I think I was scared to make the baby come out.

Several thoughts were going through my mind at once: "What if a deformed monster comes out!" "Am I ready to be a mother? To hold this baby in my arms?" "Can I push a human being through my body?" That last thought made me not want to do it. These thoughts were like walls holding me back. So I took it very slow. I needed to.

I didn't really do much during the first forty-five minutes of pushing. It was scary to try and to feel myself opening up. It felt impossible. I had to ask everyone to tell me that I could do it. And they did. I needed to hear it over and over again because I wanted to get up and say, "Sorry, I'm leaving!"

I was not used to making really deep sounds, so my husband started making them with me. His voice took me deep. He placed his arms around me during each contraction. I had to think of myself like an animal, a big mama bear.

The head kept going back in after each contraction. It was still in its sac until the very end, and when it broke it was like an explosion inside. I had been sitting on a low birth stool of the kind used in Holland. I got nervous that the baby might come too fast and I would tear. So I got off, sat on the floor, and leaned back against some pillows. When the head started coming out, I took it real slow.

After the head was out, I didn't quite realize it. One of the midwives' daughters, who was eight, was awake and sitting on the couch across from me. Her eyes were like mirrors. I don't remember feeling the shoulders coming out, but she noticed, and told my husband he could reach down and grab the shoulders. It was great watching him. He was surprised how slippery they were.

I saw it was a boy right away. A boy coming out of my woman's body! He was purple and his head was elongated, but he was all there. My husband told me later that as soon as he saw Jakub, he felt he'd known him already. I was still thinking, "How could this complete person have been inside me all this time? What was he doing in there?"

I challenged myself to my limits during Jakub's birth. Sure, I was scared. I never expected it to feel so painful, so intense. But now I can't wait to make love with my husband again.

SHOSHANA

Shoshana is a freelance editor and writer who had very difficult circumstances for a first pregnancy at age forty-four, yet created a normal birth for herself and her son.

When I was young, I didn't think I ever wanted to have a child. At some point in my thirties, I began wanting a baby, but I was never in the right relationship. Something told me I would be pregnant when I was forty-three. In the meantime, I did a lot of things that I wanted to do.

I've always been someone who made sure that I had several exits in everything I did. To me, pregnancy was the only experience I could imagine where there would be no exit. I'd have to go through with it. That's why I was so hesitant. Also, I had a great fear that a baby's head would not be able to get out of such a small opening.

On my forty-second birthday, I had a gathering with close friends and announced to everybody that I was finally open to becoming pregnant. John, the man I had been with for two and a half years, was also there. It was very frightening, but I also said that if it didn't happen, that was fine too. I performed a ceremony.

I got pregnant very soon. After the initial shock and denial, I began to feel incredible, like the cat who caught the mouse. Me, pregnant at forty-three years old!

Everybody thought I was high risk and would have lots of problems, but I didn't. I'd eaten well all my life, done yoga, exercised, and worked through a lot in therapy. Money was the biggest problem. I'd quit my job as an editor the year before to start my own business. All my savings had gone into renting an office and getting started. I had no savings and no paycheck. John agreed to support me for a while, but that all changed just a couple of months later.

He walked out. A couple months later, he was living with someone else. He had been so sure he wanted to be a father again, but he wasn't. I was scared. At first, our agreement was that we would live separately but that he would be there for me through the pregnancy—go to counseling and to birth classes with me, and be at the birth. Several months later, I was still hanging on to the idea of having a partner for this child, some financial support, and sharing parenting. Finally, I had to give it all up. John had begun to say that he didn't even believe the baby was his. He was trying to get out of any responsibility. A male friend forced me to face reality. "If you were to make a list right now of your priorities, John would be at the top. It's supposed to be the baby, and you, and the delivery, not him!"

I wrote John a letter, told him I didn't want any connection with him whatsoever, and mailed it. From that point on, I got my strength back. On August 13 I went into labor—a single mother, age forty-four, on government assistance.

I could have had a lot of complications from all the stress, but I didn't. From the beginning, I was determined to make my body and mind ready for a normal childbirth, a home birth. It took me awhile to find the right midwives, and I didn't find a backup physician until two months before giving birth. I must have called almost everyone in the county. Finally I found one who knew friends of mine. His insurance policy would not cover backing a home birth, but he did it on the agreement I wouldn't tell anyone. If I had to go to the hospital he would meet me there, on the condition I told no one I had been doing a home birth. I found a therapist who used hypnosis to help me work through all my fears. He even took me back through my own birth, and I saw clearly why I'd always been so afraid of hospitals and medical procedures. Then he had me redo my birth the way I wished it had been, and I created a wonderful birth. That was Elias's birth!

The labor was probably much longer than it needed to be, because I was very tired from working. I hadn't been able to nap for weeks, and I worked up until nine o'clock the night I went into labor. Contractions started slowly at eleven but didn't get active until one the next afternoon. He was born just before nine in the evening. I had the childbirth at the home of friends who'd gone to all the childbirth classes with me. As it turned out, I didn't want anyone with me in labor except the midwives and two friends.

I got stuck for a while at five centimeters. The one thing I had not prepared for in hypnotherapy was my cervix dilating. I had no concept of it; when one of the midwives said, "You're not dilating," I couldn't picture it. I finally let them break the waters. I had to lie on my back for it, and I couldn't believe how much contractions hurt lying on my back. It's torture! You can't imagine the difference between that and squatting.

I remember roaring at the end and shouting to one of my friends, "Sing something!" Everyone started to chant, while I yelled and grunted. I made a lot of sounds in labor. People would remind me to keep my voice low down in my throat and would make noises with me. I can't imagine what I would have done in a hospital, with strangers around, feeling inhibited.

I pushed while squatting, holding onto a rope that my friends had hung from one of the beams. I read in a book that women in some cultures used them. It felt good, and it worked. I squatted until his head was out, crawled over to the bed, turned over, and Elias was born.

His eyes were wide open. There were eight people in the room by then, and I swear he looked at every person. Then he nursed for a little bit, picked his head up, and looked around at everyone again.

I didn't tear. I had done perineal massage on myself in pregnancy, which is supposed to help, but the midwife who delivered was like an artist: she protected my tissues.

I never got taken care of after giving birth and could only take a month off from work. I stayed at different friends' houses for the first two weeks; after the first three days, everyone let me cook for myself, because they were too involved in their own lives to do it. I didn't get much rest, but people did help financially, and my mom came out for ten days.

My attitude has really come a long way. As a single mother, I could have felt like a victim. I had to say, "I'll do this in a positive way." It's taken practice. The first nine months were hard. Even now, challenges come up, and I still freak out. Every day, I have to remind myself to say, "This is what it is."

The experience of giving birth is 99 percent of what has made the difference in my life. I used to have a hard time knowing and saying what my limits are. Now, I've learned how to say what they are, because in birth it was a matter of life or death, for me and for Elias.

I really believe in the depth of our bonding. Bonding can later, at all different points, but the way I did it then was to keep him right with me, after birth, next to my skin, not wearing any clothes for four days. That and the birth established some-thing between us that's made it possible for me to do what I am doing now, as a single mother. Because I gave birth the way I did, because my body did it, no matter how tired I get there is something within me that knows that I can do it. Because I already have.

SHEILA

Sheila, a mother of four—including twins born at home—has for decades been a pioneer in childbirth education. An integral force in the British National Childbirth Trust, she developed their teacher training program. She is a prolific writer and the internationally respected author of numerous books relating to childbirth and women's sexuality.

I started life as a "Truby King baby." He was a popular pediatrician in the 1920s who gave talks all over the Western world on how to rear children. He believed that "any baby can be spoiled and made a cross, fretful little tyrant." I was kept isolated in an all-white room and fed on a strict schedule every four hours, weighed before and after every feeding. My mother was careful not to rock me or pat me, because that was said to "overstimulate" babies and lead to indigestion and "nervous disorders" later in life. King's system was based on how he'd raised dairy calves. So, I lay in my lonely cot and yelled for what must have seemed like hours. In the end my frantic mother had to give the schedule up because I made life such hell.

After I graduated from Oxford in anthropology, I did a research degree. I got married and was commuting between Edinburgh University, where I was teaching, and Strasbourg, where my husband was a diplomat. After a bit I gave up my job, because it was understood that when a woman was married she should no longer work. I can't believe now that I did that, but I did! It was the mid-1950s.

We were in France when I had my first daughter. I knew I wanted a home birth, I never considered any other way. I did not get any support for it except from my husband. I got a midwife who had been to Dr. Lamaze's clinic in Paris and taken a short course there but hadn't yet tried it. I told her about Grantly Dick-Read's work, since I'd read his books on natural childbirth. Dick-Read considered relaxation very important, and he had great confidence in women. Birth for me each time was so joyful!

I began teaching because I wanted to make good birthing information available to give women a choice. I never did believe in lecturing about techniques for giving birth. I always preferred discussion groups. I was interested in group dynamics, and I learned all the time from the women and men in those classes. I did talk about breathing and "centering," as I saw it.

A lot of what I know has come from my own personal Quaker practice, that when you "center down" into an experience you are *with* yourself, *with* your body, and have a chance to be in tune with its rhythms in a way that you can't if you are fighting your body.

When I started my work, I felt that those involved in childbirth education did not have enough knowledge, enough clarity of thinking. I felt teachers needed to have some intellectual acumen about what we were doing, that we should question and question and never be satisfied with quick answers. I did not want us to get into the trap so many doctors have gotten into.

In helping women prepare for birth it is essential to look at the whole woman as she is in her social context. It is important to explore with a woman what her experiences of pain have been and how she's coped in the past. This is not psychotherapy. It's sharing in an adventure!

I feel the central issue of birth is that of control, whether we can have control over what happens to us. Women are often afraid of what a baby can do to their lives. We need to explore what a challenge and enrichment the experience of mothering can be. Sometimes having a baby is presented as being very awful and sometimes it is seen in a romantic haze. Both are unhelpful. As a result of them, a woman is likely to feel very guilty about any negative emotions she may have about the pregnancy and birth and may think that any hostility she feels toward her baby is all her fault.

I use the term "psychosexual" regarding birth because childbirth can be part of our sexual lives, if we think of sexuality as far more than simply penetration or orgasm. It can be seen as part of the surge of exciting energy in our body and a sense of satisfaction in using our bodies well, living in and expressing ourselves through our bodies. What comes with that is increased self-awareness and the enrichment of self. That's how my births were.

What I find most hopeful today is the new alliance between radical feminism and the childbirth movement. I stand with a foot in both camps. A lot of women who focused primarily on the family and on being good mothers are now beginning to see the larger perspective. One needs to take political action to be heard.

It is *so* important that women share their experiences with each other. We've been terrorized by male professionals—and sometimes female professionals following the male-dominated structure—into thinking we cannot believe other women and so shutting our ears to them. We've been told, for example, not to believe in "old wives' tales."

But those tales are marvelous! They are foundations of our culture, and we can use them. We *should* be listening to women. It is important to listen both to those women who have had joy in childbirth and those who have been violated in birth and dare not tell their story because they know it will not please us.

For some women giving birth is as if they have been raped. They use the same language as rape, the same imagery, and have the same kinds of dreams afterward. I did a very brief television interview in the late 1980s in which I talked about what happens to so many women in the hospital as being raped, and afterward the letters just poured in—ninety-seven the first day alone! Women wanted to talk about it. They wrote about the shame they felt, how they had caused it, how it was all their fault. They felt they couldn't tell anyone.

I was amazed at the searing quality of their language. They wrote of "butchery," of their bodies feeling like "a bloody mess," and of a loss of identity and personality: "They didn't speak to me, only about me." "I was just a case to them." "The professionals were only interested in the lower half of my body."

After birth, when a woman first begins to talk about her experiences she almost always says how grateful she is to her doctor. Many women say, "If I hadn't been in the hospital the baby wouldn't be all right." Later these same women begin to talk about what it was *really* like to have an epidural, to watch the whole thing without sensation, as if it had been on television. Still later, if you keep listening over a period of time, the same woman will suddenly begin to realize the enormity of what she's been through. That's when so many talk about birth being depersonalized and feeling afterward as if something were taken away.

When a woman has been raped she will also try to rationalize the situation afterward. She may even make the man a cup of coffee! Listen to the things we tell women who have had a traumatic or dehumanizing birth experience. "Don't think about it."

"Think of the baby." "You're thinking only of yourself."

Doctors get furious at me for talking about this. "You are treating me as if I am a rapist!" But midwives usually understand. The workshops I give called "Childbirth and Rape" are the ones midwives are pouring in for. I remember one British midwife—who was not very intellectual—whose eyes grew wide as the discussion continued. She said quietly, "I realize now that I have been helping women to be raped." And she went on to describe the inhuman things happening now in her hospital.

What we will see more and more of is how to get a "perfect" baby, no matter what. We are more dependent on tests. I've seen a woman who had cysts in her baby's kidneys detected by ultrasound in utero, only to find the cysts disappeared by the time the baby was born. Meanwhile, women's anxiety levels have been raised as have the anxiety levels of everyone around them.

I had one woman who underwent three amniocenteses and a prenatal examination of the cord blood in the very best hospital and had the best specialists working with her. Her husband was a mathematician and colluded with the doctors, he was so fascinated by the technology. The woman felt very isolated. She gave birth three months prematurely to a little wisp of a thing who, except for prematurity, had no physical problem. To think of all she went through! We must reverse this trend.

WILLIAM

William, fifty-two, is a recent father and a psychotherapist and teacher. He has spent many years exploring how to recognize and deal with trauma that can occur around the time of birth, both in the United States and in Europe and India. He has pioneered treatments for adults, children, and babies who have experienced perinatal trauma.

In my doctoral program I was encouraged to do some sort of therapeutic work on myself. I happened upon a hypnotherapist who believed that going back to one's early life could help you in the present. In one of my first sessions he had me close my eyes, put me in a trance, and asked me to go back to my earliest memories. All of a sudden I found myself choking, gagging, and feeling incredibly small. I still recall the sensations.

I was lying on my right side and asking myself, why not my left? A nonverbal answer came: "Because this is the way I was lying."

I found myself arching back and upward. It hurt but my body kept doing it. The thought came, "Babies can't turn around in the birth canal!" The arching continued, I began to feel sadder and sadder and in my mind came the words: "I want to help you." My arm and hand began extending backward and down, toward my feet. I felt immense pain behind my right shoulder blade. Then I realized that I was trying to pull my sister out. Until then I had only known I had a twin sister who died at birth.

I dissolved into tears, and I suddenly knew that part of the longing I had been plagued with all my life had to do with a desire to reunite with my twin.

I'd always been compulsive about my relationships with women, going from one to another, feeling the one I was in wasn't good enough, and constantly filled with longing. I never wanted to be sexual with the woman I loved, and I turned each relationship into a brother-sister one and called each woman "Sis."

After that session something changed. This sounds unbelievable, but I really began to relate differently, and within a year I met and married the woman I've been married to for twenty years.

That first hypnotherapy session got me to look into my birth. I wrote the hospital for my records and discovered that I weighed less than a pound at birth. So I had been small enough to have turned my body, even moved my arm, while in the birth canal! And I was born first.

The pain behind my shoulder blade I felt in that regression was the same one I'd felt most of my life and which had always slowed me down as an athlete. Every day I had had to do stretches to keep that area from spasming. Now I have much more mobility of my shoulder and arm, but the pain is not completely gone, due to scar tissue from the spasming of muscles all those years. I carried fantasies of rescuing my twin all the way into adulthood. They now have a name for it: twin guilt.

I began to treat adults for birth trauma in the early 1970s. I didn't know of any other people doing it, but I felt certain it was valuable. In England I found an older psychiatrist doing birth regressions with adults, so I went and worked with him over a five-year period. We verified much of each other's observations and made two major findings. First, that the time around birth accounts for a broader range of long-term symptoms than people believe—from personality disorders to a select range of physical diseases, especially bronchia and asthmatic conditions, heart disease, cancer, and inflammatory diseases. Second, that while we all go through the same stages in development to become unique individuals, the origins come not only from heredity but from perinatal experiences.

I've found that when adults go through perinatal or birth regressions early on in their therapy, therapy proceeds much more quickly and efficiently. What Otto Rank had found in the 1930s is true: many people spontaneously recall these memories at some point in therapy. Clients will bring up many more memories if the therapist is open to them.

I've found that child abuse can also be linked to trauma around birth. Birth experiences that are trau-matic lay the patterns of actions and reactions which later permit abuse to happen to a child. A lack of trauma, a lack of abuse later. I can tell you a true story that illustrates this.

A three-and-a-half-year-old girl I was working with did a story in a sand tray, using miniature dolls and other objects, which is a standard way for getting young children to express things they cannot talk about directly. She had the little girl's daddy in her play want to touch the little girl's genitals.

I asked her what the girl doll said when her daddy did that. She said very clearly, "The little girl didn't let her daddy do it." Then she turned and looked me straight in the eyes and said, "I didn't let my daddy do it to me."

So I said, "What did you do?" She looked me deep in the eyes and gave me the most profound and intense expression and said simply, "I told him, NO!" Later her father corroborated his daughter's story. He'd felt deep remorse and shame about it and was grateful she'd said no as strongly as she did.

When I evaluated that little girl for birth trauma I found none. She was third born, born at home after a normal three-hour labor, and had no problems beginning life. I have treated lots of children who were sexually abused over the years and found in each case that something about their birth was traumatic and that a pattern of helplessness began at that point, which later got in their way of being able to stop the abuse at the outset. Babies appear to be born with a natural capacity to protect themselves. Early trauma changes that.

A major trauma is being stuck in the process of being born, unable to move. This inability to change the situation in any way leaves its mark on a child—into adulthood. What gets paired up, in associative learning of this kind, is the pressure of the contractions on the baby and the baby's inability to do anything to get away. This creates the primal boundary disorder, the inability to stop unwanted intrusive and unasked-for energy or physical contact by another person. The person cannot say no.

Several of us have developed a series of games designed to play out various kinds of traumatic experiences around birth. For one game, called "Earthquake," kids create a cave out of furniture, pillows, and adult bodies. The child is always made safe by being told in advance that they can stop the game at any time. As kids play this particular game certain ones will be more and more dramatic and will take higher and higher risks in how they do the game and allow feelings to come up.

Kids who have experienced birth trauma of some kind and contacted the original trauma through a game always want to do that game over and over again. A child who does not have any trauma doesn't get particularly excited about repeating any of the games. Children can rewound themselves by repeating a game too many times in a given day, but they can also completely work through—heal—the original trauma by repetition in this symbolic way. Children—even babies—can direct their own healing.

I always work with children with their parents present. And they notice profound changes in their kids. Most commonly, kids who previously could not tolerate much holding or hugging become overtly affection and cuddly; kids with asthmatic conditions breathe without difficulty; somewhat hyperactive kids become calm and centered.

A family brought me a two-and-a-half-week-old infant who was considered by doctors to be at risk, having strong asthmatic symptoms and "failure to thrive"—losing weight despite being breast-fed. Her parents were caring and attentive, but she did not respond.

It was 1974. I'd been developing a process called "birth-simulating massage" for several years, working with medically healthy infants, learning from and teaching mothers. I witnessed some dramatic changes in these babies after only a few sessions: sleep problems abruptly ceasing, the amount of crying in a day decreasing significantly, and feeding problems stopping.

I did this massage on this newborn in front of both of her parents. When I got to a certain spot on her head—the spot where I later learned she had been stuck during birth when they put a scalp electrode on her for fetal monitoring—she went into visible panic, bronchial sneezing, wheezing, and choking. It happened so quickly she didn't even have time to cry. I backed off immediately and her reaction stopped. I started again, got to the same spot, and she went immediately into the same reaction.

Then all three of us noticed that she would put her hand up and try to push at my hand, as if to say, "STOP!" So each time I touched the spot and she did that I stopped in response to her hand movement. Then, she would actually place my hand on her head. It sounds impossible but it's not. I have video-recorded such reactions many times in sessions.

It's clear to me that, just as adults want to be in control of their treatment, babies do, too. And they *need* to be, for healing to occur. At least half of healing has to do with a person being in control of what goes on, the timing and pacing. The other half is due to the catharsis itself, simply uncovering a memory of the trauma and allowing whatever feelings and bodily sensations and movements that come up to occur.

These are standard, well-accepted procedures in psychotherapy today. The only difference is that I apply it to infants and children with regard to an area of life most adults don't believe matters.

Trauma during the birth is not the only one that can have such long-term negative effects. Most obstetric interventions—including hormones given the mother to force fetal lung development or start or speed up or stop labor, anesthesia or narcotics given the mother during labor, the use of forceps, suctioning of the baby's throat or lungs after birth, and cesarean surgery—can cause trauma. Other early experiences that can be traumatic include being in a hospital neonatal intensive care unit, being the result of an unwanted pregnancy the mother cannot come to terms with, and being adopted.

Parents can spot possible trauma to their babies. Do they cry inordinately? (Most cry less than an hour total each day.) Are they unconsolable? Do they have continuous feeding or sleeping difficulties? Babies spend about 80 percent of their time in the womb sleeping, so sleeping is one thing a baby naturally does easily! Another sign is a baby who won't tolerate either being held and cuddled or being put down.

There aren't yet many people formally trained in perinatal trauma work in babies. However, if you think a baby might be suffering from the effects of trauma that occurred around the time of birth, look for a cranial osteopath, play therapist, midwife, nurse, or chiropractor who is sensitive to someone having emerging deep feelings and who is open to the idea that painful and shocking experiences around the time of birth can leave their mark.

As a man, I can't speak from direct experience about giving birth. However, I do know we as a culture could not have made modern birth more unnatural for women than we've made it. We've not only increased the number of complications and interventions, we have also increased the trauma for babies.

NANCY

Nancy is a social worker and veteran teacher. She has also been the director of several infant and toddler day-care programs in the United States and is deeply concerned about the problems created by full-time group day-care for babies. She has worked with private programs for the middle and upper classes as well as with government-funded programs for the poor, and has found that these problems cut across all socioeconomic groups.

When I had my daughter Rebecca, I was married. Because my husband was making enough money, I was able to stay home with Rebecca until she was two. I couldn't have done that if I were a single parent. Being with her, I learned that parenting is all about the small, day-to-day interactions between an adult and a child. I also learned that the real tasks of childhood are for parents to learn to trust their children and to bond deeply with them.

Now, women are going back to work sooner and sooner after giving birth. Many are putting their babies in full-time group day-care; they are not permitted to bring their babies with them to work, and there's usually no day-care available at the job. For many, the day-care facility is a distance from their office, making it impossible for them to visit the baby during the day.

People talk about having family quality time on the weekends. But on Monday mornings many parents are just relieved to have somewhere to leave their babies. A lot actually say, "I'm so glad to be here!" For working parents today, the weekend is a pressured time. Parents are trying to do everything around the house that they cannot get done during the week.

What I am seeing is very disturbing. Women are coming to check out day-care programs early in their pregnancy, in order to get themselves on a waiting list. For the most part these are first-time parents. They don't know what it will be like, or how it will feel after the baby is born, when they must face leaving this tiny baby for hours a day with someone else. A mother—or father—who has bonded with their baby knows how difficult it is to leave a three- or six-week-old with anyone for more than a few hours. It is physically wrenching!

It's my observation that, because these mothers know they are going to have to leave their babies just a short time after birth, they start adjusting to that emotional loss during their pregnancies.

Unconsciously, they distance themselves from the baby before they've even met it. That is how early detachment is starting!

I came to this conclusion after seeing many parents who did not display normal nurturing feelings that are part of the bonding and separation process. The risk of full-time group infant care is not simply that the infant does not attach to its mother, but that the mother—and father—do not attach to the baby. Let me tell you the incident that initiated my realization that full-time group infant care is just not workable.

There was a freak accident at the center. A nine-month-old boy put his hand on a hot floor-heater vent that ordinarily was not on. The baby burned his hand badly. He was in great pain, crying hysterically, wanting to be held. Yet he couldn't stop crying and couldn't be comforted in any way. The assistant director called his mother, who worked just a few blocks away. It would have been a two-minute walk for her. He explained the situation. She said, "I am busy. It'll be a few hours before I can get away."

When he told the mother she had to come, she got angry and said she wouldn't. I had been worrying that she would be angry that her son had burned his hand in our care. Instead she was angry that we were interfering with her workday! So we called the father and told him we needed him to come right away. He worked thirty minutes away but said he would leave work early.

A half hour later, the mother walked in, very angry. The father had apparently phoned her. She picked up her son—a baby who had by then been crying uncontrollably for almost an hour—and he stopped crying. The change in him was dramatic. She looked at his hand, which was bright red with white welts, and said, "He'll be okay until the end of the day." Then she put him down on the floor and walked out. He started sobbing again until he fell asleep in one of the teacher's arms.

This is a dramatic example but not an isolated incident. If something had happened to my daughter Rebecca when she was so young and I was not with her, I would have moved steel bars to get to her. I knew I was not unusual in this. What has to take place in order for a mother to be able to ignore her child's suffering? I began to realize it occurs when she does not have a strong bond with her baby.

The real loss in full-time early infant child care is that parents don't have the time—or energy—to bond well enough with the baby. That little boy was bonded to his mother, even though she was emotionally distant from him. I empathize with parents who leave their infants for many hours each day in the care of strangers. It would be too hard for them to do it if they allowed themselves to become fully attached to the baby in the first place. So they don't. It's just self-preservation.

When we work with very young children, the "curriculum" is establishing a relationship with the children in our care. We talk to them, we listen, we touch them, we help them express who they are, and we accept who they are. The building of trust in each other, child and adult, develops over time. That's why being with our babies and young children a lot every day is important. While I certainly loved Rebecca when she was a baby, our relationship has become much closer over time. We were closer when she was four than when she was a baby, and we keep getting closer.

Although I don't want to go back to the days when mom stayed home alone with the kids and had total responsibility for the nurturing of the family, I don't believe equality for women should mean that nobody is doing the nurturing. Both parents going to work full-time and leaving their infants in full-time group care is not working. Parenting—nurturing—can and ought to be shared by both partners, and certainly can include other people as well. What is crucial is that a child receive the nurturing it needs *when* it needs it. The question is: What will these children's capacity for attachment to their own children be if they have not experienced attachment themselves?

FAYE

Faye is a fifty-year-old grandmother and mother of three. She has worked in maternity and newborn care since she was eighteen, first as a nurse, then as a birth educator, now as a midwife. She has worked throughout the United States. Her experiences demonstrate how postpartum care services in the United States differ from those in other industrialized countries. In Europe, for example, it has never been routine to give drugs or anesthesia to women in labor, to separate mothers and babies after birth, or to put healthy babies in nurseries. Siblings and other family members have always been welcome to visit mother and baby—even in crowded wards.

One of the first things I was taught as a student nurse was that if you "baby" the mother, the mother will "baby" the baby. Today we call it perinatal care, not maternity care, because the focus is no longer on the mother but on the baby. As bad as many of our hospital birth practices have been since women were first encouraged to have babies in hospitals, at least there was a "lying-in" period of rest and support. Mothers remained in the hospital for a week to ten days after delivering and were considered deserving of care.

Of course, the downside was that fathers were not expected to do anything regarding the baby or the other kids. But there was respect—in the culture and in hospitals—for the mother's need to rest, recuperate, and develop a caretaking relationship with her baby. It was understood that time and a protected environment were needed for this to take place.

I don't mean to make light of the many problems that existed with hospital postpartum care. Many newborns suffered serious problems as a result of the massive amounts of drugs—sedation, pain relief, and anesthesia—routinely given to mothers in labor. There was no "rooming-in." Regardless of the health of the baby and of the mother's desires, all babies were kept in nurseries except during feeding times. Breast-feeding was actively discouraged; most infants were bottle-fed "on schedule," every four hours.

Because babies were kept in nurseries much of the day, they were exposed to contagious infections from other infants. Many babies died from these infections before the advent of antibiotics. There were infant diarrhea epidemics in hospitals throughout the 1940s and 1950s. And when babies got sick in the nursery, they remained isolated from their mothers for even longer. Most of that has changed, thank God! Now, most women leave the hospital within twenty-four hours after an uncomplicated delivery, and three days after cesarean surgery.

I get nostalgic when I look back at the quality of care women used to receive after giving birth. First of all, they were put in maternity wards, not in private rooms. (Private rooms came along when private insurance began paying for maternity care.) Typically, a maternity ward had four to eight mothers, of all ages and levels of experience. It was a community. Inexperienced mothers could learn from the more experienced ones, in much the same way they did before hospitalized birth.

There was a lot of camaraderie in those early maternity wards. Women swapped stories about childbirth, passed along tips to each other, and formed friendships that continued long after they left the hospital. Then it became fashionable for women with insurance coverage to choose a private or semiprivate room. Without realizing it, they had isolated themselves from the community of other mothers.

A mother's stay in the hospital has always been disruptive to the family, especially to the mother's relationship with her other children. It used to be difficult for fathers to form healthy relationships with their new babies, since most hospitals' visiting hours were very restricted. Fathers and other family members could only see the baby through the glass "viewing" window of the nursery. Nobody thought much about what happened to mothers and babies, or their families for that matter, after they went home. No one considered that hospital birth practices, including separation and isolation after birth, might damage bonding and increase the potential for abuse or neglect. Child abuse or neglect was a taboo subject! There was not even the concept of attachment, much less an awareness of its importance!

Women accepted the way the system was. Most wanted drugs, especially "twilight sleep." To give scopolamine, the most popular sedative—and the tranquilizers that went with it—it was necessary to be hospitalized. The main reason for obstetric care, for using physicians rather than midwives, was so women could be medicated during childbirth! It wasn't because hospitals were safer places to give birth. Women were routinely drugged and anesthetized, leaving them partially or fully unconscious during the delivery. It often meant that women were flat on their backs, so the doctor could pull the baby out.

When I began training, deep episiotomies, done well before the baby's head crowned, had been routine for decades. They left women painfully sore for weeks, unable to walk or even sit easily. Plus, there was always the danger of infection. Many people don't know this, but women have died from episiotomy infections.

There is a separate point I want to make. What hospitals are now doing to the mothers—ignoring them—is what they used to do to the babies. Just twenty years ago, mothers and babies actually benefited from what in medicine is called "benign neglect." The hospital staff wasn't yet obsessed with doing tests and procedures and "just-in-case" treatments, looking for pathology.

I was working in a hospital nursery during the years when breast-feeding began to become popular. Then, the question of who did the baby belong to became an issue. Until the late 1950s, the baby belonged to the nurse who ran the nursery. Then, the pediatrician took over the nursery. I still have a copy of the written policy at my hospital, which forbade breast-feeding on the delivery room table unless there was a signed order from the pediatrician. Now, babies belong to the perinatologists.

In the late 1960s and early 1970s women increasingly wanted to take back control, not only of their bodies and the act of childbirth, but also of their babies. I used to fight to get women discharged early because I saw the conflict between mothers and the hospital system. Mothers always need to be in charge of their babies, especially if breast-feeding is going to be successful. The traditional structure of a hospital, with its separate staff for babies, has never been conducive to successful breast-feeding or bonding. Hospitals have always been run for the efficiency of its staff, never for the patients. This policy never has and never will promote the long-term well-being of mothers and babies.

Today, unfortunately, women who give birth in a hospital go home a day or two, or even as little as a few hours, later and have no opportunity to form relationships with a staff member or with other mothers. Most of the women they know work, and so do their partners. Mothers have no positive role models to look up to and get no help while caring for a baby. Even women who give birth at home or in birth centers seldom receive any real nurturing afterward. The truth is, women *need* to be served long after childbirth. They do not benefit from being isolated from other mothers or being separated from their babies any more than they benefit from experts taking control of childbirth.

There used to be a feeling of protection toward women who had given birth, and a respect for their capacity to care for their own babies. As we've stopped respecting women, they have stopped passing on information and wisdom to each other.

The best learning comes from simply hanging out with one another. Now we have "experts," and the assumption is that these professionals are best equipped to know what babies need.

The nurse, the physician, the day-care person, the teacher, the child psychologist, and the social worker all think they know best. Motherhood—parenthood—has been made into another money-making business like childbirth. But it's not the mother who gets the money, it's the professionals. Women are the ones who ultimately pay the price.

When women suffer, families suffer. For women—and men—to be good parents to infants and young children, they need a number of things from the people around them. A parent of a young child must be respected and honored. People should call up or stop by, and ask what they can pick up at the store, what food they can prepare. If you want to help a new mother, offer to clean the house once a week, do the laundry, take her other children for a few hours. We must respect the process each woman goes through on her journey to finding her own way to meet the needs of her baby. Let's give mothers the support they need.

MARINA

The following true story is representative of a disturbing trend in the United States. Every year thousands of healthy newborn babies are placed in intensive care unit (ICU) nurseries simply for "observation," but they almost always end up undergoing aggressive testing and treatment in the name of "active management." These healthy babies, who could easily be observed while in their mothers' care, are subjected to the full range of current perinatal testing and technology. Parents are, for the most part, kept ignorant of what is being done, uninformed about the necessity of it, and made unnecessarily anxious. In this case, the parents are acquaintances of mine and the nurse-midwife and obstetrician are people I know to be highly competent. They did their best but were unable to buck the hospital system, in this case a major medical center connected to an internationally renowned medical school.

Marina was born after thirty hours of labor, twenty-four of which was "active." Although long, this was a normal labor: there was continuous confirmation that mom and baby were doing well, consistent progress in dilation of the cervix, and considerable progress in the baby's descent prior to the mother's pushing. The waters broke spontaneously and copi-

ously near the end and were clear, another sign that all was well.

During pushing, fetal heart tones remained excellent and Marina came out head first, in a slow, controlled delivery. Her mother had no tears. There was no cord around the baby's neck.

Still, although she was pink and had a normal heart rate, Marina was limp and made only slight attempts to breathe after being laid on her mother's belly. (This practice has been documented to be the best way to keep a baby warm.) The attending obstetrician and the nurse-midwife, who'd been with the mother throughout labor, both felt there was no reason to worry or panic. The baby was likely to be tired after such a long labor. They would observe her carefully for a minute.

The cord continued to pulse and the obstetrician specifically delayed cutting it to allow Marina more time to get breathing going on her own. (Since the placenta was still attached to her mother's uterine wall, oxygen continued to flow into Marina's body from her mother.)

Because of hospital policy, the nurse felt she had to call the neonatal staff. When they arrived, Marina was starting to respond. Nevertheless, the nurse had already taken her away from her mother's warm skin and put her under an electric warmer, which, unfortunately, was not working properly and was cold. Marina was given several whiffs of oxygen. Her Apgar scores were only 4 and 5 at one and five minutes (on a scale of 1 to 10), but at six minutes her muscle tone had greatly improved.

Unfortunately, the decision had already been made, so she was on her way to the ICU when she was just six minutes old. By seven minutes, according to the records, she was crying and had good muscle tone. Her mom and dad were told, "She's just going to be observed for a few hours, because of her slow start."

In the ICU a nurse thought she saw Marina's chest retracting (hollowing) with inhales. Although this was not confirmed by another neonatal nurse, because Marina's birth had been labeled "traumatic" by the neonatal staff (none of whom had been present for any part of it), the wheels were put in motion and she was given standard ICU protocol. Blood was drawn from her veins to be cultured in a lab, an X-ray was taken, and a spinal tap (a needle inserted into the space alongside the baby's spinal cord, withdrawing a sample of spinal fluid) was performed. A temperature sensor and a heart monitor were taped onto her skin. A metal clip was attached to her finger to record blood gas, electrolytes, and blood sugar.

Marina's parents were not asked permission to perform any of these procedures. Although her father had gone to the nursery with her to comfort her, he felt helpless to stop the flow of events. She lay on her back in a brightly lit room, naked, under a lamp. So the father returned to his wife's side, and she was wheeled to her room.

The X-ray came back showing "streaking," which was interpreted as possibly meaning fluid in the lungs, a symptom of pneumonia. Pneumonia was the diagnosis. Because the mother had no elevated temperature and no other sign of infection, there should have been no reason to suspect any infection in the baby. Since healthy babies normally don't get X-rayed, it is impossible to know how many of their lungs might also show some "streaking."

Rather than wait for more test results, the neonatologist decided to administer two antibiotics immediately. It is standard procedure to begin treatment before any test results are in, "just in case."

Marina was not held by her mother until the next morning, ten hours after birth. She was not even allowed to nurse because the staff was concerned it might be too tiring for her. When her mother was finally able to put Marina to breast, she nursed well—one more indication of a healthy newborn.

Twenty-four hours after the antibiotics had first been given, the mother was told that Marina's kidneys had become poisoned and were unable to function properly. (This is a well-known side effect of the drug gentamicin that Marina was getting.) The staff then started an IV to run fluids through her kidneys to flush the antibiotics out. They promised the mother that the IV would be taken out as soon as the medication had been flushed. She was only permitted to nurse every four hours, even though most newborn babies would naturally breast-feed about every two hours.

During the night, nurses informed her that, because the baby had urinated only once in the first twenty-four hours, they were going to increase the fluid in the IV. (Peeing only once in the twenty-four hours after birth is within the range of normal, however. The resident who made this decision either did not know this or ignored it.) The mother was appropriately concerned that if Marina got too much fluid by IV her desire to breast-feed would diminish. Sure enough, at 6:00 the next morning Marina did not nurse so well; her mother wanted to try again at 8:00, but she was not allowed to come until 10:00 because the medical rounds were beginning.

Meanwhile, preliminary reports from blood tests and cultures all came back normal. Marina had been taken off the gentamicin, but was still on another antibiotic. Despite the favorable reports, the

IV remained in, apparently due to concern that the drug had not been fully flushed from her system. It takes longer for drugs to clear from newborns' bodies because their systems are not yet able to handle drugs very well.

At this point, the mother just wanted to take her baby home. The hospital neonatal staff wanted to keep Marina there so that they could keep her on the antibiotics just in case it turned out that she did have an infection. Her private pediatrician felt uncomfortable going against hospital protocol—it is never politically wise for a physician in one specialty to question another—but did tell the parents that their baby was fine and did not need to be in the hospital. The mother thought having Marina come home and be in a normal environment, in her arms, might help them both. She asked if she could take Marina home and bring her to a private pediatrician for shots of the antibiotic, but was told it would be too difficult and that shots were too painful for a baby. She felt guilty for suggesting it.

Test results continued to come back "negative" throughout the week. A sympathetic nurse lobbied successfully on behalf of Marina's mother to cut back on the IV fluids so the nursing could go better. Marina's mother spent all of her time trying to get information about what was being done to her baby, trying to learn the rationale for each procedure, trying to be an advocate for her baby, in addition to trying to hold and nurse Marina as much as possible. The ICU was located nearly a quarter mile from the mother's room. Because Marina was doing so well she was sent to the "stepdown" nursery, which was located even farther from her mother's bed.

Five days after the birth the mother began to hemorrhage. Her OB wanted to take her into surgery to explore her uterus under anesthesia for possible retained parts of placenta. Heavy bleeding, however, is not uncommon right after birth, when a woman is on her feet too much, is under a great deal of stress, and is getting too little rest. (One of the best ways to control bleeding is to have the baby nurse frequently.) This mother was told she could not nurse because the doctor had not left orders that she could.

The obstetrician and midwife finally intervened, against the pediatric staff's orders, and insisted that Marina be brought to the mother to nurse. By the time she came, her mother was not there. She had been wheeled to the operating room, where she was made to wait outside for the next hour until the anesthesiologist showed up. Just as the mother was taken into the OR, she was told that her baby had been taken back to the ICU for observation, due to possible seizures. (It would later turn out that a nurse had seen some movement of an arm and leg she feared might be a seizure.)

There proved to be no seizures, but by the time the midwife arrived at the ICU they were doing a second spinal tap and all the standard procedures for possible meningitis, and Marina had been started on phenobarbital. The father, who was there, asked a resident if the muscle movement could be a side effect of the medication his baby had been on. He was told "definitely not." The midwife later read in the *Physician's Desk Reference* that muscle twitches, even convulsions, are common side effects of the antibiotic gentamicin, especially when the kidneys have shown toxicity.

A CAT scan was strongly recommended, because of "possible cerebral hemorrhage." It was done. The results were unclear. The neonatal physicians wondered if Marina might have bruising on the brain. They elected to continue the phenobarbital. It made Marina sleepy, so she couldn't nurse.

On Sunday, a week after the birth, the parents finally got up the courage to insist on taking their daughter home, but not before being made to watch a video on infant CPR, which made them doubt their decision. Marina was supposed to be given phenobarbital three times a day by injection. Her parents were told nothing about follow-up neurological checks. After a week of struggling with nursing and with the growing conviction that Marina was in fact healthy, they sought the support of a second private pediatrician who, after examining the records and Marina, advised them to stop the drug treatment altogether.

Once a baby is in a hospital intensive care nursery, it is considered the legal property of the nursery. Parents' wishes do not have to be considered. Because of the aggressive approach to these babies when they are in ICUs, well-informed parents and midwives—and some obstetricians—do their best to keep babies out of them altogether. Some parents choose to take their babies and sign out of the hospital AMA (against medical advice). However, you should know that doing this can result in a future investigation by child protective services.

DIANE

Diane is twenty-nine; her husband forty. They have two sons, ages four years and four months. Her approach to birth—especially toward the issues of uncertainty and pain—is unlike most North American mothers of her generation and provides insight and inspiration.

Both my pregnancies were easy, but during my second I knew more of what I wanted to experience. There was a special excitement the first time, because it was about facing the unknown. I went through certain concerns and fears as my pregnancy progressed, all the what-ifs. Somehow, early on I realized I should look at the fear as a signal of what I should pay attention to and learn from or try to resolve.

I remember consciously making the determination when I was about six months pregnant with Tyler, that my fears were just images my mind created and that I could put energy into them or not.

I had to pay attention to what my mind brought up to see what I might learn, what I needed to do—like finding a doctor I could respect and trust, taking a tour of the hospital, asking questions, and learning what I could and could not expect. But after a certain point in the pregnancy, putting attention on my what-if thoughts and fears seemed like wasted energy.

Fear did not dominate my pregnancy or my labor. I had looked at every possibility: having to have a cesarean, the baby not getting enough oxygen in labor, even the baby dying or me dying. What finally came loud and clear was my commitment to taking responsibility for this baby's birth, its life, everything. After that it really became an honor to give birth. I looked forward to it and I surrendered to the whole process.

When people talk about pain, fear is usually attached. So many times we are inflicted with pain in an injury, an accident, an illness, where everything is unknown. I'm as afraid as anyone about some things. But I saw the pain of labor as something to allow to be there and to be present.

I knew labor might hurt as much as the pain from a bad injury; but I didn't have to be afraid of it. I think our society places too much emphasis on pain, anyway, as something to be escaped. Here was the chance to feel the intensity of pain from a place of understanding. My husband and I talked about it a lot during the pregnancy—about both of us facing our fears.

When I was growing up, my mother never once complained about giving birth or talked about it as horrible or scary. That helped me when I gave birth. She had three hospital births. During each one, my dad had to wait outside, and the doctor didn't show up until the delivery. She went through her labors mostly alone. I remember her mentioning once that one of us, either myself or my brother, was almost born on the toilet in the hospital bathroom because she was unable to tell anyone she was about to deliver. She didn't take any drugs, either. My interpretation as a kid was that my mom did it on her own, so childbirth must not be too bad.

Labor was fine during my first pregnancy. I remember that it seemed long. Because it was all so new, I didn't know what I was doing and I was pretty dependent on others to help bring the baby out. The pushing stage was hard. I never had the urge to push. Up until that time, all I had to do was breathe with the contractions and ride through them. It was not easy, but it was tolerable.

In the hour it took to push the baby out, I had to consciously focus all my energy on the task. I was mainly on my hands and knees during active labor— I liked that position because it felt good getting the pressure off my back—but for pushing I squatted, supported by my husband. At first, he sat on the bed, and I squatted on the floor between his legs. Then, as the baby started crowning, my husband stood up, placed his hands underneath my armpits, and lifted me up a bit.

Right after Tyler's birth, I found myself in a trance. I felt that I was as close as I might ever get to the spiritual world, short of dying. Sometimes labor puts a woman in another state of consciousness. I had never experienced anything like it before. I completely trusted this feeling; it was like the universe had taken over, that, no matter what happened, it would be okay. During my second pregnancy, I looked forward to entering that state again.

When I gave birth to my second child, Calen, I had a midwife. She checked me and found that I was seven centimeters dilated, and I just stood up— that's what I felt like doing—and stayed standing. His head came out during the first push. Then we waited for the next contraction, and he came out all the way, just slid out like a waterfall, with all my fluid.

When Tyler came out, he made a noise right away; then he was in my arms, nursing almost immediately. It was a much different story with Calen. His labor was shorter and more intense. I was draped over Michael, my husband, afraid to move because after Calen came out, I could still feel the umbilical cord dangling from me. Then I realized he wasn't making any noise. I heard my midwife say, "There's lots of meconium." (He'd pooped inside me.) I was still in the birth trance, so her voice sounded very distant. Then I heard her say firmly, "Talk to your baby, Diane."

Right then, I became aware of what was going on. I think Calen understood, too. I said, "I love you, baby, I'm right here for you; you can make it, baby." I said, "Breathe, everybody. Breathe!" He took his first breath, about thirty seconds after he was out. In the meantime, my midwife had been suctioning out his nose and throat, clearing the meconium out.

If I had been in a hospital for Calen's birth, the doctors would have used lots of mechanical equipment and taken Calen away from Mike and me. They probably would have put him in the intensive care nursery for at least a day, taken lots of blood, and done painful tests on him. During the first days of his life, he would have been hearing the noise of monitors and strangers' voices, not our voices.

I know that babies can die—they do sometimes die—in hospitals too, even in the best hospitals. The complication with Calen's birth enlightened me. Even if he had died, I would have accepted that as what happens sometimes.

ROBIN

Robin is a mother of four, stepmother of two, and author of a well-loved self-care guide for postpartum women.

When my children and I made a home with my new husband, I discovered that his son Gabriel, who was then six, was a chronic bed wetter. At first, I tried running to him in the middle of the night whenever I heard him moan. His father, and apparently his mother, too, were such deep sleepers that they never heard him make a noise. I could usually get him up and out of bed just in time to keep him from wetting. This left us with dry sheets, but the problem didn't go away; Gabriel still needed help getting up to pee every night. Eventually, I got tired of it.

One night, I decided not to help when I heard him but just to go watch. I had noticed that when he tried to wake up so he could pee, he'd make sounds as if he were starting to panic. Sometimes when I got him up while he was still in a sleep state, he'd mutter his mother's or father's name and say something like, "You don't care about me." I didn't understand it, but I felt that his bed-wetting might be due to some unconscious anger.

I knew that both of his parents cared very much for him and showed him their love all the time, even though they had divorced. The night that I just watched him, I saw this child's hands become claw-like. He put them up against his face as if to protect it, and then frantically tried to push some imaginary object away. As he did this, his legs contracted into fetal position, and he screamed, "Don't stick it in my nose! Don't stick it in my nose! Please, please. Don't stick it in my nose. It hurts. It hurts!"

It dawned on me. I knew that Gabriel had been hospitalized for pneumonia when he was barely a week old. He must have had tubes put down his nose to feed him. It was the only time it could have happened. I climbed into his bed and held him as he continued to scream and fight in his sleep. I whispered into his ear, "Gabriel, I promise you, I am not going to put anything in your nose. I'm never going to let anyone put anything in your nose."

He stopped screaming and began to take deep breaths. He moaned and called out, "Robin, is that you? Do you really promise?" I told him it was me, and I repeated that I would never let anyone put anything in his nose. Then I asked if he wanted to pee. He got up all by himself, went to the bathroom, then came back, climbed into bed, and went to sleep.

After that night, Gabriel had only a couple more accidents. When I checked with his father, I learned that he had had tubes in his nose when he was in the hospital as a newborn, and that his hands had been strapped down so he couldn't pull them out.

ROSALIND AND MARIA

Rosalind and Maria are labor, delivery, postpartum nurses at a large health maintenance organization (HMO) that handles approximately 260 births per month. The HMO is a fully equipped and staffed "level 3" (most technically advanced) hospital and is able to care for a wide range of medical problems.

Q: Your chosen profession is working with women who give birth in hospitals; yet, both of you elected to give birth in your own homes. What is the most striking difference you find between giving birth in a hospital or at home?

Rosalind: The level of anxiety among caregivers. Honestly. In the hospital, the nurses and doctors feel responsible for your childbirth. Sure, a big part of that today is our legal liability. But it's more than that; it's hard to describe to someone who does not work in a hospital. Doctors and nurses are trained to always be on the lookout for signs of problems, to expect catastrophe. Midwives, especially those who work in people's homes, expect the normal. When you're always looking for the abnormal, it is hard to be calm and patient.

Maria: It's understandable, because hospitals, especially ones like ours, do have to deal with the abnormal. We do see placenta abruptions, eclampsia, cord prolapses, amniotic embolisms. These are all rare occurrences, but we are the ones who see them.

Q: You say that childbirth is different when you have a midwife, especially in the home. What do you mean?

Rosalind: For both of my births, when the midwives arrived at my house, it was like greeting old friends. I knew these women trusted me to do the job at hand. They saw themselves as assisting, but not managing, my childbirth. They were invited to my childbirth; let's put it that way.

Maria: For me, it's a question of who is really in control. At home, it is *your* birth. In the hospital, because of the way hospitals are set up, but also because of the propensity of women to relinquish control, the control is in the hands of the doctors and nurses. In the hospital, a woman does not have control.

Rosalind: Right. Women don't even know they have the right to ask a nurse or doctor to leave the room, or to ask for someone else if they're dissatisfied.

Maria: In a teaching hospital, whichever resident happens to be on duty attends your birth, and it's likely to be a stranger. Even if the doctor is someone you know, they usually only show up near the actual delivery. I hear from nurses who work at private hospitals that it's common for private physicians to manage a labor over the phone. They tell the nurse not to call until it's time to deliver the baby. Women don't know that. It's only when you have been there and seen a woman progress, that you know what she is capable of.

It's the nurse who knows what is going on with your labor. The nurses are the only people there long enough for you to count on, or to really support you through the rough spots. When a doctor walks in in the middle of your labor, that person's perception can be totally wrong about what is happening, and what you are feeling. And that can be very important.

One negative statement by a doctor, or anyone else, about your progress can have a demoralizing effect on your labor.

Rosalind: Right. I'm not the only nurse I know who tries to run interference for moms and attempts to keep unnecessary intervention from happening. But we can't always be there or prevent it from occurring. Many nurses care a lot, but are just too busy and have too many patients to provide that attention. And money is the bottom line in hospital administration. The first thing they cut is the nursing staff.

Women need to know when they go into a hospital for childbirth, they might not get any labor support from the nursing staff. They certainly shouldn't expect it. Every thirty minutes, one of us is required to go in and check the monitor, write down the heart rate of the baby, and give a quick glance at the patient. Sometimes we don't have the time to do anything but that. And whenever there's a cesarean, more nurses are taken away from other patients to attend the operation.

Q: What responsibility do mothers have for the way things are in hospitals today?

Maria: Many women and their partners do not want responsibility for their childbirths. They are all too happy to give it away.

Q: Why do you think that is?

Rosalind: A lot of women do not feel their bodies can actually do it. I see a lot of fear. Women hope that by walking into a hospital, it will just magically happen. Someone else will do the work.

Maria: The other day, I had a patient in active labor tell me how appalled she was that, with all that science has achieved, childbirth is still so uncivilized.

Rosalind: Many other people think that, but don't say it. I see many people who don't want to put any effort or time into giving birth. If they were better educated about the value of the natural process, I think a lot of women would put more energy into it.

Maria: So many people just want to get childbirth over with. I find it very disturbing that at least 80 percent of the women who walk through the door of our hospital want an epidural! Some are angry if their labor goes so fast they can't have one.

Q: Do nurses prefer women to get epidurals? Does it make a nurse's work easier?

Maria: It works to a nurse's advantage to let a woman be under the effect of an epidural most of her labor. The uterus usually pushes the baby down without any effort on the mother's part. It means we have to give that much less real support.

Sometimes with an epidural, a woman will reach ten centimeters just as the epidural is wearing off. She begins to feel some sensations or pain, some pressure or urge to bear down, and she can push her baby out just fine. Occasionally, she doesn't feel much sensation but still can be coached through pushing. Those are the best-case scenarios.

Q: What is the down side of epidurals?

Rosalind: I deal with many women who cannot push their baby out with an epidural. Then it's either forceps—which many hospitals aren't using now—vacuum extraction, or cesarean. You can't work with your body if you have no sensation.

When we let epidurals wear off so that women can push a lot, it *does* hurt then; the pain is worse than it would have been if they had had their full sensations the whole time, because they've not acclimated to the normal sensations. Normally, a woman's tolerance for labor pain builds throughout the labor. The epidural knocks that out. I see a lot of women who get angry when we let an epidural wear off for pushing. "Nobody told me I would have to go through this!" they say.

When a woman chooses to have an anesthetic, she probably doesn't realize she is actually preventing her body from making its *own* pain relief.

Q: What would you like to say to a woman who believes that a routine epidural is the best way to have a baby?

Rosalind: Having epidural anesthesia totally changes the nature of your labor. It automatically puts you at risk for hypotension, a drop in blood pressure that can be dangerous to your baby. There's a whole list of potential complications we have to watch out for, especially respiratory problems.

Maria: The apparent success rate for epidurals, done well, is very high, but that only means there's no apparent damage to the mother or baby when the baby is discharged from the hospital. No one is talking about long-term physical or psychological effects on either the baby or the mother.

Also, problems from epidurals, although rare, are very, very serious. For example, if the level of the anesthesia goes above the woman's nipples, she can have respiratory paralysis, which can lead to cardiac arrest. This is why a woman getting an epidural must be medically managed, and her vital signs must be watched far more closely.

People should know how serious epidural anesthesia is. Someone is putting a needle into a very delicate area, right next to your spinal cord. Even if nothing goes wrong, the epidural takes all of your control away. You can't move or even urinate on your own most of the time. So an epidural often leads to a lot of other interventions. When you have an epidural, you become a passive participant. You are bedridden and cannot respond to any signals from your body—or your baby—because you can't feel them.

Q: Do you find times when pain medication is useful?

Maria: Once in a while, such as when I see a woman in utter pain at three centimeters, I will actually recommend an epidural to her. It's a strange situation, actually advocating that a woman have something that I feel is so invasive and possibly harmful, something I would not want unless my baby or I truly required major intervention—like a cesarean.

Rosalind: There are times when a small dose of narcotics is enough to cause a very tense person to relax enough to let her body work. It can allow her to get over the hump and do the rest on her own.

Q: What is so important about experiencing the entire labor and birth?

Maria: The main problem for a woman who doesn't want to experience the sensation of her labor is that she misses out on the experience. It's not *her* birth anymore, it's *our* birth. There is also the question of what the baby is getting or missing out on.

Rosalind: Right. We cannot experience anything fully just through our minds. We experience life through our bodies. If we don't feel what is happening in our bodies, we are automatically missing out on a lot.

Maria: This is your child's entry into the world! Going through it and feeling it together connects the two of you. Most of us want our partners with us to experience the baby being born. Why *wouldn't* we want to experience it fully?

PETER

Peter is a highly revered, now-retired British obstetrician whose long career includes stints as a professor of obstetrics in several of London's most prestigious teaching hospitals as well as chairing the obstetrics department at two of those hospitals simultaneously. During his career he was a member of every committee in the Royal College, chair of two, member of the governing body, and the examiner for medical students at two other universities besides his own.

When I was considered a leader of the new discipline of perinatal medicine and a founding member of the European Society of Perinatal Medicine, I became

intensely interested through my lab research in the fetus as an individual. The fetus actually controls both pregnancy and the onset of labor! At the same time, I was becoming aware of the important responsibility I had to the teaching of medical students and was beginning to understand my responsibility, as a physician, to women. Among these arenas I soon found great conflict.

It became impossible to go on dictating to women; I had to stop talking and listen closely to what they were saying. That's when I began to change—when I realized that even though I was being paid to teach physicians, and despite my strong interest in the fetus, my primary responsibility was to serve the women who came to me. I was in a great position of power in my profession, but I became uncomfortable being used as the whiz kid who would represent the establishment's views.

The problem in our profession was not—is not—listening to the people it is meant to serve. Physicians impose their beliefs, and when women object—however nicely or graciously—we brush those objections aside with so-called logic. It is based on no evidence, merely on the built-in prejudices of a profession which is egocentric in the extreme.

Physicians are for the most part sincere people, but we're unwilling to have our opinions examined and challenged by the public. Obstetrics and gynecology are basically surgical disciplines, with surgical orientations. But the majority of the women we serve are not unhealthy, but fit, and therefore should not be considered patients, even in the orthodox terms of medicine. Yet we insist on converting these healthy women into patients, allegedly suffering from something we need to treat. What I wanted to do, and what ultimately caused me to leave my profession, was to treat women as intelligent individuals whom I respected and with whom I wanted to share responsibility.

The medical community claims that it has superior knowledge and is right. It claims the changes that humankind has perhaps benefited from in the last few decades are due to advances in medical technology. That claim may be right, but it has certainly not been proved. I could equally say the health of birthing women and babies has improved because of improved nutrition, or political changes, different social organization, or the greater availability of consumer goods.

I believe medicine has halted the ability of human beings to relate to each other in a personally and socially useful way. It has made people believe that medicine is infallible and has something to offer called "health."

Beyond that, it ignores the fact that out of suffering—and I am not promoting suffering—comes human dignity and a depth of experience worthwhile in itself. Everything in life is positive if you look at life that way. You can always find something useful in any experience. Health is an attitude of mind. There are many healthy people who are disabled almost totally in one way or another.

After I learned to listen to women I let them experience labor, experience discomfort. Colleagues have often accused me of not really caring about women. "If you care, you would step in and do something!"

I believe women should be properly informed about the choices that are available—and all the advantages and disadvantages about each choice that are currently known—and then be free to choose. The professional can perhaps also set them in the context of what their own experience has been. If you're convinced that one thing is better than the other, then you say that; but even if you feel certain, you still have to give the other person the right to choose something different without making her feel guilty. That is the most difficult thing!

It takes a lot of time to make sure a woman is well informed about her birth and her baby, and it has nothing to do with her intelligence. A professional ought to be able to communicate with any person; if we can't, that's our fault, not the woman's. When I've tried to let people take responsibility for their own health, I have been challenged by physicians. "People don't want that responsibility." I'm a realist. I know that! But unless we start trying to persuade people to take responsibility back, telling them they have a choice, we will never begin.

An obstetrician is simply a technician at the woman's service. Who could be more sensitive to the baby than the woman carrying and giving birth to that baby, especially if she has all the information she needs to make decisions? It's ridiculous for any professional to think we are the best advocates for the baby, except in rare instances.

Look at all the barriers we have put in front of women in terms of contraception, abortion, the care of pregnancy and childbearing, and the rearing of children. Look at what we do to women giving birth! Having companionship, being free to walk around, eat, drink, make noise, laugh, cry, moan—that's what life, and birth, is all about! A society that abandons home birth, normal birth, has lost its sense of adventure and romance, precious parts of life that arise from people caring deeply about each other.

Perhaps the most useful advice I could give a woman about childbirth would be: (1) think very carefully about your expectations, (2) inform yourself as much as possible about what lies ahead, and (3) keep a flexible attitude, because everything will be new. Realize that, as a woman, you have the potential within you for surmounting every obstacle. And remember, what your body tells you is usually right! Listen to yourself.

This interview was conducted in 1977. Has anything changed?

MELISSA

Melissa is thirty-eight years old, and the mother of two sons, ages five and seven. She met her husband, Bob, in junior high school. Despite her best efforts, Melissa had little control over the circumstances of her sons' births. Today, nine months pregnant, her choices for birth are once again limited by factors beyond her control. But she is prepared to overcome the politics and eager to experience the joys of birth.

When I gave birth to my first child, I went to the hospital five hours after contractions started, but I wasn't dilated at all so they sent me home again. As soon as I got home, my water broke. They had told me to come back immediately if that happened, so my husband and I got in the car and drove all the way back.

It was a huge hospital, an entire building for just women's services. Bob stayed with me. According to the doctors, my labor was not progressing fast enough, and they wanted to start me on a drip of Pitocin. I didn't want it. But then they began pressuring us, saying, "Pitocin's better than a dead baby." Finally, I gave in. They started the drip, and then I began having a real hard time with the contractions, so the nurses pushed for an epidural. Again I gave in.

I was comfortable with the anesthesia in place, but labor didn't progress after that.

Twenty-four hours passed after my membranes had ruptured, which in those days was the alarm time. It was five in the afternoon and my doctor was off-call. The new one was his office partner, and I'd met him only once before. He walked in the room, put his fingers in my vagina, and said to me and Bob, "This has gone on long enough. We're going to do a cesarean." He added, "Would you like some music? I've got anything but country." No discussion; that was it.

The baby did fine. I got to see him and nurse him in the recovery room with Bob there. After a while, the hospital staff made Bob go home, but I had my son with me during the days. We were released four days after the birth. At first, I just accepted everything that had happened as necessary; I believed that the doctors must have known best. After about a year, however, I began to consider having a normal birth the next time around. I didn't buy into the notion that it had to be another cesarean.

I got pregnant when my first son, Chase, was twenty months old. This time, I went to a different doctor. I heard from a local VBAC (Vaginal Birth After Cesaraean) group of an obstetrician who was supposedly supportive of women having vaginal births after cesareans. I went to him for three visits, and each time all he could talk about was my weight gain. "Well, gee, you really must have had a lot of Valentine's candy," I remember him telling me. "You've gained ten pounds." That was in February. In March it was, "Well, gee, you really must have had a lot of St. Patrick's Day candy. You've gained another ten pounds."

That's when I realized that this was not the care I was looking for. I knew I would have to take an alternative route. I called my doctor's office and said I'd decided to use a midwife. He was not, to say the least, happy with my decision, and tried to charge me for services that were never rendered.

Bob and I had agreed to go for a home birth. We were living in Dallas at the time and found a midwife an hour away in Ft. Worth. I'd heard about her from several women, and I found that I really liked her. I had better prenatal care—more thorough and more psychologically satisfying—than I'd ever had. She treated me as a whole person, not just a pregnant body. Bob and I were both real comfortable with her.

I couldn't believe the criticism we got from our friends and family about having a home birth. We saw Bob's and my parents often, and there was a lot of tension in the air. Bob's mother had worked in medical offices and she thought we were insane. One of my friends, whom I'd referred to my first doctor a few years earlier, told me that she and my doctor had discussed my "case" and that he thought I was taking my life in my hands.

I was angry at everyone's reaction. I had been reading up on the subject of home birth since Chase was a baby, and I knew that I was so healthy that I was capable of having a child without complications. My midwife did check me for gestational diabetes and said that some bodies react differently to pregnancy. Apparently, my higher glucose level wasn't necessarily cause for alarm; we just needed to keep an eye on it.

My body seems to take a long time in labor. For Chase's birth, I was only given twenty-eight hours to deliver—I don't know how long it would have taken naturally. Connor's took sixty hours. It took me a long time to dilate initially, and then my body took a long break at four centimeters. It picked up again, but going from four to eight seemed to take forever. Once I hit eight, though, I went to completion within an hour.

I had one major problem during Connor's birth; after a while, I was unable to urinate. My bladder was full and distended but Connor was somehow lying in a way that pinched a nerve, so I couldn't go at all. My midwife wasn't successful in catheterizing me at home and, because the bladder was blocking the baby's path, we decided to go to the hospital. We had made arrangements ahead of time with a private hospital that agreed to take me if I needed it.

Bob and I left the house, and the midwife followed us in her car. At the hospital they immediately hooked me up to a monitor, telling us it was "hospital policy" and "standard procedure." I didn't try to refuse. They also put an IV in my arm. A nurse attempted to catheterize me but couldn't. I was in a lot of pain throughout these procedures; I'd been in active labor for a long time and my bladder really hurt. Then the obstetrician told me that I needed a cesarean. I was frustrated and I felt that I was losing control of the situation. To think I'd gone all this time, just to end up with another cesarean!

Luckily, right after the doctor told us what he intended to do, Bob—who was leaning up against the door surveying the scene—said, "Melissa, we don't have to stay here." The doctor's eyes got very big. "You're right," I said, and with that, I took off the monitor belt that was strapped to my waist. "You're out of your mind!" the doctor said, but I ignored him and told the nurse to take out the IV. Then we got up and left, with me leaning on Bob.

We decided to go to the county hospital, where there was a staff shortage. Because of their gap in personnel, we felt the hospital wouldn't bother with me, and I would have the chance to labor as I pleased.

When I arrived, the hospital staff catheterized me immediately. It felt wonderful, and labor picked right up. I dilated fully on my own and was told I would be "allowed" two hours to push the baby out. In exactly two hours the nurse and doctors said time was up. They began to put me on a gurney to prep me for a cesarean. While I begged to be allowed to push one more time, they placed electrodes on my chest in preparation for anesthesia and scrubbed my abdomen with iodine. Finally, they relented. I gave one last push, and out came Connor! Nine pounds, fourteen ounces. I insisted on leaving early, so we were "allowed" to sign a special release and go home after twenty-four hours.

This time, for our third child, we wanted a home birth. But while home birth is still legal in Colorado, where we live, midwife-attended home birth apparently isn't. So I'm going to a certified nurse-midwife who works at the local hospital. She used to be a lay midwife and attended home births for ten years, but she doesn't dare do them in this town because of the political climate. We like and trust her, which is fortunate because she's really the only option here.

I'm prepared to go as many hours as it takes for this birth. I hope to find someone who will help us at home during labor so we avoid the hospital for as long as possible; once I'm there, I know they will try to perform procedures that I don't want and don't need. My sons don't want to be there for the actual delivery, so I plan to be home with them for most of the labor and have them brought to the hospital as soon as the baby is born. I plan to leave the hospital right after the birth. We will go home and have some peaceful time, and let the boys spend time with the new baby.

It may go smoothly, but it might not. I'm prepared for either case. If I had to give advice to a woman having a baby, I'd say, "Educate yourself. Read, read, read. And listen to your body."

Melissa gave birth to her daughter, Andy. Melissa and Bob stayed home until labor was well advanced. Bob checked her progress just as he had been shown. Melissa gave birth on her hands and knees in a darkened hospital room. A friend brought the older boys a few hours later. Six hours after the birth, they all went home.

BEATRIJS

Beatrijs Smulders is head of the Amsterdam midwives' association and author of an important book about home birth in the Netherlands. She and the other three midwives in her practice collectively attend four hundred births a year. In 1988 Smulders traveled to the United States to speak at hospitals about birth in the Netherlands. While in Philadelphia she mentioned that she had never seen an epidural performed, so an obstetrician in the audience invited her to see one. This is her account of it.

We do not do epidurals in the Netherlands. And cesareans are only done if nothing else will work—only five or six out of every one hundred births—and when one is needed we use general anesthesia. Anesthetics are not used during normal births. Midwives prefer to use a hot water bottle or a hot shower or bath, because the warm water helps the laboring woman to produce endorphins. That's natural anesthesia.

I've never seen a circus like that epidural I saw. The woman was talked into having it done. She'd been coping with her labor really well—she was already dilated six centimeters, and this was not her first birth. All of a sudden the whole atmosphere changed. People filled the room, gadgets were wheeled in, and then a doctor thrust a needle into the woman's back. The labor slowed down. It took five hours before she had bearing-down contractions, and the nurses didn't even notice at first because the woman was paralyzed from the anesthesia.

Suddenly there was a great deal of commotion. Wheeled to the delivery room, the woman had to be carried from the bed to the delivery table; she couldn't walk—or move—by herself. I felt so funny standing there. They made me dress in a mask and hat and shoes. Everybody was dressed like that, except the woman, and we all looked like clowns.

The anesthesiologist took charge of the woman's head, and overseeing at the other end was the obstetrician. The pediatrician was there too, waiting for the child. All I could see of the woman was her face at one end and her vagina at the other. The rest was covered by drapes. The woman was completely divided. She had no connection with her body at all.

You see, in the Netherlands we believe that pain is something you need in labor. It connects you with your body, it tells you how to cooperate with your body. Of course, nobody likes pain. It is an ugly—a difficult—friend. But we believe it helps to go through that pain, and we find that after the birth, women are that much happier with their achievement. The pain—and the need for the pain—is engrained.

In my country there is a healthy competition between midwives and obstetricians. We need ob-stetricians, but they get their referrals from us. And if an obstetrician practices too much intervention, he feels it in his pocket immediately, because we stop referring women to him. It's like a good marriage. Both people are equally necessary and equally strong. Friendships between midwives and obstetricians often spring up; we respect one another's work and we depend on each other for our livelihoods. I am trained to know when to refer a woman or bring her to the hospital. Many births that end up in a hospital are, ultimately, normal, but I know it's always better to go too soon rather than too late.

In the early 1980s in the Netherlands, midwives rediscovered the vertical birth position and began having women do it at home and in hospitals, too. Before that we did lying-down positions like in the United States. In the upright position women are much stronger, feel more in charge, and have a higher pain threshold. They don't need instruction in how to push; they feel what is happening in their pelvic floor. And when the baby is born, they know what to do.

At first obstetricians didn't like the upright position. They had to be on their knees, and it changed their relationship to the woman. It became more equal and that was difficult for doctors. But they have to do it because the women are not so willing to lie down anymore.

STEPHANIE

Stephanie was sixteen when I first met her, a friend of my daughter's. By seventeen she had a baby to raise. Stephanie became pregnant during her junior year in high school. She had a D average, but her boyfriend was a senior with his hopes on a basketball scholarship to college, not on child rearing. In some ways Stephanie was like many other pregnant girls her age. Her parents were divorced; she didn't get along with her mom, so she lived with her dad, but she was mostly raising herself. She elected to have the baby (only admitting that she might be pregnant when it was too late to choose an early abortion) and raise it by herself. But in other ways she proved to be strikingly different from her peers and more determined than many women twice her age.

My boyfriend and I didn't know what we were going to do, so we put off thinking about what would happen after the baby came. We were hoping that if we didn't talk about it, it wouldn't be a big deal. My main concern, once I knew for sure I was pregnant, was getting through high school.

My father finally caught on when I was seven months pregnant, and he took me to a clinic to get prenatal care. The woman physician didn't get on me for not coming earlier and she was open about everything. She was just very concerned about how I was really feeling about everything. I never had morning sickness, no back pains, no swelling. The only way I knew I was pregnant was that I could feel the baby moving and kicking. Plus my stomach was getting outrageously huge! The doctor loaned me some videos of babies being born. It was couples learning breathing techniques and positions to help ease labor pains, and how to focus attention in labor and what you could do to relax yourself. My boyfriend and I watched them together.

The birth was in May. I'd almost finished the year, with a home teacher. I was very anxious because the people I had talked to who had babies all told me horror stories. Mom had anesthesia with me. My aunt said it was excruciating, to be sure to take drugs to numb me. My friend Stacy had a baby two years old and said, "If they offer a drug, take it!"

I read some books that gave tips on how different positions in labor can make the pains less difficult to handle. It made me feel better knowing there was something I could do rather than take a drug. Also, I talked to my ob-gyn about drugs. She said if I felt I could do it naturally she preferred it, that giving drugs in labor is not good for the baby. I didn't want anything to affect the baby. My mother had spinal anesthesia for my birth and she didn't breast-feed my brother or me. I knew I wanted to breast-feed. I thought, "If I'm going to experience this, I want to do it all, naturally.

I talked about my plans with mostly my male friends. The girls were just, "Ooooh, my god! You're

gonna have a baby!" The guys were thinking about what would happen to me after the baby. One of them, John, told me that if the baby's father ever left and I needed anything, to call him, even if I needed a coach in labor. He even gave me all the telephone numbers where he would be every day toward the end of the pregnancy, so I could be sure and reach him. I'd watch him run track after school, and he would come sit next to me and rub my tummy and talk to the baby. It was really sweet.

Labor began in the evening. I was at my boyfriend's mother's house and he was at his night class. I knew it was labor. All of a sudden it came on. It hurt real bad. My boyfriend's brother and I went for a walk to the park across the street because I remembered reading that walking helped labor.

The hospital room was very comfortable—with a bed that didn't look or feel like a hospital bed. There were two chairs and a window with a really nice view of the city lights. And a radio. I turned on classical music. My mom, my stepfather, my dad, and my boyfriend and his mother were all there during labor. I had called them all. I said, "I'm doing it, and I don't want to do it alone." They all took turns holding my hands and talking me through contractions.

Two positions seemed to work best, standing up and lying on my side. So I alternated. The breathing technique I found most helpful was breathing in through my nose and letting the air fill my belly like a balloon and then breathing out through my mouth, very slowly. I did this each contraction, no matter what position I was in. A nurse came in every forty-five minutes or so to examine me and see how far along I was. It was very painful to be examined, and I lost my cool with the nurses a couple of times. I told one, who was really cold toward me, that if she came near me I was going to hit her.

I didn't panic at all. I think it was because I had everyone with me, so I felt really safe. My mom had not met my boyfriend until she was introduced to him in the labor room. That was kind of stressful at first. I could also feel the tension from people knowing I was going through so much pain and feeling there was nothing they could do to fix it. Every time I got a contraction I would look at either my mom or my dad—they usually didn't get along, but they put all their aggression aside in that room—and I would stare into their eyes until it was over, and they would tell me it was going to be okay.

During hard labor they hooked me up to an electronic fetal monitor. It had a wide band pulled tight around my abdomen. No one asked my permission, which would have saved a lot of time, because I didn't want it. I couldn't switch positions without having it move around, and then the nurse would come in and yell at me for moving each time I did. So I unhooked it and gave it to my boyfriend to hold, and when the nurse came back in I told her what she could do with it.

Pushing felt like a relief, it was a lot easier than the other contractions. Each time I felt like I would just have to do one more push and that would be it. It didn't hurt. I could feel the baby move as I pushed. With every push I felt it go lower and lower. When I saw the crown of the baby's head in the mirror—I was sitting back and my mom and dad were on each side of me, holding my hands, and my boyfriend was behind the bed rubbing my shoulders and neck— everyone got excited. I couldn't believe it! I was high just seeing this head coming out! The final two pushes I watched his head emerge and not go back inside. He just popped right out. Physically it was a relief that this thing was out of me and labor was over. Mentally, I was in shock. I was so happy that he was okay. And I could not believe that I had actually done this, that there was actually a baby inside me all that time.

As soon as he was out and they wiped his nose and mouth and eyes, the doctor handed him to me. She just put a blanket over him, so his skin was against my skin. It made me happier than anything in the world. I wasn't aware of anyone else in the room but him. He had cried when he came out, but once he was against my chest he got very quiet. I held him for a long time. Everyone backed off and let me just be with him.

The doctor had done an episiotomy, without asking me. When she began stitching me up, it hurt more than the early labor pains and made it very hard to concentrate on the baby. A nurse came to take the baby and weigh him and all that. I told her, "No. I want to hold him longer." She just looked at me. I think the look in my eye said: Don't push it!

After the episiotomy was stitched, I told the nurse she could take Kyle to check him and do a heel stick for some test she wanted to do. I was wheeled to my room. My mother and father had gone to the nursery with Kyle, and my boyfriend went out and told everyone it was a boy. I told a nurse to get my baby. She did and left us alone. It was wonderful.

I tried going back to high school in the fall after he was born, but he was only four months old and we were breast-feeding, and I didn't want to be separated from him. I could pump my breasts and leave my milk, but Kyle was already on his own feeding schedule. He liked to feed every couple of hours all day long, but he only woke once each night. I thought it would be easier if I stayed home with him a while longer and did my studying at home. After two months I quit school, took a test, and got my GED.

I breast-fed for seven months and didn't put Kyle into day care until he was two. I took a part-time job and went back to school. I decided to become a paralegal. It is interesting work and you can earn a lot of money. I got straight A's and finished last May. Kyle is four and a half now. His father is not around anymore, but I still talk to his father's mother and Kyle still sees her pretty often. I have never gotten any child support, but my mom and stepdad let me live at home for free—Kyle and I share a room—and she and my dad split the cost of day care while I was in school. I paid for my own schooling though. I was tired all the time, but I was glad I did it.

I've learned what responsibility is, and Kyle's birth had a great deal to do with it. I think I felt closer to Kyle because I dealt with the pain of his labor and did not drug it out. And breast-feeding— I had the ability and felt I should do it, because it was so much better for him. There was a special bond that came with nursing. A month after the birth my home teacher had me do a paper. I made it a letter to Kyle about pregnancy and my labor with him. I want him to know what it was like.

JANINE

Janine, a thirty-five-year-old childbirth educator and doula, gave birth to her second son eleven years after her first son was born, and one year after a miscarriage. Although she has lived for the past twenty years a few minutes away from one of the most prestigious medical centers in the United States, for her first birth she chose to use an out-of-hospital birth center founded by a group of consumers. For her second, she and her husband—a doctor—elected to birth at home.

It was the pain of my second son's birth that was the biggest surprise for me. When I had my first son I didn't consider the labor that painful, just intense. I loved the dilation phase, felt I was dancing with my contractions! I did dance, I moved with the rhythm of them. In the beginning I'd just lean on things and sway. Then as it progressed I'd let myself drop to the floor, get on all fours, and sway in that position. That went on for twelve hours, once I started to dilate. Before that, I'd had what they call prodromal labor for about forty-eight hours. Contractions were five minutes apart all day and all night, so I couldn't sleep, but they weren't strong enough to dilate my cervix. I used visualizations, relaxation exercises, listened to music, even resorted to milk and whiskey, but nothing helped. If I'd gone to the hospital I'm sure they would have admitted me and induced labor, put an IV in and strapped a fetal heart monitor on. I might even have had a cesarean.

I have supported probably around two hundred and fifty women in labor—at the birth center, in women's homes, and in various hospitals in our area. Labor assisting is most valuable when a woman is having a hospital birth. As much as I prefer a birth center or home birth, I'm most needed in the hospital.

Let me think how to say this. I think being able to help a woman stay centered in the choices she wants to make makes all the difference in terms of a woman's experience. What I see happening is women going into their birth clear about the kind of birth they want to have—the women who choose me are unusual because they actually want a natural birth. But what I see happening when they go into the hospital is they're in an environment where it is normal for birth to be handled in a medical way, and they tend to lose sight of what they really wanted.

I help women embrace their pain by facing it and staying in the moment—which is the only place they can be if they are going to cope with it. It's been the women who do not stay in the moment, who fight the pain and try to run away from it, who need their pain taken away. In my second labor, which was very painful, I couldn't even allow myself to think about the last contraction—much less the one that was about to come—or the pain would have been too intense to bear.

Back labor, I found from this birth, does hurt more. I thought about all the women I'd helped who had back labor and who I had thought were just overreacting, and I found myself apologizing to all of them. But a lot of my pain was emotion and had to do with having had a baby die in a miscarriage a year earlier. Now I really understand how it happens that women fall apart in labor, come unglued, and end up with a C-section. A lot of it, I think, has to do with their not being encouraged to look inside. Had my midwife not pulled my feelings out of me, so I could express them and let go of them, I don't know if I could have gotten to them.

This birth—Lucas's—was wonderful, even though it hurt so much. There is something about the pain. It's very powerful. I honored myself more after this birth than I did after the first birth, and I think it had to do with this one being more difficult. I was very proud of myself, and yet I was also real thankful to my body for doing it.

There has been a lot of ups and downs this post-partum. I've been crying a lot the past few weeks since he was born, I've been angry. There've been points where I've felt pretty crazy—Mark's three other boys are with us half the time, and that's hard on me. Sometimes I fall into feeling like a victim of my circumstances; but Lucas always pulls me back.

I know—how can I put it into words—that I can learn to experience the joy of living, regardless of what is going on around me. And that's what I want to do. I make life so complex, but it's really simple. The more I can stay in the present moment, the more I can be in a state of simple joy. And it's been my births that have taught me that.

My back is so sore these days from carrying this little guy around. Sometimes Mark says to me, "You know, one day you're going to have to put that baby down!" And I say, "When he wants to get down, I'll let him down." But I can't put him down—not yet!

Resources

ORGANIZATIONS FOR EDUCATION, TRAINING, ADVOCACY, AND SUPPORT

ALACE (Association of Labor Assistants and Childbirth Educators), P.O. Box 382724, Cambridge, MA 02238. (617) 441-2500.

American Academy of Husband-Coached Childbirth (The Bradley Method), P.O. Box 5224, Sherman Oaks, CA 91413-5224. (800) 423-2397, (818) 788-6662. Focuses on natural childbirth, breastfeeding, and the family; it offers teacher training, a newsletter, videos, and teaching supplies.

American College of Nurse Midwives (ACNM), 1522 K Street NW, Suite 1000, Washington, DC 20005. (202) 728-9860.

ASPO/Lamaze, 1200 19th Street NW, Washington, DC 20036. (800) 368-4404.

Association for Pre- and Perinatal Psychology and Health (APPAH), P.O. Box 516, Geyserville, CA 95411. (707) 857-3359.

BirthWorks, 42 Tallowood Drive, Medford, NJ 08055. (609) 953-9380. This approach to birth preparation is holistic, incorporating the wisdom of many leaders in the alternative birth movement.

Doulas of North America (DONA), 1100 23rd Avenue E., Seattle, WA 98112. Fax (206) 325-0472.

The Farm, P.O. Box 48 (clinic), P.O. Box 42 (publications), Summertown, TN 38483.

Global Maternal/Child Health Association, Waterbirth Information and Referral Center, P.O. Box 366, West Linn, OR 97068. (503) 682-3600.

Informed Homebirth/Informed Birth and Parenting (IH/IBP), P.O. Box 3675, Ann Arbor, MI 48106. (313) 662-6857. This approach to childbearing and early childhood education (based on Waldorf principles) provides parents with information on alternatives. A regular newsletter by midwife/founder Rahima Baldwin is highly informative. Training courses for certification are available.

International Association of Infant Massage, 5560 Clinton Street, Ste. 2, Elma, NY 14059. (716) 684-3299.

International Cesarean Awareness Network (ICAN), P.O. Box 276, Clarks Summit, PA 18411. (717) 585-4226. Provides information on preventing unnecessary cesareans, planning for VBACs, and helping women to recover from traumatic births.

International Childbirth Education Association (ICEA), P.O. Box 20048, Minneapolis, MN 55420-0048. (612) 854-8660. ICEA offers an interdisciplinary approach to birth education. Members remain autonomous, creating their own policies and programs.

International Lactation Consultants Association (ILCA), P.O. Box 4031, University of Virginia Station, Charlottesville, VA 22903.

La Leche League International, P.O. Box 1209, Franklin Park, IL 60131. (708) 455-7730.

Midwives Association of North America (MANA), P.O. Box 175, Newton, KS 67114. (316) 283-4543. Holds regional and national conferences, publishes a newsletter, and aims to build cooperation among midwives to promote midwifery as a standard of health care.

National Association of Childbearing Centers, 3123 Gottschall Road, Perkiomenville, PA 18074. (215) 234-8068.

National Association of Childbirth Assistants and Birth Support Providers (NACA), 205 Copco Lane, San Jose, CA 95123 or P.O. Box 12307, Santa Rosa, CA 94503. This group is geared to training skilled doulas and birth assistants.

National Association of Parents and Professionals for Safe Alternatives in Childbirth (NAPSAC), Route 1, Box 646, Marble Hill, MO 63764. (314) 238-2010.

National Association of Postpartum Care Services (NAPCS), 8910 299th Place SW, Edmonds, WA 98026.

National Organization of Mothers of Twins Clubs, P.O. Box 23188, Albuquerque, NM 87192-1188. (505) 275-0955.

National Women's Health Network, 514 10th Street NW, Ste. 400, Washington, DC 20004. (202) 347-1140.

NOCIRC, P.O. Box 2512, San Anselmo, CA 94979. (415) 488-9883. An organization dedicated to ending all circumcision.

Primal Health Resource Center, Dr. Michael Odent, 59 Roderick Rd., London NW3 2NP, England. (071) 485-00-95.

MAGAZINES AND JOURNALS

Birth, a journal published four times a year by Blackwell Scientific Publications, 238 Main Street, Cambridge, MA 02142. (800) 215-1000, (617) 876-7000. Provides up-to-date research on alternatives to standard American medical maternity care.

Birth Gazette. 12 The Farm, Summertown, TN 38483. (615) 964-3798.

The Complete Mother: The Magazine of Pregnancy, Birth and Breastfeeding. P.O. Box 209, Minot, ND 58702. (701) 852-2822.

The Doula: A Magazine for Mothers. P.O. Box 71, Santa Cruz, CA 95063. (800) 693-6852.

Midwifery Today, published four times a year. P.O. Box 2672-26, Eugene, OR 97402. (800) 743-0974. This is one of several fine periodicals for aspiring or practicing midwives; it also hosts national and international conferences for midwives and their supporters.

Mothering Magazine, published four times a year. P.O. Box 1690, Santa Fe, NM 87504. (800) 827-1061. Takes a strong, and often alternative, position on parenting. You may prefer it to other parenting magazines because of the controversial issues it covers. It is available in most natural food stores. *Mothering* also publishes useful books on related topics.

MUM: Honoring the Feminine. 3922 N. Ridgeway, Chicago, IL 60618. (312) 463-6040.

Special Delivery. c/o ALACE, P.O. Box 382724, Cambridge, MA 02238. (617) 441-2500.

PAMPHLETS

"Bonding." Available from ICEA, P.O. Box 20048, Minneapolis, MN 55420-0048. (612) 854-8660.

This small pamphlet by Diony Young describes how parents become attached to their babies.

"The Cultural Warping of Childbirth." Available from ICEA, P.O. Box 20048, Minneapolis, MN 55420-0048. (612) 854-8660. This pamphlet describes in simple detail how the hospitalization of childbirth has deformed the natural process.

"Why Breastfeed Your Baby?" Available from Pennypress, 1100 23rd Ave. E, Seattle, WA 98112. This four-page pamphlet by childbirth educator Henci Goer is full of information on breast-feeding that anyone can understand.

VIDEOS AND FILMS

Babies Know More Than You Think. Suzanne Arms and David Chamberlain. Available through Touch The Future, 4350 Lime Ave., Long Beach, CA 90807. (310) 426-2627.

Five Women Five Births: A Film About Choices. Suzanne Arms. Available through Birthworks.

Gentle Birth Choices. Barbara Harper, Global Maternal/Child Health Association. (For address, see listing on previous page.) Shows half a dozen normal births that include some unusual occurrences. Woven into its inspiring yet realistic vision of birth is a great deal of information not generally known by birthing women and their partners.

Home Birth in Holland. Netherlands Association of Midwives, Highlight Productions. Available from Birth and Life Bookstore (see listing below).

Push: A Women's Western. Suzanne Arms. Available through Impact Productions, 1725B Seabright Ave., Santa Cruz, CA 95062. (408) 427-2624.

MAIL-ORDER BOOKSTORE AND BIRTHING SUPPLIES

Birth and Life Bookstore and Moonflower Birthing and Herbal Supplies. (Cascade Health Care Products) 141 Commercial Street NE, Salem, OR 97301. (800) 443-9942. This complete mail-order business offers extensive catalogs on books, pamphlets, videos, and personal and professional supplies related to conception, pregnancy, birth, babies, midwifery, parenting, and nutrition.

Selected Bibliography and Recommended Reading

HISTORY AND SOCIETY

Berman, Morris. *Coming to Our Senses: Body and Spirit in the Hidden History of the West*. New York: Bantam, 1990.

Carter, Jenny. *With Child: Birthing Through the Ages*. Edinburgh: Mainstream Publishing, 1986.

Davis-Floyd, Robbie. *Birth as an American Rite of Passage*. Berkeley: University of California Press, 1992.

DeMause, Lloyd. *The History of Childhood*. London: The Psychohistory Press, 1974.

DeMause, Lloyd, ed. *The History of Childhood: The Evolution of Parent-Child Relationships as a Factor in History*. London: Souvenir Press, 1976.

Edwards, Margot, and Mary Waldorf. *Reclaiming Birth*. New York: The Crossing Press, 1984.

Ehrenreich, Barbara, and Dierdre English. *For Her Own Good: 150 Years of the Experts' Advice*. New York: Anchor Books, 1979.

Englemann, George. *Labor Among Primitive People*. New York: J. H. Chambers, 1883.

Fehlinger, J. *Sexual Life of Primitive People*. New York: A. C. Black, 1921.

Findley, Palmer. *Priests of Lucina: The Story of Obstetrics*. Boston: Little, Brown, 1939.

Goer, Henci. *Obstetrics Myths vs. Research Realities*. New York: Bergin and Garvey, 1994.

Goldsmith, Judith. *Childbirth Wisdom: From the World's Oldest Societies*. Brookline, MA: East West Health Books, 1990.

Greven, Philip. *Spare the Child*. New York: Alfred A. Knopf, Inc., 1990.

Haggard, Howard, M.D. *Devils, Drugs and Doctors*. New York: Harper and Brothers, 1929.

Leavitt, Judith W. *Brought to Bed: Childbearing in America, 1750–1950*. New York: Oxford University Press, 1986.

Martin, Emily. *The Woman in the Body*. Boston: Beacon Press, 1987.

Melendy, Mary, M.D., Ph.D. *Perfect Womanhood for Maidens—Wives—Mothers: A Complete Medical Guide for Women*. California: Occidental Publishing Company, 1901.

Meltzer, David, ed. *Birth: An Anthology of Ancient Texts, Songs, Prayers, and Stories*. New York: Ballantine, 1973.

Merchant, Carolyn. *The Death of Native Women, Ecology and the Scientific Revolution*. San Francisco: Harper and Row, 1983.

Michelet, Jules. *Satanism and Witchcraft: A Study in Medieval Superstition*. New York: Walden Publications, 1939. (Reissued New York: Citadel Press, 1971.)

Oakley, Ann. *The Captured Womb: A History of the Medical Care of Pregnant Women*. Oxford and New York: B. Blackwell, 1984.

Ploss, Bartels, and Bartels. *Woman: An Historical Gynaecological and Anthropological Compendium*. C. V. Mosby, 1938.

Rich, Adrienne. *Of Woman Born: Motherhood as Experience and Institution*. New York: W. W. Norton, 1976.

Rothman, Barbara Katz. *Encyclopedia of Childbearing*. Phoenix: Oryx Press, 1993.

———. *Recreating Motherhood: Ideology and Technology in a Patriarchal Society*. New York: W. W. Norton, 1989.

Sagov, Stanley, Richard Feinbloom, Peggy Spindel, and Archie Brodsky. *Home Birth*. Maryland: Aspen Systems Corporation, 1984.

Scovil, Elisabeth. *Preparation for Motherhood*. New York: Henry Altemus, 1896.

Shaw, Nancy Stoller. *Forced Labor: Maternity Care in the United States*. New York and Oxford: Pergamon Press, 1974.

Speert, Harold, M.D. *Iconographia Gyniatrica: A Pictorial History of Obstetrics and Gynecology*. Chicago: F. A. Davis, 1973.

Starhawk. *The Fifth Sacred Thing*. New York: Bantam, 1993.

Waring, Marilyn. *If Women Counted*. San Francisco: HarperCollins, 1988.

Wertz, Richard, and Dorothy Wertz. *Lying-In: A History of Childbirth in America*. New York: Macmillan, 1977.

Woolger, Jennifer Barker, and Roger Woolger. *The Goddess Within: A Guide to the Eternal Myths That Shape Women's Lives*. New York: Fawcett Columbine, 1989.

PREGNANCY AND WOMEN'S HEALTH

Arms, Suzanne. *Seasons of Change: A Photographic Journal of the Year of Pregnancy, Birth and New Motherhood*. Colorado: Kivaki Press, 1994.

Baldwin, Rahima, and Terra Palmarini Richardson. *Pregnant Feelings: Developing Trust in Birth*. Berkeley, CA: Celestial Arts, 1986.

Boston Women's Health Book Collective Staff. *The New Our Bodies, Ourselves*. New York: Simon and Schuster, 1991.

Davis, Elizabeth, *Energetic Pregnancy*. Berkeley, CA: Celestial Arts, 1988.

Davis, Elizabeth, and Carol Leonard. *The Women's Wheel of Life*. New York: Viking Arkana, 1996.

Eastman, Nicholson J., M.D., and Keith P. Russell, M.D. *Expectant Motherhood,* 5th ed. Boston: Little, Brown, 1970.

Enkin, Murray, Marc Keirse, and Ian Chalmers. *A Guide to Effective Care in Pregnancy and Childbirth*. Oxford and New York: Oxford University Press, 1989.

Friedman, Rochelle, and Bonnie Gradstein. *Surviving Pregnancy Loss*. Boston: Little, Brown, 1982.

Rothman, Barbara Katz, ed. *Encyclopedia of Childbearing*. Phoenix: Oryx Press, 1993.

Simkin, Penny, Janet Whalley, and Ann Keppler. *Pregnancy, Childbirth, and the Newborn*. Deerhaven, MN: Meadowbrook Press, 1991.

LABOR AND CHILDBIRTH

Balaskas, Janet. *Active Birth: The New Approach to Giving Birth Naturally* (Boston: Harvard Common Press, rev. 1992), *Natural Pregnancy* (Brooklyn, NY: Interlink Publishing Group, 1990), and *Water Birth: The Concise Guide to Using Water During Pregnancy, Birth, and Infancy* (San Francisco: Thorsons, 1992).

Baldwin, Rahima. *Special Delivery: The Complete Guide to Informed Birth*. Berkeley, CA: Celestial Arts, 1987.

Bradley, Robert, M.D. *Husband-Coached Childbirth*. New York: Harper & Row, 1965, rev. 1981.

Chard, Tim, and Martin Richards, eds. *Benefits and Hazards of the New Obstetrics*. Philadelphia and London: Lippincott and Heinemann, 1977.

Cohen, Nancy, and Lois Estner. *Open Season*. New York: Bergin and Garvey Publishers, Inc., 1991.

———. *Silent Knife*. New York: Bergin and Garvey Publishers, Inc., 1983.

Dick-Read, Grantly, M.D. *Childbirth Without Fear: The Principles and Practice of Natural Childbirth*. New York: Harper, 1959, rev. 1972.

Dunham, Caroll. *Mamatoto: A Celebration of Birth*. London and New York: Penguin, 1991.

English, Jane Butterfield. *Different Doorway: Adventures of a Cesarean Born*. Mt. Shasta, CA: Earth Heart, 1985.

Heinowitz, Jack. *Pregnant Fathers*. New York: Prentice Hall Press, 1982.

Jones, Carl. *Birth Without Surgery: A Guide to Preventing Cesareans*. New York: Dodd, Mead, 1987.

———. *Mind Over Labor*. New York: Viking Penguin, 1987.

Jordan, Brigitte, Ph.D., revised and expanded by Robbie Davis-Floyd. *Birth in Four Cultures: A Cross-cultural Investigation of Childbirth in Yucatan, Holland, Sweden and the United States*. Prospect Heights, IL: Waveland Press, 1993.

Kahn, Robbie Pfeufer. *Bearing Meaning: The Language of Birth*. Chicago: University of Illinois, 1995.

Karmel, Marjorie. *Thank You, Dr. Lamaze*. New York: Harper & Row, rev. 1981.

Kitzinger, Sheila. Of particular note are *The Midwife Challenge* (San Francisco: Pandora Press, rev. 1991) and *The Place of Birth: A Study of the Environment in which Birth Takes Place with Special Reference to Home Confinements* (with John Davis; Oxford and New York: Oxford University Press, 1978). Other titles include *Being Born* (New York: Grosset & Dunlap, 1986), *Birth at Home* (Oxford and New York: Oxford University Press, 1979), *Breastfeeding Your Baby* (New York: Knopf, 1989), *Complete Book of Pregnancy and Childbirth* (New York: Knopf, rev. 1989), *Homebirth* (New York: Dorling Kindersley, 1991), and *Women as Mothers* (New York: Random House, 1978).

Klaus, Marshall, M.D., Phyllis Klaus, C.S.W., and John H. Kennell, M.D. *Mothering the Mother: How a Doula Can Help You Have a Shorter, Easier, and Healthier Birth*. Reading, MA: Addison-Wesley, 1993.

Korte, Diana, and Roberta Scaer. *A Good Birth, a Safe Birth: Choosing and Having the Childbirth Experience You Want,* 3rd ed. Boston: Harvard Common, 1992.

Lang, Raven. *The Birth Book*. Ben Lomond, CA: Genesis Press, 1972.

Leboyer, Frederick. *Birth Without Violence*. New York: Fawcett Book Group, 1990.

Lim, Robin. *After the Baby's Birth: A Woman's Way to Wellness*. Berkeley: Celestial Arts, 1993.

Limburg, Astrid, and Beatrijs Smulders. *Women Giving Birth*. Berkeley: Celestial Arts, 1992.

Mitford, Jessica. *The American Way of Birth*. New York: Penguin Group, 1992.

Noble, Elizabeth. *Childbirth with Insight*. Boston: Houghton Mifflin, 1983.

Odent, Michel, M.D. *Birth Reborn*. Illinois: Livingstone, 1994.

Peterson, Gayle. *Birthing Normally: A Personal Growth Approach to Childbirth*. Berkeley: Mindbody Press, 1983.

Ray, Sondra. *Ideal Birth*. Berkeley, CA: Celestial Arts, 1985.

Rooks, J. P., et al. "Outcomes of Care in Birth Centers—The National Birth Center Study." *New England Journal of Medicine,* Dec. 28, 1989.

Rosen, M. G., and J. C. Dickinson. "The Paradox of Electronic Fetal Monitoring: More Data May Not Enable Us to Predict or Prevent Infant Neurologic Morbidity." *American Journal of Obstetrics and Gynecology,* Mar. 1993.

Rothman, Barbara Katz. *In Labor: Women and Power in the Birthplace*. New York: W. W. Norton, 1982, rev. 1991.

Savage, Beverly. *Preparation for Birth: The Complete Guide to the Lamaze Method*. New York: Ballantine Books, 1987.

Scaer, Roberta. *A Good Birth, A Safe Birth*. 3rd Revision. Boston: Harvard Common Press, 1992.

Simkin, Penny. *Birth Partner: Everything You Need to Know to Help a Woman Through Childbirth*. Boston: Harvard Common Press, 1989.

Tew, Marjorie. *Safer Childbirth? A Critical History of Maternity Care*. London: Chapman and Hall, 1988.

Wagner, Marsden. *Pursuing the Birth Machine*. Australia: ACE Graphics, 1994.

MIDWIFERY

Armstong, Penny. *The Midwife's Story*. New York: Ivy Books, 1986, 1988.

———. *Wise Birth*. New York: Morrow Publishing, 1990.

Davis, Elizabeth. *Heart and Hands: A Midwife's Guide to Pregnancy and Birth*. 2nd ed. Berkeley: Celestial Arts, 1993.

DeVries, Raymond. *Regulating Birth: Midwives, Medicine, and the Law*. Philadelphia: Temple University Press, 1985.

Donnison, Jean. *Midwives and Medical Men*. London: Schocken Books, 1977.

Ehrenreich, Barbara, and Dierdre English. *Witches, Midwives and Nurses*. New York: Feminist Press at CUNY, 1993.

Gaskin, Ina May. *Spiritual Midwifery*. Summertown, TN: Book Pub. Co., 1978, rev. 1990.

Jacobs, Sandra. *Having Your Baby with a Nurse-midwife: Everything You Need to Know in Order to Make an Informed Decision*. New York: Hyperion, 1993.

Klein, Susan. *A Book for Midwives: A Manual for Traditional Birth Attendants and Community Midwives*. Hesperian Foundation, 1995. P.O. Box 1692, Palo Alto, CA 94302. (415) 321-9017.

Leap, Nicky, and Billie Hunter. *The Midwife's Tale*. London: Scarlet Press, 1993.

Myles, Margaret. *Textbook for Midwives,* 11th ed., edited by V. Ruth Bennett and Linda K. Brown. London and New York: Churchill Livingstone, 1989.

Steiger, Carolyn. *Becoming a Midwife*. Oregon: Hoogan House, rev. 1994.

Towler, Jean, and Joan Bramall. *Midwives in History and Society*. London and New York: Croom Helm, Ltd., 1986.

BREAST-FEEDING

Fildes, Valerie, R.N. *Breasts, Bottles and Babies: A History of Infant Feeding*. Edinburgh: Edinburgh University, 1986.

Huggins, Kathleen. *Nursing Mother's Companion*. Boston: Harvard Common Press, rev. 1991.

Palmer, Gabrielle. *The Politics of Breastfeeding*. London and Boston: Pandora Press, 1988.

Renfrew, Mary, Chloe Fisher, and Suzanne Arms. *Bestfeeding: Getting Breastfeeding Right for You*. Berkeley: Celestial Arts, 1990.

Torgus, Judy, ed. *The Womanly Art of Breastfeeding*. Franklin Park, IL: La Leche League International, 1987.

BABIES AND CHILDCARE

Arms, Suzanne. *Adoption: A Handful of Hope*. Berkeley: Celestial Arts, 1989.

Baldwin, Rahima. *You Are Your Child's First Teacher*. Berkeley: Celestial Arts, 1989.

Chamberlain, David, Ph.D. *Babies Remember Birth*. Los Angeles: Tarcher, 1988.

Grof, Stanislav, M.D. *The Holotropic Mind: The Three Levels of Human Consciousness and How They Shape Our Lives*. San Francisco: HarperCollins, 1990.

Huxley, Laura Archera, and Piero Ferrucci. *The Child of Your Dreams*. Rochester, VT: Inner Traditions, 1992.

Klaus, Marshall, M.D., and Phyllis Klaus, C.S.W. *Amazing Newborn: Making the Most of the First Weeks of Life*. Reading, MA: Addison-Wesley, 1985.

Leach, Penelope. *Your Baby and Child*. New York: Knopf, rev. 1989.

Leidloff, Jean. *The Continuum Concept*. Reading, MA: Addison-Wesley, 1986.

McClure, Vimala Schneider. *Infant Massage*. New York: Bantam, rev. 1989.

Miller, Alice, M.D. *The Drama of the Gifted Child and the Search for the True Self*. New York: Basic Books, 1981.

Montagu, Ashley. *Touching: The Human Significance of the Skin*. 3rd ed. New York: Harper and Row, 1971.

Pearce, Joseph Chilton. *Evolution's End: Claiming the Potential of Our Intelligence*. San Francisco: HarperCollins, 1992. Also *The Crack in the Cosmic Egg, Magical Child: Rediscovering Nature's Plan for Our Children* (New York: Dutton, 1977), *Magical Child Matures* (New York: Dutton, 1985), and *The Bond of Power* (New York: Dutton, 1981).

Stern, Daniel, M.D. *The Interpersonal World of the Infant: A View from Psychoanalysis and Developmental Psychology*. New York: Basic, 1985.

Winnicott, Donald Woods, M.D. *Babies and Their Mothers*. Reading, MA: Addison-Wesley, 1987.

Index

Attention-deficit disorder, 86
Attitude
    importance of, 24, 25, 26, 261
      fear related to, 24
      stress vs. distress, 180
Ayurvedic medicine, 100

B

Babies Are Human (Aldrich), 175
Back labor, 234, 267
Backup plan, importance of, 134
Baldwin, Rahima, 152, 272, 273, 276
Barbiturates, use of in labor, 79
Benign neglect
    in infant care, 193
    "just-in-case" medicine vs., 250
"Bikini incision," 91
Bing, Elizabeth, 150
Birth as reward, 128
Birth (journal), x, 270
Birth attendant, choice of, 217
The Birth Book (Lang), 153
Birth centers, 154-156
    advantages of, 107
    breast-feeding success and, 202
    cost considerations, 155
    current trends, 109
    historical background, 154-155
    obstacles to, 154
    proliferation of, 5
    recommendations for, 218
    safety of, 155
Birthing beds, 106, 107
Birthing Normally, 237
Birthing rooms, 107, 156, 220
Birthing stools, 47, 107
Birth memory, 174-175. *See also* Birth trauma, lasting
        impact of
"Birth plans," 108
Birth Reborn (Odent), 203
"Birth-simulating massage," 246
Birth stories
    of author, 2-3
    of author's mother and grandmother, 1
    Diane, 254-255
    Gabrielle, 238-240
    ICU problems, 251-254

Janine, 267-268
    "Marion" (1963/1968), 63-76, 84
    Melissa, 261-263
    "Sarah Hanley," (1853), 29-36
    Shoshana, 240-242
    as source of strength, 25-26
    Stephanie, 264-267
    tribal customs, 9-17
    Vicki, 236-238
Birth trauma
    asthma and, 246
    attachment disorders and, 206-207, 208, 214
    child abuse and, 245
    effect on mother of, 235-236
    healing from, 184, 191-192
      by breast-feeding, 195-196
      by taking leave from work, 194
      therapy for, 244-247
    lasting impact of, 174, 175, 181-182, 185-186,
      214-215
    newborn's sensitivity to, 175, 177
    observing for effects of, 192, 246-247
    prevalence of, 186
BirthWorks, 269
Bleeding. *See* Hemorrhage
Blood pressure of mother, epidural anesthesia and, 82,
    258-259
Blood sugar
    gestational diabetes, 262
    labor progression and, 138
Blood transfusions, for jaundice, 192
Bonding, 204-205
    early day care and, 247-248
    ICU effects on, 99
    importance of, 183
    labor as preparation for, 77
    policies for fostering, 220, 221
    separation as impediment to, 207
    by single mother, 242
    specialization risks and, 100-101
Bottle feeding
    drying up mother for, 69
    illness and, 22
    long-term effects of, 86
    on schedule, 69
    sociopolitical issues and, 94, 196-197
Bradley, Robert, 151

doula presence and, 162
effects on baby of, 69, 76, 77, 78, 82, 84-87, 237
effects on mother of, 69, 132
historical background, 55-56, 78-80, 83-85, 123, 127
indications for, 78
Lamaze method and, 150-151
in 1963 birth story, 66-67, 69
in 1968 birth stories, 71, 73-74, 237
as reason for hospitalization, 250
routine, 76, 84, 123, 127
Dutch midwives. *See* Netherlands

E

Eastman, Nicholson, 64, 78, 79, 84, 86, 87, 273
Eating in labor, 138, 188-189
Ecology of birth, 167, 170-171
Ectopic (tubal) pregnancy, 140
Education
of doulas, 233-234
in infant and child care, 221
of midwives, 219
of parents. *See* Childbirth preparation
EFM. *See* Electronic fetal monitor
Electronic fetal monitor (EFM), 93-96
accuracy issues, 95
alternative birth movement and, 95-96
cesarean rate and, 93, 95, 96
device described, 94-95
historical background, 93, 94
as "hospital policy," 113-114
marketing of, 94
nursing issues, 95, 96
refusing, 270
risks of, 96, 114
Endorphins, 179-180, 263
Enema, 68
Engelman, George, 52-53, 271
Environment for birth
negative impact of, 167, 170-171
recommendations for, 107, 131-132
Environment for newborn, negative impact of, 167, 170, 184-186
Epidural anesthesia, 80
cesarean delivery and, 80, 82, 92, 93, 261
complications of, 82, 258-259
current use of, 80
doula presence and, 162

effects on baby of, 82, 98-99, 258-259
effects on mother of, 80, 82, 84, 129, 258-259
insistence of women on, 258
intensive care and, 98-99
interventions required by, 82
midwife's view of, 263-264
mother's blood pressure and, 82
nurses' view of, 258-259
pain sensation and, 258-259
socioeconomic class and, 93
Episiotomy
historical background, 54
in 1963 birth story, 69, 70
in 1968 birth story, 74, 75
refusing, 146
routine, examples of, 74
Equipment, recommendations for, 107
Ethical issues, 221-222
Evil, concept of, attitudes toward women and, 38-39

F

"Failure to progress," 81, 106, 132-133
"Failure to thrive," birth trauma and, 246
Family life. *See* Parenting
Family physicians, need for, 219
Far Eastern medicine, holistic principles in, 100
Far Eastern religions, good and evil in, 38
The Farm, midwifery at, 153, 269
Father
See also Support
birth classes and, 144
effect of traumatic birth on, 235, 236
fear instilled in, 114
labor role of
doula and, 163
in 1960s hospital birth, 68
nurturing role of, 217
postpartum role of, in 1960s hospital birth, 69-70, 75
Fear, 111-114
attitude toward birth and, 24
birth trauma resulting from, 181-182
chronic states of, 112-113
control needs and, 113
cultural sources of, 118
dealing with, 118-123, 237, 254
by breathing, 120-121
by support, 102

Informed Homebirth (Informed Birth and Parenting), 152, 269
Inhalation anesthesia, 66, 69, 83-84
Insurance. *See* Health insurance
Intensive care unit (ICU), 98-99
    aggressive interventions in, 251-254
    bonding research and, 183
    as cesarean risk, 92, 98
    epidural anesthesia and, 83
    improvements in, 194-195
    labor intervention and need for, 98
    lasting impact of, 256
    legal issues, 254
    for meconium staining, 189, 191
    need for parent contact in, 185
    recommendations for, 179, 219-220
    risks to baby in, 92, 98-99
    as stressful environment, 167, 185
International Cesarean Awareness Network (ICAN), 91, 269
International Childbirth Education Association (ICEA), 151, 269
International Congress on Home Birth, 154
Intervention
    See also Labor, noninterventive aids to
    actual rate of need for, 116-117
    aggressive model of, 138-139
    in birth centers vs. hospitals, 155
    chain of, 189
    for dehydration prevention, 188-189
    "just-in-case," 188-189, 191
        benign neglect vs., 250
        "maxi-min" theory, 228-229
    labor delayed by, 165, 166
    for meconium, 189, 191
    newborn care cautions, 179, 229-230
    panic as cause of, 229
    recommendations for, 222
    newborn resuscitation, 229-230
    support vs., 27
Intubation, routine use of, 189, 191
"Iron hands," 53-54. *See also* Forceps
Islam, attitudes toward women in, 40

J

Janov, Arthur, 182
Jaundice, 192, 229
Joan of Arc, 40

Judaism
    attitudes toward sexuality in, 41
    attitudes toward women in, 40
"Just-in-case" medicine. *See* Intervention

K

Kaiser, cesarean rate at, 92
Karmel, Marjorie, 150
Kennell, John, 162, 183
Klaus, Marshall, 162, 183, 275, 277
Klaus, Phyllis, 162, 275, 277
Kloosterman, G. J., 164, 234
Kneeling position. *See* Position in labor
Knowledge, importance of, 25-26

L

Labor, 124-125
    active, 81, 125
    altered state of consciousness in, 24, 117, 127, 255
        of baby, 178
        danger of disrupting, 131
        hormonal changes and, 77, 129-130, 180, 263
    benefits of
        for baby, 20, 77, 178
        for mother, 77
    birth attendant choice for, 217
    complications in, 133-141
        alternative corrections for. *See* Labor, noninterventive aids to
        hospital backup for, 134
        self-correcting, 137
    drug use in. *See* Anesthesia; Drug use
    early, 124
    "failure to progress" in, 103, 106, 132-133
    glucose IV in, 188-189
    hormonal changes in, 77, 129-130, 180, 263
    induced. *See* Induced labor
    length of
        doula presence and, 162
        environment and, 81, 132-133
        fear and, 164, 165
        variations in, 81, 103, 106, 262
    need for fluids in, 138
    noninterventive aids to, 60-61
        blood sugar elevation, 138
        breathing, 121
        calm observation, 130

changing position, 137
environmental, 131-132
rest, 137
touch, 130
visualization, 122-123
"normal" vs. "average," 103, 106
pain in. *See* Pain
positions for. *See* Position in labor
problems of standards for, 81, 103, 132
real risks in, 133-141
self-correcting, 134, 137
sensations preceding, 12
stress vs. distress in, 179-180
support persons for. *See* Support
visualization in, 122
La Leche League, 152-153, 200, 270
Lamaze, Fernand, 149, 150
Lamaze movement, 150-151
Lang, Raven, 153, 275
Lavage, routine use of, 189, 191
Lay midwives
alternative birth movement and, 153
legal battles of, 156, 158-159, 160
legal status for, 160, 161
nurse-midwives vs., 156, 158
LDR rooms, recommendations for, 220
Learning, postnatal period and, 174-175
Learning disabilities, childbirth anesthesia and, 85, 86
Legal considerations
in newborn care, 109, 254
in midwifery, 156, 158-161
Lifestyle, healthy outcome and, 17-18, 24-25
Lister, Joseph, 57
London Royal Free Hospital, women's march on, 154
"Lying-in," 249

M

Male midwives, forceps used by, 53-54
Malpractice issues
cesarean delivery and, 91
electronic fetal monitoring and, 95, 96
hospital practices and, 108, 109, 212-213
jaundice treatment, 192
recommendations for, 221
MANA (Midwives Association of North America), 155, 270
Marketing issues
electronic fetal monitoring, 94

formula manufacturers, 94, 196-197
Massage, "birth-simulating," 246
Maternal and Child Health Foundation (MCHF), 152
Maternal mortality
childbed fever and, 30-31, 56, 57, 58
social reform movement and, 42-43
Maternity care, 168-169
Maternity homes and hospitals, 154
Maternity leave. *See* Parental leave
Maternity wards, 249
MCHF (Maternal and Child Health Foundation), 152
Meconium aspiration syndrome, 189
Meconium staining, 189, 191, 230
Medical advances, 48, 51-59
Medical education, exclusion of midwives from, 46
Medical model of childbirth
aggressive intervention in, 138-139
current trends, 155-156, 211
emphasis on abnormal in, 43, 59, 212, 257
fear as basis for, 26-27, 37, 113-114, 257
fear as result of, 130-131, 243
locus of control in, 58-59
in nineteenth century cities, 29-37
origins of, 58-59
pain and, 129
physician's criticism of, 232-233
Mental imagery, 121-123
Midwives, 155-161
See also Lay midwives; Nurse-midwives
breast-feeding success and, 203
grassroots movement of, 153-154
healthy view of childbirth among, 26
historical background, 43-48
in the Netherlands, 48, 263-264. *See also* Netherlands, birth practices in
hospital privileges denied to, 158, 159
in hospitals, 101, 102
benefits of, 101, 102, 108-109
legal problems of, 156, 158-161
male, forceps used by, 53-54
nursing confused with, 47-48
physician backup denied to, 158, 160
physicians' appreciation of, 230, 232-233
postpartum care by, 232-233
professionalization of, 45, 48, 109, 153-154, 160
prosecution of, 158-159
recommendations for, 218, 219

networking by, 154

    practice problems, 158

Nurse practitioners, recommendations for, 219

Nursery, environmental stress in, 167, 184-185.
    See Intensive care nursery; Separation of baby
        from mother

Nurses, interview with, 256-259

Nursing

    midwifery confused with, 47-48

    specialization in, 102-103

    staffing inadequacies, 257

O

Observation, as source of support, 130

Obstetricians, ideal role of, 218, 231-233, 260

Obstetric nurses, interview with, 256-259

Obstetrics, historical background, 48, 51-59

Odent, Michel, 129, 130, 203, 270, 276

O'Driscoll, Kieran, 81

Older mother, birth story of, 240-242

Opiates, effect on baby of, 85. *See also* Demerol

Overdue labor, 61, 262

Ovulation, recurrence of, in tribal societies, 19

Oxygen availability, epidural anesthesia and, 82

Oxytocin, jaundice and, 192

P

Paganism, midwifery seen as, 44-45

Pain

    cesarean to avoid, 91

    childbirth classes focused on, 142

    cultural attitudes toward, 127-128

    epidural anesthesia and, 258-259

    fear related to, 65, 128, 130, 149, 254

    focusing on, 127-128

    medical model of childbirth and, 129

    perception of, 24

    physiology and, 23-24

    pleasure related to, 128-129

    positive role of, 264

    religious view of, 39, 55

    sense of well-being inhibited by, 117

    support as relief for, 129

    viewed as abnormal, 87

Panic, feeling of

    over-intervention caused by, 228-230

    in transition stage, 129

Pankhurst, Sylvia, 43

Paracervical block, 83

Parental leave

    healing process and, 194

    recommendations for, 220, 221

Parenting

    birth experience and, 214, 230

    decline in quality of, 206-207

    doula presence and, 163

    support recommendations, 220, 221

    working parents and. *See* Work, returning to

Partner. *See* Father; Support

Patient advocates, doulas as, 163, 233-234

Pavlov, Ivan, 150

Pelvic structure, birth process and, 20-21, 140

Perinatal experiences, lasting impact of, 176, 204-208,
    214, 215. *See also* Birth trauma

Perinatologists, 99

Pethidine. *See* Demerol

Phototherapy, 229

Physician assistants, recommendations for, 219

Physicians

    opposition to midwives by, 158, 160

    resistance to change by, 213

Physician specialization, 99-101, 190

    historical background, 99-100

    midwives and, 158

    recommendations for, 218

Physiology, birth process and, 19-21, 23

Pittsburgh, Pennsylvania, out-of-hospital ICU in, 195

Placenta, 173

    delivery of, in tribal birth, 16

    labor complications, 130

    postpartum complications, 140

Pleasure, pain related to, 128-129

Podalic version, 35, 53

Political issues, in bottle feeding, 94, 196-197

Pollution, birth problems and, 18-19

Populist health movement, 32-33

Position of fetus

    mother's physical activity and, 18, 52

    turning, 35, 52-53, 140

Position in labor

    advantages of upright position, 58, 125, 268

    class differences and, 58

    for fetal heart rate correction, 137

    ideal, 18

feeding practices and, 197, 206
hospital practices, 22, 101, 207, 249-250
immune system and, 200
in intensive care, 194
for meconium staining, 189, 191
need to avoid, 191-192
by return to work, 194, 204-205
"Septic workup," 98-99, 229
Seventh-Day Adventists, healthy view of childbirth
among, 26
Sexuality, Puritan view of, 40-41
Shame, 25
Shaving in labor, 68, 73, 191
Sibling, presence of at birth, 226-227
Silver nitrate, routine use of, 75
Simpson, Sir James Young, 55
Single mother, birth story of, 240-242
Sleeping of infant with parent
advantages of, 21, 22-23
in tribal societies, 17
Smulders, Beatrijs, interview with, 263-264
Social reform movement, 42-43
Socioeconomic class
breast-feeding and, 200
cesarean delivery and, 92-93
epidural use and, 93
Sociopolitical issues, in bottle feeding, 94, 196-197
Spacing of pregnancy, in tribal societies, 19
Special-care baby unit. *See* Intensive care unit
Specialization
of hospital staff, 102-103
of physicians, 99-101
midwives and, 158
recommendations for, 218, 231-232
Spinal anesthesia, 3, 79-80
in 1968 birth story, 71, 73-74
pushing inhibited by, 74
Spinal headache, 3, 82
Spinal tap
danger of, 230
for meconium staining, 191
Spiritual Midwifery (Gaskin), 153
Spontaneous abortion, as pregnancy risk, 139
Spotting in pregnancy, as self-correcting, 137
Squatting position. *See* Position in labor
Standing position. *See* Position in labor
Status of women. *See* Women, attitudes toward

Stewarts, NAPSAC founded by, 152
Stress
distress vs., 180
in newborn, 191-192
in hospital nursery, 167
newborn's responses to, 184-185
positive, labor as, 179-180
Suction device, preferred to forceps, 54
Suctioning of baby's mouth, as routine practice, 75
Sugar water, as first feeding, 75
Support
See also Doulas; Father; Midwives
as alternative to drugs, 87, 129
as antidote to fear, 102
for breast-feeding, 202, 203-206
EFM as substitute for, 95
hospital staff practices and, 106, 107
for infant care, 194
intervention vs., 27, 87
for learning breast-feeding, 202
postpartum need for, 232-233
types of, 130
Support person, fear instilled in, 114
Symbiosis of mother and baby, 173-174, 221

T

Technology. *See* Intervention; Medical model of childbirth;
specific technologies
Teenage mother, birth story of, 264-267
Thank You, Dr. Lamaze (Karmel), 150
Thich Nhat Hahn, on breathing, 120-121
Touch, as source of support, 130, 131
Tranquilizers, 79
Transient tachypnea of the newborn. *See* Breathing problems
in newborn
Traumatic birth. *See* Birth trauma
Tribal customs, 9-17
delivery of placenta, 16
delivery position, 15-16
infant care, 17, 19, 193-194
labor position, 14, 15
postpartum care, 16-17
Trilene, 84
Trust
breast-feeding and, 201
fear vs., 116-118
as first developmental task, 174, 193

Trust, *continued*
    of mother by midwives, 260
    newborn care and, 193-195
Tubal pregnancy, 140
"Twilight sleep"
    common use of, 55, 66, 228, 250
    components of, 78
    effects on baby of, 69, 228
    effects on mother of, 69, 78-79
    reason for popularity of, 78
Twin birth, 136

U

Ultrasound, 97-98
Umbilical cord prolapse
    interventions for, 137-138
Unassisted birth, fear and, 117
Uterine fever. *See* Childbed fever

V

Vaginal birth after cesarean (VBAC), 90, 91, 261-263
Vaginal examination, childbed fever and, 57
Valium, 79
VBAC. *See* Vaginal birth after cesarean
Vegetarianism, Victorian beliefs and, 41
Vellay, Pierre, 150
Victorian customs, 29-36, 41-42
Victoria, Queen, chloroform used by, 55-56
Visualization, 121-123

W

Walking around, as labor aid
    advantages of, 18
    in tribal birth process, 14

Water, as labor aid, 124, 131
Watts, Alan, 128
Weight of newborn, birth process and, 20, 21
Well-baby clinics, recommendations for, 220
Well-being, feeling of
    in breast-feeding, 117
    in childbirth, 117
    pain sensation and, 128
Wet nurses, 30, 36, 54
Witch-hunts, 40, 44-46
The Womanly Art of Breastfeeding (La Leche League), 152
Women, attitudes toward
    childbirth practices and, 37, 59-60
    religion and, 37-41, 44
    witch-hunts and, 44-46
Women's Cooperative of England, 42-43
Women's work, childbirth as, 23-26
Work, taking leave from
    healing process and, 194
    recommendations for, 220, 221
Work, returning to
    attachment problems and, 206-207, 247-248
    breast-feeding and, 230-231
    current practices, 111, 206-207
    workplace recommendations, 221
World Health Organization, parenting trends noted by, 206
World War II, hospital practices in, 1, 21-22

Y, Z

Yale University Hospital, midwife policy, 159
Zoroastrianism, 38